Janelle Gonsalves

C **Callahan**
5349 Laurel Dr
Concord, CA 94521

Prosthetics and Orthotics

PROSTHETICS AND ORTHOTICS

SECOND EDITION

Donald Shurr, C.P.O., P.T.
Director of External Relations
American Prosthetics and Orthotics, Inc.
Iowa City, Iowa

John W. Michael, M.Ed., C.P.O., F.A.A.O.P., F.I.S.P.O.
President, CPO Services, Inc.
Chanhassen, Minnesota

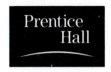
Prentice
Hall

Upper Saddle River, New Jersey 07458

Library of Congress Cataloging-in-Publication Data

Shurr, Donald G.
    Prosthetics and orthotics / Donald Shurr, John Michael—2nd ed.
      p.   cm.
    Includes index.
    ISBN 0-8385-8133-1
    1. Prosthesis.   2. Orthopedic apparatus.   I. Cook, Thomas M. (Thomas Michael), 1944-
II. Title

RD130.S53   2000
617.69—dc21   00-062369

Publisher: Julie Alexander
Executive Editor: Greg Vis
Acquisitions Editor: Mark Cohen
Production Editor: BookMasters, Inc.
Director of Manufacturing and Production: Bruce Johnson
Managing Editor: Patrick Walsh
Manufacturing Buyer: Ilene Sanford
Design Coordinator: Maria Guglielmo
Marketing Manager: David Hough
Editorial Assistant: Melissa Kerian
Cover Design: Eve Siegel
Cover Art: Diana Ong/Superstock
Composition: BookMasters, Inc.
Printing and Binding: RR Donnelley & Sons, Harrisonburg, VA

Notice: The author and the publisher of this volume have taken care that the information and recommendations contained herein are accurate and compatible with the standards generally accepted at the time of publication. Nevertheless, it is difficult to ensure that all the information given is entirely accurate for all circumstances. The publisher disclaims any liability, loss, or damage incurred as a consequence, directly or indirectly, of the use and application of any of the contents of this volume.

Prentice-Hall International (UK) Limited, *London*
Prentice-Hall of Australia Pty. Limited, *Sydney*
Prentice-Hall Canada Inc., *Toronto*
Prentice-Hall Hispanoamericana, S.A., *Mexico*
Prentice-Hall of India Private Limited, *New Delhi*
Prentice-Hall of Japan, Inc., *Tokyo*
Prentice-Hall Singapore Pte Ltd.
Editora Prentice-Hall do Brasil, Ltda., *Rio de Janeiro*

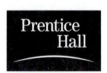

1 0 9 8 7 6 5 4 3 2
ISBN 0-8385-8133-1

This book is dedicated to Marilyn, Carrie, Molly, Linda, David, and Kate: our infinitely supportive spouses and children who patiently endured the long hours of "homework" needed to produce this volume.

It is also dedicated to the unfinished work ahead, begun with one of our mentors, Mr. Harold E. Miller, CPO, whose untimely death did not allow us to learn from him all that he desired to teach.

Brief Contents

Contents

Foreword

Too frequently, an amputation is assumed to be the final event in the care of a patient instead of the beginning of a critical phase in functional restoration and improvement of quality of life by the use of modern prosthetic and rehabilitative methods.

Again too frequently, adults and children with neuromusculoskeletal disorders may be relegated to a life of disability instead of receiving attempts to overcome impairment by contemporary orthotic and restorative techniques.

This deplorable state of affairs results from two major problems in the education of health professionals: the lack of emphasis on the subject in curricular design and the heretofore absence of a thoughtfully prepared text designed to provide a coordinated overview for the serious student who needs an understandable distillate of an evolving, fragmented, and complex discipline.

The authors of this text deserve congratulations for undertaking the formidable task of helping correct these aberrations. I am honored to have worked with them and I have learned much from them over past years. I can attest to their comprehensive knowledge of the subject, their ability to teach, and their tireless dedication to the care of patients.

This inclusive volume with chapters on materials, mechanics, upper and lower limb prosthetics and orthotics, and spinal orthotics presents an overview and a method of approach that reflects, in a superb manner, both the art and science of the subject. It will be of great benefit not only to the beginning student but also to those who want to extend their working knowledge of the fascinating, dynamic, and increasingly important topic of prosthetics and orthotics.

I, and many of my colleagues, express deep appreciation to the authors for their time and effort in providing yet another service to patients through those whose education will be greatly enhanced by this text.

Reginald R. Cooper, M.D.
Department of Orthopaedics
The University of Iowa
Iowa City, Iowa

Preface

This volume was initially developed while the senior author was teaching prosthetics and orthotics to entry-level physical therapy students over a period of many years. During that time our students and others asked repeatedly for a *single* resource around which they could focus their learning. This book is our response to their prodding.

Although developed primarily for physical therapy students, this book should be useful for many with limited experience or background in prosthetics and orthotics. It should be appropriate for other health care professionals including nurses, physicians, occupational therapists, vocational counselors, and more recently, managed care providers. The text assumes only a basic understanding of anatomy, kinesiology, and to some extent, pathology.

The primary objective of this volume is to provide a sound overview of the principles underlying the art and science of prosthetics and orthotics as currently practiced in the United States. We fully recognize that there are distinct regional differences and preferences in prostethics and orthotics (P&O) practice throughout this country and others. The reader should know that he or she may never encounter some of the devices described in this text and is very likely to encounter devices, which vary significantly, or even drastically, from those presented herein. This book is not intended as an encyclopedic treatise of every possible P&O device. Such a work, if possible, would be overwhelming in size and outdated before it appeared in print. Rather, our intention is to address the fundamental concepts underlying the rational selection and application of common prosthetic and orthotic devices. Our hope is that the interested reader will use this information as a foundation for informed dialog to enhance the quality of patient care.

A final comment must be made about the concept of integrating both prosthetics and orthotics into one volume. Although traditionally considered as somewhat distinct topics, we have found an integrated approach to teaching these subjects to be very logical and effective. Recent developments in materials and fabrication methods and common functional goals for applying these external devices appear to blur some of the long-standing distinctions between these two disciplines. Although comments and techniques from both prosthetics and orthotics may be integrated, the reader is reminded that chapters dealing with anatomical levels of both disciplines appear as separate entities. This allows the text to be used as a quick reference by simply accessing the chapter dealing with the relevant question. Perhaps future editions of this or similar texts may include chapters entitled "Prosthotics"!

Donald G. Shurr
John Michael

Acknowledgments

The authors and publisher gratefully acknowledge the following individuals who reviewed the manuscript for the Second Edition of *Prosthetics and Orthotics* and provided comments and suggestions for improving it.

Martha Walker, MS, PT
Associate Professor of Physical Therapy
Old Dominion University
Norfolk, Virginia

Deborah A. Nawoczenski, PhD, PT
Associate Professor, Department of Physical Therapy
Ithaca College-University of Rochester Campus
Adjunct Assistant Professor
Department of Orthopaedics-University of Rochester
Rochester, New York

Cheryl D. Ford-Smith, PT, MS, NCS
Assistant Professor in Physical Therapy
Department of Physical Therapy
Virginia Commonwealth University

CHAPTER 1

Introduction to Prosthetics and Orthotics

From very early historical recordings, wars and battles dramatically increased the number of people in need of prosthetic and orthotic devices. Such activities also contributed to the development concepts in the field and eventually to the financial backing for research and development of new designs and materials. Blas de Lezo is said to have freed Columbia and his statue stands at the city gate of Cartagena, Columbia. He lost his left leg, his right arm, and one eye in the battles to free the city.

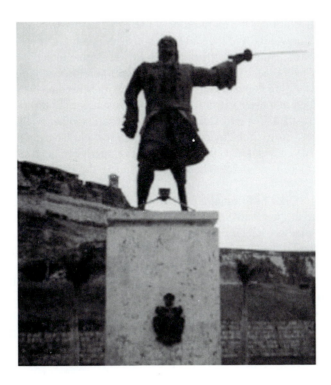

Following completion of reading this chapter, the student will be able to:

1. Discuss a brief history of orthotics and prosthetics.
2. Discuss the roles and respective functions of the rehabilitation team members.
3. Describe the causes of amputation, and the need(s) for orthotic care.
4. Discuss the comparative preparation and necessary skills of a certified orthotist/prosthetist.

This chapter will present a brief historical perspective on the development of the fields of orthotics and prosthetics followed by a description of orthotic and prosthetic services as currently provided in the United States. Overviews of prostheses and orthoses include discussions of those factors common to all amputees and users of orthotic devices. The chapter concludes with a description on the prosthetic/orthotic clinic team.

HISTORICAL PERSPECTIVE

Brief History of Prosthetics

Historically, amputation was often the only medical option for the definitive treatment of complex fractures or infections of the extremities. Although even Neolithic man was thought to have the necessary knowledge and tools to accomplish amputations, most did not survive the procedure. By the sixth century BC, the physician Susruta wrote in detail about proper surgical procedures that had become standard technique. The more precise the procedures and the faster the amputations were done, the higher the survival rates became because blood loss and shock were minimized in these early days before the discovery of anesthesia.

Historically, prosthetists were blacksmiths, armor makers, other skilled artisans, or often amputees themselves. Early limbs manufactured in Europe and later in America used metal, wood, and leather. Articulated knee and ankle joints eventually replaced stiff joints, and gradually metal was replaced by wood. These changes made the devices more functional and lighter in weight.

In 1860, A. A. Marks substituted a hard rubber foot for a wooden one. Soon after, J. E. Hanger, an amputee in the Confederate army, placed rubber bumpers on solid feet and thus produced an articulated prosthetic foot. Hanger also popularized skin suction as a method of suspending a transfemoral (above knee) prosthesis. The prosthetic industry grew tremendously during the Civil War, as over 30,000 amputations were performed on the Union side alone. Wooden socket limbs from Marx of New York sold at that time for $75 to $150 each and were available by mail order.

War continued to provide the major impetus for research and development in prosthetics. Details and materials have changed considerably since 1900, but little change has occurred in the basic designs of limb prostheses. Following World War II, the Department of Veterans Affairs (VA) financially supported the development of the patellar-tendon bearing and quadrilateral sockets for transtibial (below-knee) and transfemoral amputees respectively. These designs and techniques were taught to all prosthetists so that both veteran and civilian amputees would benefit. Following Vietnam, renewed funding by the VA led to further refinements in prostheses, including the provision of myoelectrically controlled upper limb prostheses and endoskeletal, modular prostheses.

Brief History of Orthotics

The development of the art and science of splinting and bracemaking, now referred to as the field of orthotics, paralleled developments in the field of prosthetics. Pictorial examples of splints and various assistive devices can be found among early civilizations, including ancient Egypt and Greece. The same metal, leather, and wood materials found in early prosthetic devices were also used in orthotic devices; and the same artisans, namely blacksmiths, armor makers and patients, were the first orthotists.

By the eighteenth and nineteenth centuries, the manufacture of thin steel had reached such a refined state that splints and braces were sometimes mass produced and described in catalogues often published by enterprising "appliance makers." Pioneers in this early period were Ambroise Pare (1509–1590); Hugh Owen Thomas (1834–1901); and Sir Robert Jones (1859–1933), a nephew of Hugh Owen Thomas, who is considered the "father of orthopaedic surgery." All were accomplished and innovative bracemakers, as well as "bonesetters." Eventually surgery replaced manipulation and bracing as the cornerstone of the practice of orthopaedics. Bracemakers then became professionals distinct from physicians.

The term *orthotics* has recently replaced the use of the word *bracing* to describe the control of body segments by external devices. *Orthotics* is meant to include dynamic control of body segments compared to the more limited, static connotations of the word "brace." The term was first used in the early 1950s and was officially adopted in 1960 by orthotists and prosthetists in America when they formed the American Orthotic and Prosthetic Association from the original Artificial Limb Manufacturers' Association.

Just as the wars of this century have caused a renewed interest in the development of prostheses, the polio epidemics of the 1950s spurred increased interest in the field of orthotics. Since 1970, many innovations in orthotic designs were made possible by the adaptation of industrial techniques for vacuum-forming sheet plastics. Because of the continuing introduction of new materials and methods, present-day orthotic practice is a growing, rapidly changing discipline.

PROSTHETIC AND ORTHOTIC SERVICES

Need for Services

The National Health Interview Survey published in 1969 indicated that those using prosthetic legs numbered 0.6 per thousand. By 1977, the figures had jumped to one per thousand using an artificial leg. Total people reported to be using either artificial legs or arms in 1977 were 275,000.

For the same population survey, Furst and Humphrey reported that 6,250,000 people in America used orthoses, wheelchairs, canes, or special shoes in 1969. By 1977, the number had grown to 6,500,000, or about 3 percent of the American population. Specifically, people using leg orthoses increased from 233,000 in 1969 to 400,000 in 1977. This represents roughly

1.2 people per thousand population in 1969 and 1.9 people per thousand in 1977, nearly twice the number using prostheses.

By comparison, orthopaedic impairments were reported in 16 percent of all activity limitations published in the National Health Interview Survey for 1983–1985. Of the 16 percent, deformities of the back and lower extremities accounted for 86 percent. Back and spine injuries occur 50 percent plus in ages 18 to 44. Thirty-eight percent of users of all orthoses in age groups less than 25 wore foot orthoses.

In 1990, 3,514,000 wore some orthosis. User numbers doubled between 1980 and 1990. Back orthoses accounted for one-third of all reported orthoses. By 2020, Nielsen predicts the number of persons using an orthosis to rise to 7.4 million.

Concomitantly, the incidence of spina bifida is decreasing. The cases reported reduced from 6.0 per 10,000 in 1970 to 3.5 per 10,000 by 1988. Recent breakthroughs in understanding the importance of folic acid in the diet during pregnancy is expected to reduce this incidence further.

Using the same data source, the number of persons with amputation of a major part of the arm or leg is expected to increase 47 percent between 1995 to 2020, paralleling the increase in the total population. According to Nielsen, if 75 percent of all amputees wear prostheses, the need for prostheses will grow from 1,211,895 in 1995 to 1,786,810 by the year 2001.

Professional Organization and Certification

Certification of professionals and facilities is administered by the American Board for Certification (ABC) in Orthotics and Prosthetics, Inc. This board was established in 1948 through a combined effort of the orthotic and prosthetic industry and the American Academy of Orthopaedic Surgeons. The ABC establishes rigorous professional conduct and facility standards and develops and administers national qualifying examinations for both practitioners and assistive staff. Additionally, the organization serves as an appeals committee for alleged violations of established standards of practice, ethics, or law.

Educational Programs

There are currently eight practitioner-level accredited programs in the United States [National Commission on Orthotic and Prosthetic Education (NCOPE, 2001)]: offering education in orthotics and/or prosthetics. According to published enrollment figures, 232 students will graduate per year from these eight schools. There are 272 approved residencies. It should be noted that graduates from the Army orthotic school, where no formal education is required prior to admission, do not qualify to sit for the ABC board examination and therefore will not increase the ABC credentialed workforce in the field for the future.

New on the educational horizon for orthotic and prosthetic education is the entry-level Masters. St. Ambrose University, in Davenport, Iowa, admitted the first Masters of Orthotic Science (MOS) class in Fall, 2001.

Currently there are two subprofessionals in orthotics and prosthetics: the technician and the assistant. Technician and practitioner education programs are accredited by NCOPE, while the individual practitioners, technicians, and assistants are credentialed by ABC.

Number and Distribution of Prosthetists and Orthotists

Since 1949 there have been more than 1,720 certified prosthetists/ orthotists (CPO), 2,814 certified orthotists (CO), and 2,585 certified prosthetists (CP) certified by the ABC. On January 1, 2001, there were 1,059 COs, 1,048 CPs, and 1,138 CPOs in good standing. This total of 3,265 represents the current ABC certified workforce in orthotics and prosthetics. Assuming the present total of 3,265 professionals, together with an addition of 9 to 10 percent per year and a 2 percent annual retirement rate, Nielsen estimated in 1998 that by 2000 there would be less than 3,400 orthotic/prosthetic practitioners in the United States. This is in contrast to 577,000 physicians, 2,079,000 nurses, and 120,000 physical therapists.

At this time in the United States, orthotists and prosthetists practice in several major settings. The first and most common of these settings is the private office. Beginning in the late 1880s, Nickel reported that many orthotists began moving out of individual physicians' offices and hospital settings, and became independent providers of services and devices to many physicians and patients.

The second most common practice setting for the delivery of prosthetic and orthotic services is the institutionally based service/consultation. Many large institutions such as general and children's hospitals, rehabilitation centers, or rehabilitation and research institutes provide orthotic/prosthetic services from an internal staff.

The third type of practice in which a prosthetist/orthotist might be involved is that of a supplier and fabrication manager. The use of a central production laboratory, physically distant from the site of measuring and fitting, has grown rapidly in recent years and will probably continue to increase in the United States. The economic and professional advantages and disadvantages of this type of arrangement will be discussed more fully in chapter 2.

In the eight accredited orthotic or prosthetic entry-level programs, full-time professional faculty are required. According to a 1976 report from Ponte, there were 17 full-time certified prosthetists, 24 full-time certified orthotists, and 13 full-time certified prosthetists/orthotists in this area of practice. Current figures include 7 full-time CPs, 12 full-time COs, and 14 full-time CPOs.

Finally, there are almost no opportunities to do basic research in orthotics/prosthetics full time. Many practitioners, however, are working on the cutting edge of materials, design, or rehabilitation engineering as an integral part of their daily clinical practice.

The Prosthetics/Orthotics Clinic Team

Due to the complexity of many prosthetic/orthotic cases, referral is often made to a clinic team. This team is likely to include the physician, prosthetist/orthotist, nurse, physical therapist, occupational therapist, social worker, vocational counselor, and most importantly, *the patient*. It is impossible for this clinic team to function meaningfully without the active participation of the patient in making decisions.

Clinic teams provide evaluation, prescription, delivery, and followup for prosthetic/ orthotic services. Followup is important because changes in the functioning of the device or the patient necessitate regular reevaluation by the experienced team. This is particularly important when caring for growing children, because the sometimes rapid changes in their body size and configuration will require concomitant changes in the prosthesis or orthosis. All mechanical devices require maintenance or replacement due to normal wear and tear and for that reason should be evaluated regularly to assure they continue to function properly.

AN OVERVIEW OF LIMB PROSTHETICS

The term amputation refers to the process whereby a part is severed from the body. The term prosthesis refers to an artificial device used to replace a missing part of the body. The portion of the limb remaining following the amputation is referred to as the residual limb, and the portion of the prosthesis that is fitted over the residual limb is called the prosthetic socket. With proper care, the amputee (the individual who had undergone an amputation) can return to a useful life, and amputees can be found in nearly every occupation. When the proper surgical techniques have been employed and when sound training methods and components are used in providing the prosthesis, the amputee can be expected to participate in many of his or her previous activities.

The Amputee Population

Figures 1-1 to 1-3 summarize statistics on the relative incidence of amputation as reported by Kay and Newman in their classic study in 1975. This study reported only amputees fitted with prostheses. No similar, more recent study exists. Figure 1-1 shows the relative distribution of amputees by site of amputation, and it is clear that the large majority of amputations occur in the lower limbs. As a general rule, Kay and Newman report that it is estimated that there are about 11 lower limb amputees for every upper limb amputee. Figure 1-2 shows the distribution of amputees by sex and cause of amputation. It can be seen that the leading cause of amputation is vascular disease, with an approximate equal incidence between males and females. It is also clear that most vascular amputations occur to people aged 61 to 70 years, with approximately equal occurrence in ages 51 to 60 years and 71 to 80 years.

Lower limb ischemia, secondary to peripheral vascular disease, remains the most common cause of amputation. Most experts also agree that about 50 percent of these patients also have diabetes. In some areas of Europe, up to 90 percent of all amputations performed are secondary to vascular disease.

Lind reported a 2.5 times greater incidence of postoperative infection and revision in 165 primary above knee and below knee amputations done for vascular reasons.

Level of Amputation

Amputation may occur through joints or through bone. In general, the site of amputation is described by the joint or long bone through which the amputation has been made. Common descriptors of sites of amputation are shown in Figure 1-1. The reader is reminded that this study was published before the ISO terminology was developed. An amputation of the lower limb makes standing and walking difficult, while an amputation of the upper limb poses a different set of problems related to activities of daily living (ADL).

Causes of Amputation

Causes of amputation may be grouped into four major categories: trauma, disease, tumor, and congenital malformation. Amputation may be the result of trauma or the result of a life-saving surgical procedure intended to arrest a disease. Additionally, a small percentage of individuals are born without a limb or limbs or with deformed limbs that require surgical conversion to a more appropriate level.

Trauma. In some accidents or trauma, part or all of the limb may be removed or autoamputated during the initial incident, or the limb may be damaged to such an extent that removal

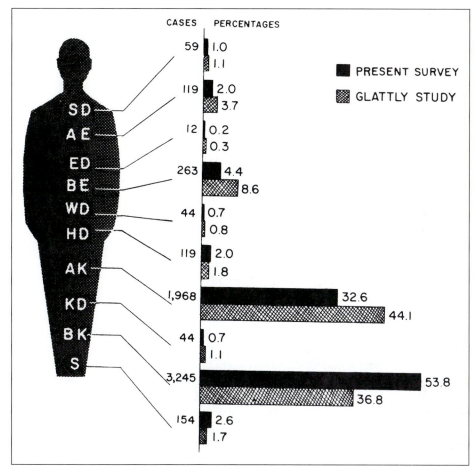

Figure 1-1. Distribution of amputees by site of amputation, comparing studies done in 1975 with 1964 (SD = shoulder disarticulation; AD = above elbow; ED = elbow disarticulation; BE = below elbow; WD = wrist disarticulation; HD = hip disarticulation; AK = above knee; KD = knee disarticulation; BK = below knee; S = Syme's). (*Source:* Kay HW, Newman JD. Relative incidence of new amputations. *Orthot Prosthet.* 1975; 29:8, with permission.)

of the limb is required following the accident. Figure 1-2 from Kay and Newmann demonstrates a 22.4 percent trauma-related cause for amputation. Current data from Nielsen suggest little change at 23 percent. Common accidental causes of traumatic amputation include the following: automobile accidents, farm machinery accidents, firearms, freezing, electrical burns, and power-tool accidents. In some cases, as in severe brachial plexus injuries, damage to the nervous system results in paralysis to the limb that is debilitating enough to require amputation. These levels are said to be elective, because they are usually not life threatening emergencies and may therefore be performed at a time elected by the surgeon and patient. The amputating physician must have sufficient knowledge about prosthetic restoration to be able to elect the most functional level for the patient under the circumstances.

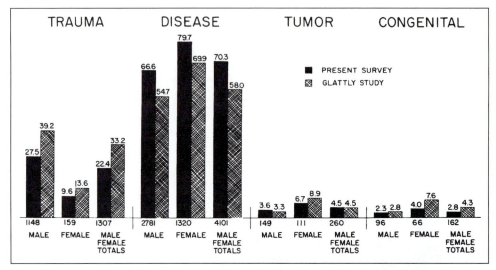

Figure 1-2. Distribution of amputees by cause and sex, comparing studies done in 1975 with 1964. (*Source:* Kay HW, Newman JD. Relative incidence of new amputations. *Orthot Prosthet.* 1975; 29:8, with permission.)

Disease. Vascular disease may lead to amputation. Diseases that may cause vascular or circulatory problems include diabetes, arterial sclerosis, and Buerger's disease. In these instances, the blood supply to the limb is inadequate, so necrosis or dry gangrene of the tissues can occur. Circulatory disorders are more common among the elderly, and thus the majority of amputations for vascular reasons occur in the lower limbs of these persons. Kay and Newman reported 70.3 percent of all new amputees to be of vascular disease origin. Furst and Humphrey reported an 85 percent vascular or metabolic origin for 5,000 amputations annually in England and Wales. Of these 85 percent, men were two times as likely as women to need amputation, and overall 70 percent of all new amputees were 60 years of age or older. On another note, Furst and Humphrey surveyed the wives of transtibial amputees to identify their perceptions of the commonest causes of amputation. Four of five wives felt that trauma was the leading cause and that the average age for amputation was 40 years less than it actually was. Often although younger, non-dysvascular, transtibial amputees may be the most visible amputees in our society, they are also a small minority of the entire amputee population. Infection is also a potential cause for amputation, although more recently, with the advent of more effective antibiotic drugs, the number of amputations for this cause has been reduced.

Although the Kay and Newman study was published over 25 years ago, it remains a meaningful comparison and is cited here for that reason. Nielsen reported current figures for amputation for vascular reasons to be 70 percent. The most frequent age group was 61 to 70. In addition, she reported that 50 to70 percent of this group also had diabetes. Smoking has been reported to increase the likelihood of amputation as much as sevenfold. According to the American Diabetes Association, 56,000 amputations are performed annually on diabetics (2001).

Tumor. Amputation may also be undertaken as treatment for tumorous conditions. Primary bone tumors occur frequently in adolescents but can occur at any age. Figure 1-2 from Kay and Newman shows that about 4.5 percent of all reported limb fittings are due to tumors. Figure 1-3

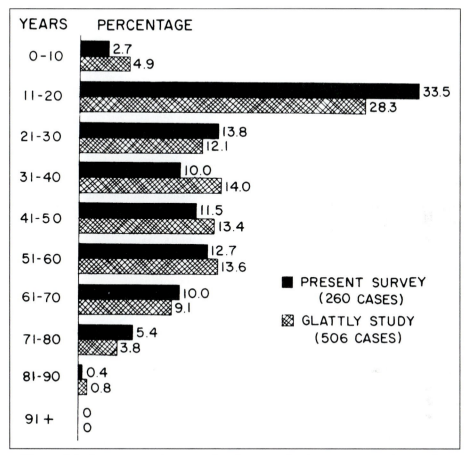

Figure 1-3. Occurrence of tumor-related amputation by age, comparing studies done in 1975 with 1964. (*Source:* Kay HW, Newman JD. Relative incidence of new amputations. *Orthot Prosthet.* 1975; 29:8, with permission.)

further demonstrates that 33.5 percent of these amputations occur between the ages of 11 and 20. Of further concern is the fact that bone tumors tend to occur more proximally in the limb making high-level limb ablation necessary. Nielsen reported a current incidence of less than 4 percent. The advent of limb salvage techniques, including custom total joint replacements at the knee and hip, are largely responsible for the decline in incidence of this cause for amputation.

Congenital Malformation. In some instances, all or part of a limb is deficient at birth. These absences may be either the result of a congenital amputation or a limb deficiency or defect. Congenital amputations, although rare, connote the one-time presence of the limb and its amputation, in utero, often the result of a constriction band or ring. Limb deficiencies are malformations of the limb bud, occurring around day 28 in utero, yielding something less than a normal extremity. Although both may be treated in a similar manner prosthetically, limb deficiencies tend to require nonstandard prostheses and are often surgically converted to more standard anatomic and/or prosthetic levels. One such common condition is the congenital absence of the left forearm, the so-called terminal-transverse-congenital-limb deficiency of the forearm. Limb deficiencies, however, can occur anywhere and in any combination. Incidence of congenital deficiencies has remained steady at 3.6 per 10,000 infants.

Reactions and Adjustments Associated with Amputation and Use of a Prosthesis

Amputation of a body segment results in problems that are physical, psychological, social, and often economic in nature. These various problems are closely interrelated, and often require simultaneous solutions because addressing one area may affect other problems. Careful listening on the part of the health care professional may hasten the rehabilitation process or may prevent problems from ever occurring. Good, complete communication with the amputee and family is essential to facilitate adjustment to a new way of life or at least to a different way of doing things.

Nicholas et al surveyed 94 amputees about their feelings, perceptions, and problems concerning their prostheses and their lives as amputees. Additional tests were given to assess depression and ADL. The average age of participant was 57; levels of amputation included most upper and lower levels.

Findings of interest included:

84 percent perceived no choice in prescription of prosthesis.

74 percent reported wearing their prosthesis 8 or more hours per day.

72 percent perceived themselves less able to defend themselves post amputation.

98 percent were satisfied with their rehabilitation physician.

97 percent were satisfied with their prosthetist.

Depression appeared to be negatively correlated with time: The longer the time post-amputation, the less the depression. Those wearing their prostheses for longer periods of time were less depressed.

Physical Factors. The most obvious problems associated with loss of a limb are the functional limitations that result. There is a primary satisfaction enjoyed by all individuals who are able to control their body and perform a variety of desired activities. In addition to the satisfaction derived from the use of one's physical faculties, there are other satisfactions that are achieved only through the use of prehensile or ambulatory functions as intervening steps or prerequisites to other activities.

When the amputee approaches a physical task, the following alternatives are available: avoid performing the task, compensate for the lost segment by increased use of the remaining segments, or perform the activity by utilizing an artificial replacement for the missing segment. Depending on the particular task and the patient's level of amputation, any one or a combination of these alternatives may be used. In any event, at least some minor restrictions and limitations occur in accomplishing the activity so that total normal satisfaction is never achieved.

As a general rule, lower limb prostheses replace lost function more completely than upper limb prostheses. Varying amounts of difficulty will be manifest depending on the level of amputation, the adequacy of the prosthetic device, the patient's general condition, and the patient's motivation. Because hand functions tend to be inherently more varied and complex than the repetitive task of walking, upper extremity prostheses cannot be expected to provide near normal function. The loss of function in the upper limb increases very rapidly with each more proximal level of amputation. Bilateral amputation results in a drastic increase in loss of function compared to unilateral amputation.

In addition to the loss of motor function resulting from amputation, the amputee is also deprived of important sensory information normally present with an intact limb. This lack of direct sensory feedback is important in the lower limb but is probably even more useful in the upper limb and is one barrier to the effective use of artificial hands and hooks.

Because the artificial limb is not attached to the skeletal elements of the residual limb, there is a false joint between the skeletal system and the prosthesis. This insecure attachment commonly results in feelings of instability and uncertainty in the control of the prosthetic device. This phenomenon is particularly important for weight bearing in the lower extremity. A secondary consequence of this unstable attachment to the skeletal system is the feeling that the artificial limb is heavier than an intact limb, even though, in fact, it may be considerably lighter.

Because the socket may be fitted over tissues that are not normally weight-bearing tissues, a number of secondary physical problems may occur related to the socket fit. These problems include edema resulting from a socket that is too tight at the proximal end, pressure problems leading to atrophy of muscle and subcutaneous fat, osteoporosis as a result of reduced skeletal weight bearing, bony spurs, allergic reactions to the socket material, cysts, infections, reduced blood flow, and neuroma at the site of amputation.

In addition to the problem of heat buildup within the socket, the amputee may have a problem with central body temperature regulation due to the loss of body mass and its related surface area. Because of the lost body segment, perspiration over the rest of the body tends to increase, further compounding skin problems.

A general problem experienced by amputees is the overall increase in fatigue associated with "normal" activities. This factor is particularly important for lower limb amputees because it has been clearly shown that ambulation using a prosthetic device considerably increases the energy required for this activity. Because the amputee must expend more energy for ambulatory functions, he or she has less energy available for other activities. This additional energy requirement is likely to have an impact on the amputee's motivation and willingness to participate in such activities.

For the amputee, conscious attention must often be paid to functions that are carried on more or less automatically with an intact limb. In other words, many functions that are controlled subcortically with an intact neuromusculoskeletal system require cortical attention by the amputee. Such attention requires additional motivation by the amputee and also limits the attention that can be given to concurrent activities. This problem tends to be more important in upper limb tasks where the amputee must use vision as a substitute for normal sensory feedback for prehensile activities.

Another problem experienced by the prosthetic wearer is general discomfort associated with wearing the prosthetic device. What is referred to as a comfortably fitting prosthesis is in reality one offering the minimum tolerable degree of discomfort for the amputee. Prosthetic devices are fitted over tissues that are performing atypical functions, primarily weight bearing in the lower extremities. Until these tissues become adjusted to these new functions, significant discomfort may be experienced by the amputee.

A physical problem associated with amputation is the presence of phantom sensations in the limb that has been removed. Phantom sensation is defined as a painless awareness of the presence of the amputated part, and often includes a mild tingling sensation. Phantom sensation is frequently incomplete and the segments felt most often are those with the greatest sensory representation in the cerebral cortex. The sensory homunculus, or little person, acts as a switchboard of pain signals. The foot and hand are usually felt more than other parts of the limb, and the thumb and great toe are usually areas of high awareness. If phantom sensation is painful and disagreeable, it is then referred to as phantom pain.

According to Sherman and Arena, phantom pain may be constant or intermittent and may vary greatly in intensity. The three most commonly described types of phantom pain are (1) postural cramping or a squeezing sensation, (2) burning sensation, and (3) sharp, shooting pain. Some patients report feeling a mixture of these three types of pain. Sherman reports that 80 percent of 7,000 responses to a questionnaire revealed enough phantom pain to elicit problems for 1 week each year. The reported episodes last from a few seconds to several weeks. In time, phantom pain tends to diminish for most amputees, but the presence of phantom sensation tends to remain indefinitely for many individuals.

Sherman likens phantom pain to a larger group of referred pain syndromes. He believes that burning and tingling phantom pain is caused by decreased blood flow to the end of the residual limb. The cramping or squeezing phantom pain is due to spasms in the residual limb.

Bach reported favorable results using preoperative lumbar epidural blocks on vascular, transtibial amputees who reported preoperative pain. A course of 72–hour preoperative bupivacaine and morphine resulted in fewer cases of phantom pain at 1 year, when compared with a control group.

Phantom sensation and pain are typically not present in individuals with congenital amputations or deficiencies. In instances of crushing injuries or among older amputees, phantom pain tends to remain longer and pose a greater problem. Once phantom pain becomes a problem, treatment is quite difficult, and treatment successes are limited. One report by Sherman lists 43 individual treatments for phantom pain, from lobotomies to injection, to reexploration/reamputation. Most treatments were reviewed by one author as successful and by another as being unsuccessful.

Psychosocial Factors

For some individuals, the psychological and social problems associated with amputation are of greater consequence than the physical problems. Grief is considered to be the universal reaction resulting from the loss of a limb segment. The grief reaction follows a predictable course that can be conveniently divided into the immediate impact phase, the recall phase, and the reconstruction or psychological rehabilitation phase. All grief reactions are not the same, and each amputee's reaction is dependent upon his or her basic personality type. An essential factor in the grief process is the acceptance of the limb loss and the realization that the loss is permanent. Denial of the importance of the handicap or limb loss is not an uncommon phenomenon. Anger is also a common manifestation of the grieving process and this anger may be directed to anyone who attempts to help the individual accept his or her loss. Anger may also be directed at parents whom they blame for "giving them" diabetes, or other vascular diseases.

The sense of loss is dependent upon the significance of the physical loss to the amputee. Feelings of increased dependence as a result of amputation present further complicating factors. Changes in behavior and evidence of depression are also common reactions to limb amputation. During the recall phase, the patient learns to talk about the loss and, in some cases, to make light of his previous reactions. In the final reconstruction phase, the amputee adjusts to a new self-image and begins to direct his or her energies towards more constructive and satisfying activities. Most amputees work through all three phases of the grieving process, although some individuals remain fixed in the first or second phase.

Breakey reported the results of his doctoral dissertation dealing with the effects of body image on psychological well-being of the 90 male, unilateral, traumatic, transtibial and transfemoral amputees who served as subjects. Using the amputee body-image scale (ABIS), the 110–item instrument included questions concerning body image, self-esteem, nonpsychotic depression, anxiety, satisfaction with life, and demographics. Results for the 60 transtibial and 30 transfemoral amputees indicated that there is a significant relationship between how an amputee perceives his body and psychosocial well-being, specifically in the areas of anxiety, depression, self-esteem, and life satisfaction. Breakey recommends focusing more positively on attitudes toward the body following amputation.

Because the amputee is dependent upon a mechanical prosthetic device, he or she must learn to live with the awareness that the device may fail at any time. The amputee must anticipate some instances when he or she will fall down during ambulation or fail in simple acts of prehension using a prosthetic device. These failures are sources of embarrassment for the individual and have significant psychological and social implications, because most societies have a relatively negative attitude toward people who fail.

Loss of acceptance by one's peers is another psychosocial factor affecting amputees. Social prejudices against disabled individuals have been reflected in literature by depicting amputees as Captain Hook, Long John Silver, and other devious characters. These attitudes toward amputees are ingrained at an early age and are changed only very slowly. Parents of young children to be fitted with hook terminal devices commonly react negatively when first shown such devices.

The term cosmesis refers to the visual appearance of the prosthetic device. Cosmetic problems tend to be of greater importance for the upper limb amputee than for those having lower limb amputations because the leg is more easily covered with clothing than is the hand. Young children tend to be less conscious of appearances than adolescents or adults. Because our society places great importance on the quality, adequacy, and conformity of one's physical appearance, individuals not meeting society's standards often suffer loss of group acceptance. Along with feelings of group rejection, the amputee may develop problems of an interpersonal nature.

Because artificial limbs are, in essence, mechanical devices, they are subject to a variety of low-level sounds associated with their operation. These sounds draw attention to the amputee, and again are a cue to others that the amputee is unusual in some way.

Vocational and Economic Factors

The occurrence of a limb amputation may have significant impact on an individual's ability to earn a living. Unskilled or semiskilled laborers tend to rely more on their physical abilities for gainful employment. The employability of these individuals is particularly affected by amputation and it is this group of individuals who are least able to adjust to skilled or managerial positions. For individuals whose duties are professional, managerial, or executive, the economic adjustments to amputation are less significant. The large majority of unemployed and marginally employable amputees come from lower socioeconomic groups. Hence, an important adjustment to be made by amputees in this group is the need to relearn vocational skills. This often entails a major change in life style. State offices of vocational rehabilitation were designed to help just such individuals.

Individual Reactions

For any given individual amputee, it is impossible to make generalizations about the relative significance of the physical, psychosocial, vocational, and economic problems associated with amputation. In most cases, effective treatment results in the reduction of the number of the amputee's problems, but fails to completely irradicate any one of them. Likewise, during the amputee's lifetime, different problems will assume greater and lesser importance depending upon other factors.

Gauthier-Gagnon reported on factors predisposing to prosthetic use among 396 adults with unilateral, transfemoral or transtibial amputations: 85 percent were prosthetic wearers, 77 percent of vascular origin, or 42.5 percent in the adult population. The factors included level of amputation, absence of respiratory problems, and adaptation to prosthesis wear. Predictors of active use outdoors included residence, claudication pain, delays in prosthetic fitting, and duration of prosthetic training.

Prosthetic Preoperative Evaluation

Ideally the clinic team begins its work as soon as it is determined that an amputation is necessary. The preoperative evaluation of any patient attempts to both gain and transmit information. The information gained helps in determining the nature and severity of any potential problems that may be encountered during the postoperative course. The preoperative evaluation also serves as a time when the prospective amputee may ask any questions that have been harbored during the process of making the decision to proceed with the amputation. Questions may arise as to components, cosmesis, or other concerns about perceptions, taboos, or media images, all of which are of concern to the patient and family.

In order to document the service aspect of the modern orthotic and prosthetic practice, Billock published his system for defining the different levels of service involved in the delivery of an orthosis or prosthesis: minimal, brief, limited, intermediate, extended, and/or comprehensive. The key to all definitions of all terms involves the length of time necessary to perform the evaluation, the difficulty of the problem to be addressed, and the number of times the patient is expected to return. The comprehensive level involves the previous plus the need to consult with or document such consultation in the permanent medical record.

Patient Expectations

Questions concerning the expectations of the patient are important. This information, when coupled with the diagnostic and other team input, assists the members of the clinic team in developing a reasonable and workable treatment plan. It is also important to ascertain how the impending amputation will affect the patient's lifestyle. In the process of collecting necessary information concerning the patient's future, it is often helpful to contact a significant other, whether this person is a family member or not. Any person in the patient's life in whom trust may be placed, both by the clinic team members and the patient, may serve in this role. This significant other often plays a role in the decision-making process and may be invaluable in effecting a successful transition back into the home and/or work environment once discharge from the hospital or care facility occurs.

Many decisions made by the amputee about the future will involve his or her vocation or avocation. The degree of motivation that the amputee brings to the postoperative situation will help determine the goals to which the ultimate prosthetic fitting may lead. Additionally, the type or intensity of the patient's vocation may assist the clinic team in making decisions about the type and strength of the components of the prosthetic device.

It is very important to assure the patient at the preoperative meeting that all questions are important and that all will be answered. It is important to deal with the subject of pain and the sensations of the lost limb and to communicate the normal and usual nature of these feelings. One of the questions usually asked by the soon-to-be amputee is when all these things are going to happen. It is common for the patient and his or her significant other to begin to focus on the prosthesis and the events following the amputation. This allows the physical therapist and other team members to enumerate the events and goals associated with both the early and late prosthetic phases and to put them in their proper time sequence.

Physical Examination

Along with a thorough review of the medical record and discussions among the members of the clinic team, the physical examination occurs. The discussion with the attending surgeon should reveal the anticipated level of amputation and any potential medical problems that may lead to a less-than-optimal result.

Before the amputation, the physical therapist needs to know the patient's abilities with whatever walking aids have been used prior to surgery. If the patient is a good crutch user, teaching him or her to use a new gait in expectation of the amputation saves some time and gives the patient an idea of what to expect following surgery. If the patient is unaccustomed to using crutches or a walker, it is best to teach him or her while there are no pain or balance problems. Because balance may be affected in the early postoperative days, balance routines may be demonstrated to educate the patient about what to expect following surgery. This is also a good time for the physical therapist to establish a helping rapport with the amputee and to demonstrate how future goals will be addressed together.

As a part of the overall preoperative evaluation, it is important to evaluate the strength and range of motion of both the involved and uninvolved limbs and joints. Normal prosthetic ambulation requires good range of motion and strength on both sides. The presence of fixed deformities limits the expectations for the patient, but also assists in setting realistic goals. Accurate evaluation of proximal joint strength allows early exercise programs to target these areas, preparing them for later use.

It is not uncommon for patients to develop flexion contractures in the early postoperative days following amputation. It is therefore necessary to know that the contracture was not present prior to surgery and that it may be quickly dealt with and remedied. In cases of extreme flexion contractures, the patient should be given information concerning the nonstandard nature of the finished prosthesis. Often the managing surgeon will delay the elective procedure until all conservative measures of managing the contracture have been exhausted or until sound medical evidence indicates that a life-threatening situation exists.

AN OVERVIEW OF ORTHOTICS

Orthosis Users

The 3 percent of the American population who may benefit from application of an orthotic device includes individuals who have been affected by a wide spectrum of neuromusculoskeletal diseases, trauma, and congenital problems. Although pediatric and geriatric applications are somewhat more prevalent, orthosis wearers include all age groups: 3.5 million Americans use some type of orthosis. In patients under 25 years, 38 percent use foot orthoses and 24 percent use leg orthoses, according to Nielsen's research. Orthotic applications for specific problems will be discussed in chapters 8, 9, 10, and 11.

Orthotics (and Prosthetic) Nomenclature

Just as in prosthetics, as various orthotic devices have been developed there has been a tendency to name them after the developer. This is especially widespread in regard to spinal orthoses. The need for a standardized nomenclature had been recognized for many years, but not until the 1960s was a joint effort to develop a system undertaken by the American Academy of Orthopaedic Surgeons, the Committee on Prosthetics-Orthotics Education of the National Academy of Sciences, and the American Orthotics and Prosthetics Association. A series of workshops resulted in the development of a nomenclature and its attendant terminology for orthotic devices and systems that has become accepted in many parts of the world and now forms the core for the International Standards Organization (ISO) official descriptors for orthoses. The core of these descriptions is acronyms based on the major joints that an orthosis is intended to control or effect. For example, an ankle-foot orthosis is referred to as an AFO, and an orthosis that extends from the foot to the thigh is referred to as a knee-ankle-foot orthosis, or KAFO. Table 1-1 presents a summary of this nomenclature.

TABLE 1-1. Orthotics Nomenclature

Upper Limb Orthoses

HO	Hand orthosis		
WO	Wrist orthosis	WHO	Wrist-hand orthosis
EO	Elbow orthosis	EWHO	Elbow-wrist-hand orthosis

Spinal Orthoses

CTLSO	Cervical-thoracic-lumbosacral orthosis		
CO	Cervical orthosis	TLSO	Thoracic-lumbosacral orthosis
TO	Thoracic orthosis	LSO	Lumbosacral orthosis
LO	Lumbar orthosis	SIO	Sacroiliac orthosis

Lower-Limb Orthoses

FO	Foot orthosis	AFO	Ankle-foot orthosis
KO	Knee orthosis	KAFO	Knee-ankle-foot orthosis
HpO	Hip orthosis	HKAFO	Hip-knee-ankle-foot orthosis

In 1993, the American Academy of Orthotists and Prosthetists (AAOP) and the American Orthotic and Prosthetic Association (AOPA) adopted and endorsed ISO terminology. This terminology had previously been accepted by the American Academy of Orthopaedic Surgery (AAOS) and the International Society for Prosthetics and Orthotics (ISPO). Although this new system included some old terms (TLSO, AFO), it changed some long-standing terms substituting transtibial for below knee and transfemoral for above knee. Syme amputation became ankle disarticulation while congenital limb deficiencies are described as either transverse or longitudinal. The transverse deficiencies are named as amputation-type conditions and are named at the point of deficiency (Figure 1-4). Longitudinal deficiencies are named for the absence of skeletal anatomy within the long axis of the bone (Figure 1-5). Longitudinal deficiencies are named by the bones affected in a proximal to distal sequence using terms that indicate whether each

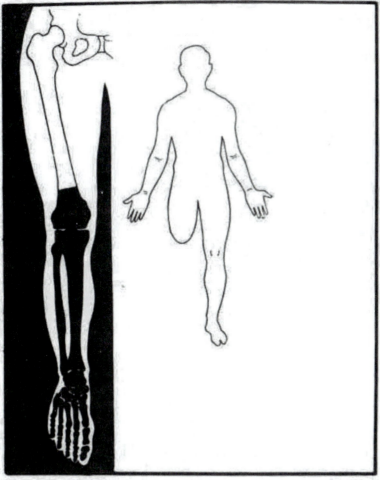

Figure 1-4. ISO transverse deficiency. (*Source: J Prosthetics Orthot.* 6(1), 1994; 29–33.)

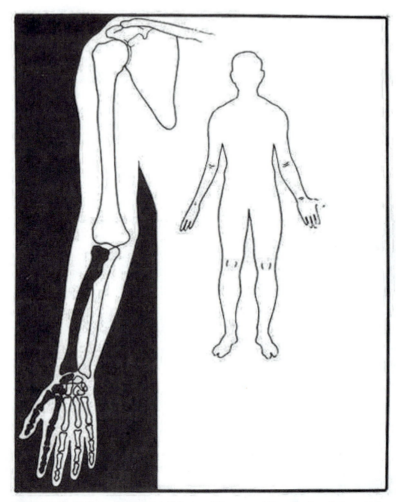

Figure 1-5. ISO longitudinal deficiency. (*Source: J Prosthetics Orthot.* 6(1), 1994; 29–33.)

affected bone is totally or partially absent. A congenital transfemoral deficiency is a transverse deficiency of the thigh, lower third. A proximal absence of the fibula is a longitudinal deficiency of the fibula, partial.

Reactions and Adjustments to Orthotics Use

The reactions and adjustments to wearing and depending on an orthotic device are similar to but often less dramatic than those associated with amputation and using a prosthesis. They are, nonetheless, important factors that must be taken seriously and dealt with conscientiously.

Unlike most prosthetic fittings, orthoses may be viewed by the user as something optional, as in the case of diabetic shoes and inserts, or an AFO in the early stages of multiple sclerosis (MS), amyotrophic lateral sclerosis (ALS), or any number of pediatric diseases. Often wearing time for these orthoses may be measured in weeks or months rather than years. Orthoses play an important role in the treatment and prevention of future problems or deformities.

The nonsurgical treatment of (DDH) Developmental Dysplasia of the Hip, scoliosis, Legg-Calve-Perthes (LCP), and/or acute spinal fractures afford parents and children an option. It is the team's responsibility to teach each family to follow prescribed wearing regimens in order to afford the patient the best possible, nonsurgical option when using orthoses.

REFERENCES

1. American Board for Certification (ABC). Personal communication 2001.
2. American Diabetes Association *(www.diabetes.org)*, 2001.
3. Bach S, Noreng MF, Tjellden NU. Phantom limb pain in amputees during the first 12 months following limb amputation, after preoperative lumber epidural blockade. *Pain.* 1988; 33:297–301.
4. Benson V, Marano MA. Current estimates for the national health interview survey, 1993. National Center for Health Statistics, *Vital Health Statistics.* 1994;10(190).
5. Billock, JN. Clinical evaluation and assessment principles in orthotics and prosthetics. *Jour of Prosth and Orth.* Spring 1996; 8(2):, 41–44.
6. Breakey JW. Body image: The lower-limb amputee. *Jour of Prosth and Ortht.* Spring, 1997; 9(2): 58–66.
7. Furst L, Humphrey M. Coping with the loss of a leg. *Prosthet Orthot Int.* 1983; 7:152–156.
8. Gauthier-Gagnon C, Grise M-C, Potvin D. Predisposing Factors related to prosthetic use by people with a transtibial and transfemoral amputation. *Jour of Prosth and Orth.* Fall 1998; 10(4): 99–109.
9. Kay HW, Newman JD. Relative incidences of new amputations. *Orthot Prosthet.* 1975; 29(2):3–16.
10. Lind J, Kramhoft M, Bodtker S. The incidence of smoking on complications after primary amputations of the lower extremity. *Clin Orthop.* 1991; 267:11–217.
11. National Health Survey. *Use of special aids-1969.* Rockville, MD: US Dept. of Health, Education, and Welfare publication; 1969. HSM 73–1504.
12. National Health Survey. *Use of special aids—1977.* Rockville, MD: National Center for Health Statistics; 1974. US Dept. of Health, Education, and Welfare publication, 126 series 10.
13. Nicholas JJ et al. Problems experienced and perceived by prosthetic patients. *Jour of Prosth and Orth.* January 1993; 5(1): 36–39.
14. Nickel V. Orthotics in America. *Clin Ortho.* 1974; 102:10–17.
15. Nielsen C. Issues affecting the future demand for orthotists and prosthetists. A study prepared for the National Commission on Orthotic and Prosthetic Education, November 1996.
16. Ponte Vedra II. Orthotic/Prosthetic Future. Washington, DC: American Orthotic and Prosthetic Association, 1976.
17. Practitioner Level Programs. *Orthot Prosthet.* 1984; 38(2):20–68.
18. Schuch CM, Pritham, CH. International standards organization terminology: application to prosthetics and orthotics. *Jour of Prosth and Ortho.* Winter 1994; 6(1):29–33.
19. Sherman RA, Arena J. Phantom limb pain: Mechanisms, incidence, and ireatment. *Critical Reviews in Physical and Rehabilitative Medicine.* 1992; 4:1–26.

CHAPTER 2

Methods, Materials, and Mechanics

Over the years, the recognition of the value of prosthetic and orthotic care has increased whenever well-known people acquired disabilities that required the services of an orthotist or prosthetist. One of the best-known examples is the rehabilitation center established in Warm Springs, Georgia, thanks to President Franklin D. Roosevelt. In 1926, President Roosevelt spent two-thirds of his personal fortune to purchase the Meriwether Inn and the warm springs and 1,200 acres surrounding it to establish a polio aftercare facility. A monument to his generosity stands today at the gate of the Roosevelt Warm Springs Institute for Rehabilitation.

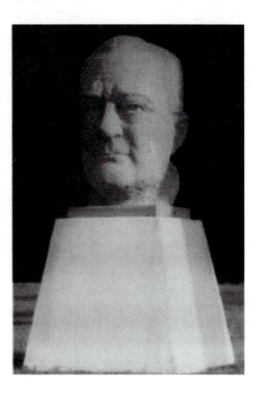

Following completion of reading this chapter, the student will be able to:

1. Describe the elements and chronology involved in the provision of an orthosis or prosthesis.
2. Discuss the options involved in fabrication and production of orthotics and prosthetics.
3. Describe the options available in materials and differentiate among those options relative to physical characteristics and patient needs.
4. Discuss the importance of mechanics in the decision of design and materials used in orthotics and prosthetics.

This chapter presents an overview of the processes and materials used to produce prosthetic and orthotic devices. Also presented are some common biomechanical considerations that must be taken into account when making and applying these devices. Although there are some factors that are specific to either prosthetic or orthotic practice, there are many more commonalties than differences in the methods and materials used to produce these devices. Therefore, this chapter will focus on methods, materials, and mechanical concepts that apply to both prostheses and orthoses.

FABRICATION METHODS

Steps in the Provision of an Orthosis/Prosthesis
The provision of any prosthetic or orthotic device, whether a simple finger splint or a complex design such as lower limb prosthesis, includes the six steps outlined in Table 2-1. As was briefly discussed in chapter 1, the prescription specifying the type of device desired should, ideally, be the result of consultations among the members of a multidisciplinary clinic team and should be based on a thorough, client-centered, evaluation of the patient's needs, functional goals, and desires.

Once consensus has been reached on the optimal approach to be taken, the prosthetist/orthotist then proceeds to take the measurements and/or impressions needed to provide the device. Measurements are likely to include such items as the lengths and circumferences of body segments, locations of bony landmarks and tendons, and joint ranges of motion. According to

TABLE 2-1. STEPS IN PROVIDING AN ORTHOSIS/PROSTHESIS

1. Evaluation/prescription
2. Measurement/impression taking (casting)
3. Fabrication/bench alignment
4. Fitting/static alignment
5. Modification/dynamic alignment
6. Reevaluation/follow up

Quigley, careful attention is also paid to potential complications such as the presence of scar tissue, neuromas, edema, and weight problems. When a custom-molded design is desired, the measurement process includes an impression of the body segment (or residual limb in the case of a prosthesis). Although electronic digitization techniques are now available, most commonly this is achieved by taking an impression of the segment, making certain that the impression is in close contact with the limb segment at biomechanically significant anatomical sites. Figures 2-1a and 2-2a illustrate impressions taken using plaster bandages.

The third step is the fabrication of a tangible device. In the simplest case, this step may consist of selecting the proper size of prefabricated device that will be modified based on the measurements taken from the patient. In the case of a custom-made device, the prosthetist/orthotist uses the measurements and impression to produce a positive model of the affected body segment. Figures 2-1b and 2-2b illustrate this step in the process. The finished positive model is not simply a duplicate of the body segment but is skillfully modified by the prosthetist/orthotist so that the final device will have specific areas of increased contact (pressure) and other areas of reduced contact (relief) so that it will be biomechanically effective and comfortable to wear. If the device being fabricated is a lower limb prosthesis, the prosthetist will initially arrange or "align" the foot and other components of the device based on established clinical guidelines referred to as static alignment, which will be discussed in chapters 4 and 5.

Once the device has been fabricated, the next step is fitting it to the patient: trying it on to see how it fits and feels. At this stage, the practitioner must carefully evaluate whether the forces and pressures applied by the device are in the desired locations and of magnitudes that the patient can comfortably tolerate. If the device is for the lower limb, this fitting step includes an assessment of whether the components are adequately aligned for static standing and weightbearing.

The fifth step in the provision of an orthosis or prosthesis is to modify or fine-tune the device after the patient has tried to function with it. This step may include relatively minor adjustments such as the addition of padding, localized thermal remolding, or the removal of material by grinding or trimming. It might also consist of more major changes such as the substitution of different components or re-fabrication of part of the device that does not perform satisfactorily. For lower limb, prosthetic applications, this step includes the process of dynamic alignment wherein fine adjustments are made to the device while the patient is walking on it to optimize the gait pattern.

The final and equally important step in providing a device is to schedule regular reevaluation and followup by the clinic team to verify that the patient's needs continue to be met by the device. Not only is it expected that the device will function differently over time due to mechanical wear and tear, but the patient's biomechanical needs may fluctuate due to changes in functional ability, lifestyle, body weight, and proportions.

CAD-CAM (COMPUTER AIDED DESIGN-COMPUTER AIDED MANUFACTURING)

Perhaps the most exciting new technology in this industry is CAD-CAM. Dr. James Foort is given credit for theoretically likening music to shapes and proposing that prosthetic and orthotic shapes should be able to be stored on magnetic tape like songs. It would follow that if

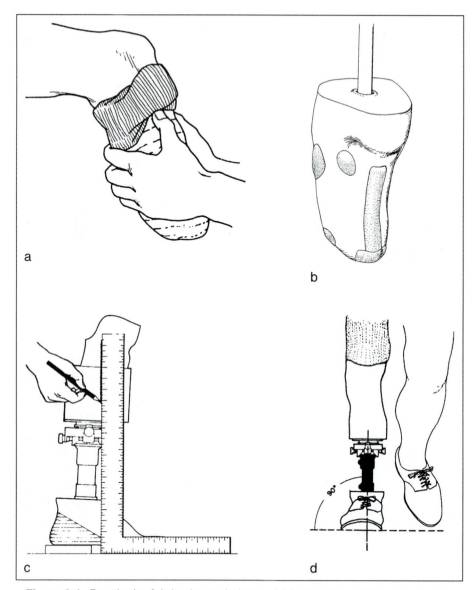

Figure 2-1. Prosthetics fabrication techniques: (a) impression taking using a plaster cast; (b) modified positive plaster model of residual limb; (c) bench aligning a below-knee prosthetic limb; (d) dynamic alignment.

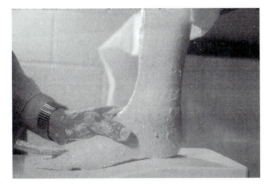

a

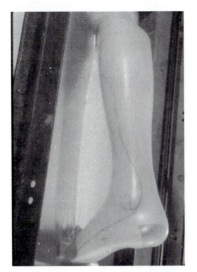

c

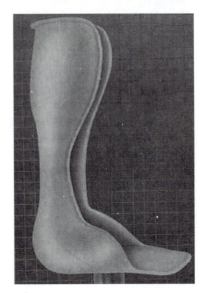

b

d

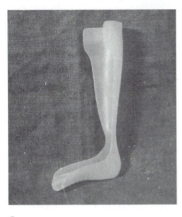

e

Figure 2-2. Orthotics fabrication techniques: (a) impression taking using a plaster cast; (b) positive plaster model of limb segment; (c) heated plastic sheet being vacuum-formed over plaster model; (d) trimlines being marked on cooled plastic; (e) finished plastic molded ankle-foot orthosis.

stored, they could also be recalled and reproduced by some sort of machine. Foort later developed the first prosthetic CAD-CAM system in the early 1980s. This system produced prosthetic sockets and reference modeled shapes and is credited to Foort, Dr. Ron Davies of the University College of London, and Dr. Geoff Fernie from the University of Toronto.

The first useable CAD-CAM system in orthotics and prosthetics was unveiled to the world in 1983 at the ISPO Congress in London, England. The system, pioneered by the University College of London, combined a scanner (data input unit) with an industry-grade cutter, which slowly produced a positive model using a computer-aided, 6-degree of freedom lathe. This approach created the modified positive model of the limb without the first two conventional steps: it eliminated the need for negative impression taking and positive model rectification.

Current CAD-CAM systems incorporate a number of different methods including lasers to digitally capture body surface topography. These digitizers are responsible for transmitting surface contour data to the software that the practitioner uses to rectify or modify the model on the computer screen (see Figure 2-3). The data depicting the modified shape is electronically transmitted to a commercial milling machine that carves the rectified model from a blank of plaster or rigid foam material.

The reported advantages of CAD-CAM include exactness of image; rectification using computer software rather than manually sculpting plaster positive models; references to a standard developed over time from many images; quick storage and retrieval of past images; time savings to the practitioner due to automation.

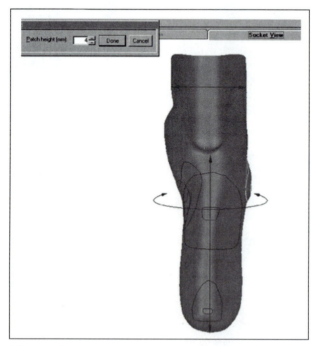

Figure 2-3. An example of a computer-rectified model of a translibial residual limb.

Most commercially available CAD-CAM systems in use today were originally developed to create prosthetic sockets (see Figure 2-1). Because of the simple and generally symmetric shape of many residual limbs, CAD-CAM often works well for such uncomplicated cases. Some of the newer systems have limited orthotic capabilities, and because of the inherent difficulty in carving the right angle formed by the ankle and foot, progress has been slow in this area. Foot orthoses and shoe lasts are more easily produced using CAD-CAM because they do not extend above the ankle.

Dr. Michael Vannier and his associates at the University of Iowa have begun using spiral-computed tomography (SXCT) as the data input source, with the scanning taking approximately 10 seconds. Vannier, a radiologist and engineer, compared three-dimensional electromagnetic point digitizers with spiral X-ray computed tomography (SXCT) andthree-dimensional optical surface scanning (OSS) with caliper measurements and evaluated the precision and accuracy of each system. After each system measured 13 transtibial adult amputee residual limbs, the results demonstrated the precision and accuracy of the surface scanner and SXCT. Compared with plaster models, the SXCT and OSS were found to be accurate to within 2 mm.

Kohler et al studied comparisons between handmade sockets and CAD-CAM produced sockets and could not demonstrate any significant differences in comfort.

Staros and Schwartz reported on the use of CAD-CAM in the development of custom footwear. Nelson, in New York, enhanced their concepts and now regularly provides custom footwear for veterans using this technology.

Magnetic sensing technology allows data access/input to be done by using an electromagnetic wand and laptop computer. The TRACER-CAD system allows the prosthetist to manually move the wand to collect surface contour data from the residual limb and to rectify the on-screen image to create a three-dimensional model of the rectified shape desired. These data may then be transmitted via modem to a geographically distant central fabrication facility for positive model production and socket fabrication.

Otto Bock uses the same type of electromagnetic input in the creation of custom seating systems. Wand-type digitizers capture the shape of a temporary seat and back produced using a special seating simulator. Once this data has been transmitted via modem, the rectified positive models are produced and the device manufactured (see Figure 2-4).

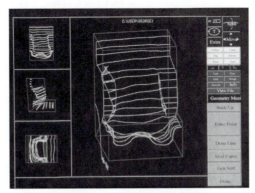

Figure 2-4. Otto Bock Seating System. (Copyright owned by and photo reprinted with permission by Otto Bock Health Care.)

Otto Bock also markets the Electronic Test Socket (ETS) system. This simplified CAD-CAM approach uses referenced sizes and shapes to produce a clear plastic test socket based on patient measurements. Shurr reported on 53 consecutive ETS test socket fittings at a symposium in Nürnberg in May 1997. All patients were able to stand comfortably once the test sockets were modified during the usual fitting process. This ETS system currently applies only at the transfemoral level; however transtibial applications will soon be available to certified prosthetists and their patients.

Fabrication Options

There are several different fabrication options and terms that need to be understood. The distinction between off-the-shelf prefabrication and custom fabrication has already been mentioned. In concept, devices and components that are industrially mass produced are likely to be of a more consistent quality, less expensive, and faster to deliver to the patient than devices and components that are individually manufactured one at a time. Similarly, standardized, interchangeable, off-the-shelf components should make replacement and repair of devices easier and faster. For these reasons, there has been a clear trend in prosthetic and orthotic practice worldwide to use as many pre-manufactured modular components and devices as possible. In many cases, however, a portion of the device (and sometimes the entire device) must be custom made in order to properly fit the patient and to fully accomplish the intended goals. Precise impression taking (casting or digitizing) is, and will likely continue to be, an integral part of the delivery of most prosthetic and orthotics devices.

Another important distinction is between local and central fabrication. Costs associated with the manufacturing of prostheses and orthoses, including purchasing sheet plastics, forming ovens, vacuum molding equipment, and complying with Occupational Safety and Health Administration regulations encouraged the development of central fabrication, or production of devices from a more industrial location separate from the clinical site where measurement, delivery, and fitting of the devices occur. When several offices use the same central fabrication services, complex and expensive technology may be utilized without the need for each facility to purchase, use, and maintain expensive, modern, high technology equipment such as CAD-CAM. Other advantages of the division of labor where technicians perform the central fabrication tasks include making it possible for the certified practitioner to serve more patients and to provide clinical care in a more professional setting free from the smell, dust, and congestion inherent in a fabrication site.

Some disadvantages of central fabrication include increased chances for communication problems with the technicians who actually make the devices, particularly with nonstandard applications, and time delays for shipping of rectified positive models and finished devices. Central fabrication is a natural extension of prefabrication. If an entire device needs custom fabrication, it can be manufactured at a centralized location from a cast or digitization taken by the certified practitioner and sent to the laboratory. This system is analogous to the current production of dentures, eyeglasses, and other medical or dental devices. In the future, central fabrication may become mandatory to allow the practitioner to survive economically, as profit margins are eroded by shrinking health care reimbursements.

Specifications for the "Ideal" Prosthesis/Orthosis

In producing a prosthetic/orthotic device, there are certain "ideal" design specifications that are rarely all achievable. Table 2-2 lists some of these specifications. Foremost among these specifications is the desire to have the device function precisely as it is intended to do. This includes being simple in design and easy for the patient to learn to use. It also includes having a

TABLE 2-2. SPECIFICATIONS FOR THE "IDEAL" PROSTHESIS/ORTHOSIS

Function	meets user's needs, simple, easily learned, dependable
Comfort	fits well, easy to put on and take off, lightweight, adjustable
Cosmesis	looks, smells, sounds "normal," cleans easily, stain-resistant
Fabrication	fast, modular, readily and widely available
Economics	affordable, worth cost of monetary investment

device that will continue to function dependably with little need for repair or replacement. Comfort is also of great importance when using the device. If the device continually causes areas of high skin pressure, irritation, or reaction, it is unlikely that the patient will wear it long term. The device should also be easy to put on (don) and take off (doff) as well as be lightweight and able to accommodate minor fluctuations in the patient's size.

Cosmesis, or the appearance, smell, and sound of the device, is also important. As was mentioned in the previous chapter, many individuals in our society do not want to call attention to themselves by making sounds that are abnormal or unusual. Some devices may provide good function but go unused because of these factors. Also because they are often in constant contact with body tissues, most prosthetic and orthotic devices need to be stain-resistant and easily cleaned.

Ideally, prostheses and orthoses are fabricated and delivered quickly; use a maximum number of prefabricated, modular components; and are widely and readily available to those who need them. Similarly, the ideal is for these devices to be affordable by those in need and worth the cost for the improved function they provide.

MATERIALS

Material Characteristics Important in Prosthetics and Orthotics

There are several characteristics of materials that determine their suitability for use in prosthetics and orthotics. Table 2-3 lists the most important of these characteristics.

Certainly strength, or the maximum external load that a material can sustain, is important. This is particularly critical in lower limb and spinal applications where force levels may be quite high. Stiffness is an equally important material characteristic that determines the amount of bending or

TABLE 2-3. IMPORTANT CHARACTERISTICS OF PROSTHETIC AND ORTHOTICS MATERIALS

Strength	maximum external load that can be withstood
Stiffness	stress/strain or force-to-displacement ratio
Durability (fatigue resistance)	ability to withstand repeated loading
Density	weight per unit volume
Corrosion resistance	resistance to chemical degradation
Ease of fabrication	equipment and techniques needed to shape it

compression (strain) that results in response to the load (stress) applied. In some applications, such as lower limb prostheses and orthoses, very stiff and rigid materials that allow virtually no flexion or bending when loaded are required to support weightbearing stresses. At the same time, however, it may be highly desirable to include some very flexible materials which conform to body contour changes or absorb shock and store "elastic" energy. Both the strength and stiffness of a given portion of a prosthetic or orthotic device depend on the thickness and shape of the device as well as the material selected. Cylindrical and semicircular shapes and sections with ridges, flanges, or corrugations are inherently stronger and stiffer than flat thin sections of material.

Durability, or fatigue resistance, refers to the ability of a material to withstand repeated loading and unloading cycles. In nearly all materials, repeated loading reduces the maximum strength and ultimately causes failure or fracture. Because orthotic and prosthetic devices may be loaded hundreds of thousands and sometimes millions of cycles, Henshaw learned that fatigue resistance is an important characteristic. The intersection between two materials that have significantly different properties, such as plastic and metal, is one location where fatigue stresses may be increased. Some materials are also especially prone to failure at sites where the surface has been scratched or "notched."

Density, or weight per unit volume, is a continual concern in selecting prosthetic and orthotic materials. The goal is to make the device as lightweight as possible to minimize the energy required to support and move it, possibly hundreds or thousands of times each day.

Two additional material characteristics to be considered are corrosion resistance and ease of fabrication. Limitations due to either one of these factors can severely limit the applicability of a particular material. Ease of fabrication is especially important in custom molded applications because materials must be readily transformed into a soft, malleable state in order to conform to a model of a body segment. There are many "space age" materials with several desirable characteristics that are not easily formed, shaped, or tooled for prosthetic and orthotic applications.

A final practical consideration is cost and availability. Ideal materials are readily available at reasonable costs. Research from Redford shows clearly that no one material has the required characteristics for all applications or for all the different components of a single device.

Classes of Materials

Based on consideration of the material characteristics discussed previously, several classes of materials are commonly used in prosthetics and orthotics. These materials are listed in Table 2-4.

Wood. Wood (principally maple and hickory) is used in many prosthetic feet. Research by Quigley reports that basswood, willow, poplar, and linden wood are often used for prosthetic knees and shins. These wooden components are lightweight, strong, inexpensive, easily shaped, and consistent in texture. Use of wood in orthotic systems is rare.

Leather. Leather is a material that has traditionally been, and continues to be, in common use in both prosthetic and orthotic devices. Leather (principally vegetable-tanned cowhide) is used for suspension straps, waist belts, socket liners, and protective coverings (fairings) over knee and hip joints in prosthetics. In addition to its use in the construction of quality footwear, leather is also used for molded arch supports, cuffs, straps, laces, linings, and coverings for orthoses.

**TABLE 2-4. CLASSES OF MATERIALS
COMMONLY USED IN PROSTHETICS
AND ORTHOTICS**

Wood
Leather
Fabric
Rubber
Metal
   Steel
   Aluminum
   Titanium
   Magnesium
Plastics
   Thermoplastics
   Thermosets
Composites

Fabric. Wool, cotton, silk, and a number of synthetic materials such as nylon, olefin, polyester, rayon, or vinyl may be woven or knitted for prosthetic and orthotic applications, although some may be molded with pressure, heat, or chemicals. Whenever a fabric must be fitted to a complex three-dimensional shape, Redford's research shows that knitting is usually the preferred technique. In prosthetic applications, fabrics are used for waist belts, straps, harnesses, and, most prevalently, for prosthetic socks. Fabrics also cover the new comfort liners to retard wear of the more fragile elastomers, gels, and silicones. Like athletic socks, prosthetic socks help keep the skin dry, cushion impact, and reduce shear, and act as a filler to make wearing the item more comfortable. Prosthetic socks are commonly made of wool, cotton, or blends of these with nylon or other synthetic materials, according to Quigley. Redford has shown that in orthotic applications, fabrics are used primarily for fastening or for less rigid supports, such as corsets, belts, and stockings.

Rubber. The elastic properties and high friction coefficient of rubber materials make them useful for padding in prosthetic and orthotic devices, for seals in hydraulic and pneumatic mechanisms, and for heels and bumpers in prosthetic feet and special footwear.

Metal. The three types of metals most commonly used in prosthetics and orthotics are steel, aluminum, and alloys of titanium and magnesium. Figure 2-5 shows a comparison of their maximum strength, stiffness, and weight per unit volume (density).

Steel, including corrosion-resistant stainless steel, has the advantages of low cost, ready availability, and relative ease of fabrication. It is strong, rigid, and fatigue resistant but, unfortunately, it is also relatively heavy. Steel is widely used in prefabricated prosthetic and orthotic joints, metal bands, cuffs, cables, springs, bearings, and hydraulic and pneumatic components.

Aluminum is a much lighter metal than steel with a high strength-to-weight ratio that is particularly useful in upper limb, pediatric, and other applications where weight is a major

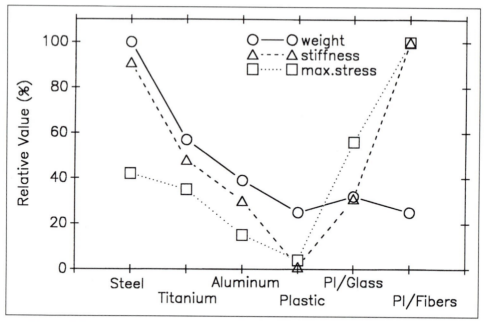

Figure 2-5. Comparison of weight, stiffness and maximum stress of materials commonly employed in prosthetic and orthotic devices. (*Source:* adaptation of data presented by Henshaw in *The Advance in Orthotics*, p. 146.)

consideration. The primary disadvantage of aluminum is its relatively poor resistance to fatigue at high load levels or at high rates of repeated loading.

Titanium and magnesium alloys have strengths comparable to steel but are substantially lighter in weight with good corrosion resistance. According to Redford, the principal disadvantage is their relative high cost.

During the 1990s, most component manufacturers adopted a system of classification consistent with patient weight and functional activity level. This allows the practitioner to order components optimized for each patient's weight and functional activity level. Otto Bock, a leader in the industry, has developed a color-coded grid that allows easy selection and visual verification of the proper parts. It also facilitates identification of the lightest weight and least expensive components appropriate for the needs of each individual patient (see Figure 2-6).

Plastics. The increased availability and use of plastic materials in recent years has had a dramatic impact on prosthetic and orthotic practice. Redford defines the term plastic as any synthetic material that can be molded, extruded, laminated, or hardened into any form. Such plastic materials are lightweight, can be readily formed into complex anatomical shapes, tend to be nontoxic, and are generally impervious to body fluids. There are two major types of plastics, thermoplastics, and thermosets.

Thermoplastics become soft and malleable when heated and then become hard again when cooled. Their potential uses in prosthetics and orthotics in the United States were first realized in

Modular Lower Limb
Otto Bock Classification System®

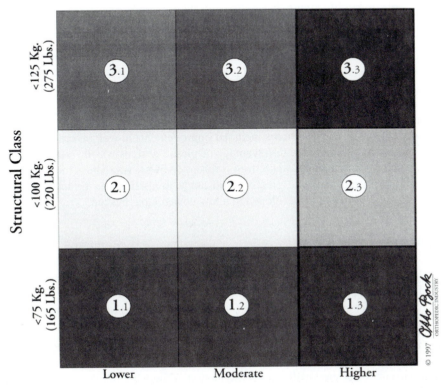

Figure 2-6. Otto Bock Classification Matrix. (Copyright owned by and photo reprinted with permission by Otto Bock Health Care.)

the late 1960s. They can be repeatedly reheated and re-molded. According to Compton and Edlestein thermoplastic materials that become workable below 80° C (180° F) are generally referred to as low-temperature thermoplastics and, with care, can usually be formed directly on a body segment. This type of material is most useful for upper limb orthotic applications and for temporary use such as in fracture braces because they usually have limited strength and fatigue resistance. High-temperature thermoplastics (malleable above 80° C or 180° F) must be shaped over a model and include materials such as acrylic, polyethylene, polypropylene, polycarbonate, ABS, and PVC. They are usually used in the vacuum-forming of permanent prosthetic and orthotic devices. Showers and Strunck report that there are also a number of soft foam interface plastics such as Pelite, Plastazote, and Aliplast that are used principally as liners or padding.

In contrast to thermoplastics, thermosetting materials develop a permanent shape once they solidify and cannot be reheated and reformed. Because of their curing temperature, thermosetting plastics such as polyester resins must be formed over a heat-resistant model. They are usually laminated with layers of natural or synthetic cloth and can be sanded, trimmed, drilled, and riveted. They also can be pigmented in an attempt to match a patient's basic skin color. As can be seen from Figure 2-5, the addition of glass or carbon fiber elements to plastic material dramatically increases its maximum strength and stiffness. Newer materials used in both orthotics and prosthetics include composites such as graphite. Graphite may be used as a primary material for limb, socket, or orthosis and is lightweight and very strong. It is difficult, if not impossible, to modify after being heated and shaped.

Silicones, thermoplastic elastomers, and urethanes are used for prosthetic socket liners or comfort liners, and will be further described in chapters 4 and 5.

The uses of plastics in the construction of prostheses and orthoses are evolving quickly. In a recent survey conducted by Nader and Boenick, 17 percent of the responding practitioners indicated that all of their patients in need of leg orthoses received plastic devices. Sixty-one percent indicated that three quarters of their patients received plastic orthoses. Only 15 percent of the practitioners reported using metal orthoses predominantly. Reasons cited for using plastic rather than metal orthoses included improvements in weight, cosmesis, and versatility. The most commonly cited disadvantage of plastic designs was the inability to adjust the ankle angle in non-articulated ankle-foot orthoses (AFOs). To address this concern, several variations in metal or plastic prefabricated ankle joints that can be incorporated into molded plastic AFOs have been developed to allow controllable motion.

MECHANICS

Before proceeding to a discussion of lower limb biomechanics and specific prosthetic and orthotic devices in subsequent chapters, it is important that consideration be given to three general biomechanical topics that are applicable to nearly all prosthetic and/or orthotic such devices.

Moments and Force Couples

When an orthosis is attached to a body segment, it is usually intended to exert a force on that segment to limit or control an abnormal or unwanted motion. Although some of the applied force may be directed along the axis of the segment, a significant element is almost always present tending to affect rotation of the anatomical joint. This rotational control effect is referred to as a three-point force system or sometimes a three-point pressure system. Rotational control forces or moments across joints are not effective unless there are at least three points of contact between the device and the limb segment(s). Figure 2-7 illustrates some examples of three-point force systems.

Amputees use their remaining limb segments to apply forces and moments to an external device, their prosthesis, to control it or make it move. When the leverage from the long bones of the skeleton are used to move or prevent motion of a prosthesis, a force couple must be exerted. This force couple usually has a distal component in the direction of the intended moment and a proximal component in the opposite direction. Figure 2-8 illustrates common sites of force application in lower limb prostheses.

In both prosthetic and orthotic applications, it is desirable to use the longest possible lever arms when applying moments to or from a device. A longer lever arm means that the same moment can be generated with a smaller force because the moment is equal to the product of the force and the lever arm. Reducing forces is the principal means of minimizing pressures on body tissues and thereby increasing patient comfort while wearing these devices.

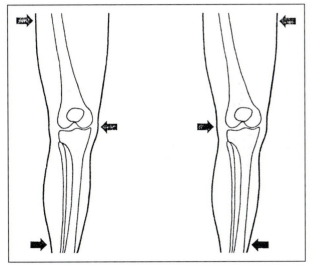

Figure 2-7. Example of a three-point force system used in knee orthotics.

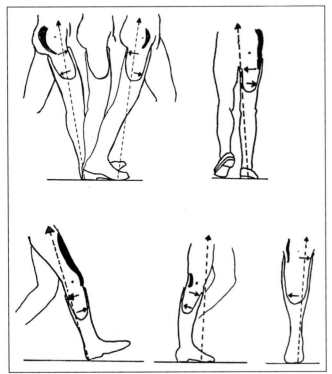

Figure 2-8. Examples of force couple application in lower limb prosthetics.

Pressure Tolerance of Tissues

Different biological tissues have markedly different tolerances for the application of external pressure. Anatomical sites with substantial muscle and fat tissue can tolerate higher pressures than bony prominences or areas containing superficial blood vessels and nerves. Contouring and padding to utilize pressure tolerant areas and to avoid pressure intolerant areas is an important element in the skillful fabrication of prosthetic and orthotic devices.

Pressure is defined as force per unit area. Besides reducing the applied force (by maximizing lever arms), the other strategy for reducing tissue pressure is to increase the area over which the force is applied. This is an important consideration when decisions are made regarding the location and size of the bands or cuffs of an orthosis or regarding the level at which a limb segment should be amputated.

Alignment of Joint Axes

Congruency between the anatomical joint axis and the mechanical joint axis of the prosthesis or orthosis is very important. If the axes do not coincide, undesirable forces are generated as the joints go through their range of motion. Compton and Redford show these unwanted forces may include both compression and shearing. Figure 2-9 illustrates some possible effects of such malalignment between the mechanical and anatomical joint axes.

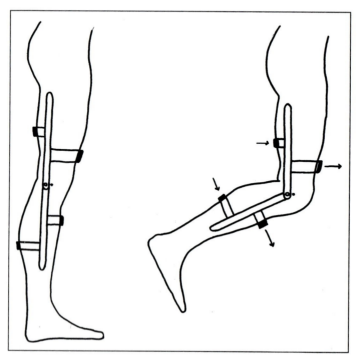

Figure 2-9. Example of malalignment between an anatomical and orthotic joint axis.

REFERENCES

1. Nader M, Boenick U. *CAD/CAM Systems in Pedothics, Prosthetics, and Orthotics.* Nürnberg: Otto Bock Press; 1997.
2. Compton J, Edlestein J. New plastics for forming directly on the patient. *Prosthet. Orthot. Int.* 1978; 2:43.
3. Condie D. The mechanics of lower limb bracing. In: *The Advance in Orthotics.* Murphy G, ed. Baltimore: Williams & Wilkins; 1976.
4. Henshaw J. The design of the orthotic appliance. In: *The Advance in Orthotics.* Murphy G, ed. Baltimore: Williams & Wilkins; 1976.
5. Kohler P, Lindl L, Wetz P. Comparison of CAD-CAM and Hand Made Sockets for PTB Prostheses. *Prosthet Orthot Int.* 1989; 13:19–24.
6. Pritham C. Analysis of the results from the questionnaire on metal vs. plastic orthoses. *Clinical Prosthetics & Orthotics.* Summer 1983; 7(3).
7. Quigley M. Prosthetic methods and materials. In: *Atlas of Limb Prosthetics.* St. Louis: CV Mosby; 1981.
8. Redford J, Licht S. Materials for orthotics. In: *Orthotics Etcetera.* Redford J., ed. Baltimore: Williams & Wilkins; 1986.
9. Showers D, Strunck M, Sheet plastics and their applications in orthotics and prosthetics. *Orthotics and Prosthetics.* 1985; 38(4):41–48.
10. Smith E, Juvinall R. Mechanics of orthotics. In: *Orthotics Etcetera.* Redford J, ed. Baltimore: Williams & Wilkins; 1986.
11. Staros A, Schwartz RS. Custom footwear: The role of computer-aided engineering. *J Test Eval.* 1988; 16:417–420.
12. Vannier MW, Commeam PK, Smith KE. Three-Dimensional Lower-Extremity Residual Measurement Systems Error Analysis. *Jour of Prosth and Orth.* Spring 1997; 9(2): 67–76.

CHAPTER 3

Biomechanics

Biomechanics and kinesiology underpin the practices of prosthetics and orthotics, as well as orthopaedic surgery. Many early pioneers in these fields understood the need for these sciences and established laboratories to study and teach these concepts to students, while caring for patients in need of such services. Early laboratories for prosthetics and orthotics often existed near or within such institutions. Dr. Arthur Steindler worked within the Children's Hospital on the campus of the University of Iowa from 1936 until 1968. It was here that he trained many early orthopaedic surgeons and orthotists whom he brought over from Austria to work alongside these surgeons in training.

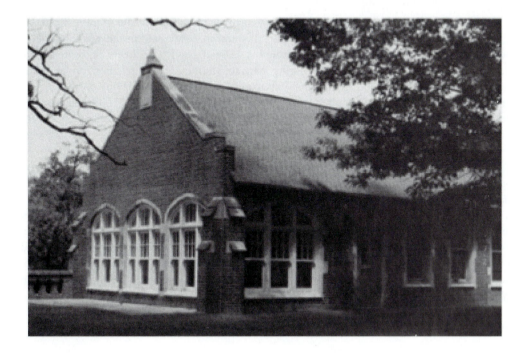

Following the completion of reading this chapter, the student will be able to:

1. Describe the gait cycle and discuss the importance of speed and energetics of gait.
2. Describe the role of the foot and ankle in gait.
3. Discuss the role of the knee and the muscles around it in the stance phase of gait.
4. Differentiate among the three planes acting around the hip and the functions they prescribe.

BIOMECHANICS OF THE LOWER LIMB

Because of its special role in weight bearing and mobility, orthotic and prosthetic devices for the lower extremity must be based on a sound understanding of lower limb biomechanics. This chapter considers the biomechanical functions of the lower limb especially as they relate to human ambulation. It is not intended as a comprehensive treatise on human gait but as a review of those functions that compose "normal" gait and of the factors to be considered when trying to restore or substitute for normal functioning by means of an orthotic or prosthetic device.

FUNCTIONAL ROLE OF THE LOWER EXTREMITIES

The primary function of the lower extremities is to provide mobility, a means of travel from one place to another in order to perform manual tasks and to participate in the whole range of human activities. While continuously opposing the force of gravity, the lower limbs must provide controlling and supporting forces during starting, stopping, and movement on level and uneven surfaces as well as during the transitions to and from the seated and lying positions. Safe and efficient accomplishment of all these tasks requires a neuromusculoskeletal system that is structurally sound, highly articulated, capable of a wide range of force development, and regulated by a sensitive and adaptable control system. Because of inherent differences in body proportions, level of coordination, motivation, and similar factors, each individual's movement pattern is unique. Yet, because everyone is subject to the same physical principles and because everyone has the same basic anatomical and physiological makeup, "normal" human movements are accomplished in very much the same way by most healthy individuals.

When any one or more components of the lower limb mobility system is altered or absent because of pathological, traumatic, or congenital factors, external devices may be provided in an attempt to maximize the individual's functional abilities. To understand the prosthetic and orthotic components that are intended to substitute for normal abilities, the major factors related to lower extremity mobility must be understood. Walking represents the most common dynamic functional activity.

THE GAIT CYCLE

The sequential repetition of (approximately) the same movements of the major joints of the body during ambulation is referred to as the gait cycle. Figure 3-1 presents some of the terminology that

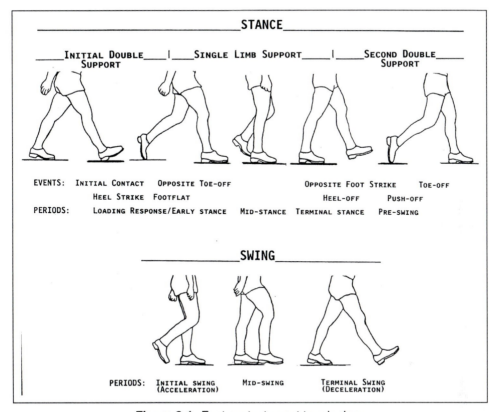

STANCE

_____INITIAL DOUBLE____|____SINGLE LIMB SUPPORT_____|____SECOND DOUBLE_____
        SUPPORT   SUPPORT

EVENTS: INITIAL CONTACT   OPPOSITE TOE-OFF   OPPOSITE FOOT STRIKE   TOE-OFF
          HEEL STRIKE   FOOTFLAT   HEEL-OFF   PUSH-OFF
PERIODS: LOADING RESPONSE/EARLY STANCE   MID-STANCE   TERMINAL STANCE   PRE-SWING

SWING

PERIODS: INITIAL SWING   MID-SWING   TERMINAL SWING
           (ACCELERATION)   (DECELERATION)

Figure 3-1. Foot contact event terminology.

is used to describe the foot contact events that occur during normal gait and to differentiate the various periods or phases that occur. The gait of healthy individuals is characterized by near symmetry in the temporal and distance aspects of the contact of the feet with the supporting surface. Although achieving a normal foot contact pattern is a worthwhile general treatment objective, this goal cannot realistically be met by patients whose locomotor system is substantially different from normal as the result of disease, trauma, or congenital abnormality. A compromise is usually reached that includes such factors as gait efficiency, safety, discomfort, and cosmesis. Often the symmetry of gait is abandoned as the individual attempts to compensate for a unilateral sensorimotor deficiency.

WALKING SPEED

Energy cost studies have indicated that, for normal individuals, a symmetrical gait of approximately 1.3 meters per second (3 mph or 78 m/min) is an optimal method and speed of walking. However, a wide range of available speeds exists among healthy individuals depending on the location of, and motivation for, the activity. An individual's self-selected or walking speed velocity (SSWV) also tends to vary directly with height and somewhat inversely with age, although the influence of these two factors is highly variable. When there is a neuromuscular, or skeletal deficit, the walking speed that may be optimal from an energy cost viewpoint is often compromised for the sake of greater stability, less pain, and/or an enhanced feeling of security. This compromise is almost always exhibited as a decrease in walking speed. In general, slower walking speeds require reduced ranges of joint motion and slower movements as well as reduced forces and reduced rates of change of forces. To "slow down" is the most common general strategy used by patients to cope with locomotor deficits and is related to the severity of impairment.

ENERGETICS OF GAIT

The major consequence of a slow and/or asymmetrical gait is reduced efficiency; that is, increased energy expenditure for each meter walked. In normal gait, the body's center of mass (located just anterior to the second sacral vertebra) progresses almost smoothly on a nearly sinusoidal path throughout the gait cycle. The movement of the center of mass is the result of all the summated forces and motions of the major joints of the body. The center of mass moves in three dimensions with a speedup and slowdown, a vertical rise and fall with each step, and a lateral cycle of motion during each stride. The general rule is that the smoother the path of the center of gravity, the less energy expended by the walker. Unnecessary, increased, or abrupt movements of the body's center of mass during gait are the result of less than optimal joint motions and less than optimal use of muscle power. Each time the center of mass goes down, it must be raised. Each time there is an exaggerated lateral movement, muscular energy must be expended to restore the system. Each time there is an abrupt decrease in forward speed, muscle power must be used to regain forward progression. To traverse the same distance at the same speed with an altered movement pattern will require a greater rate of energy expenditure and a greater energy expenditure for each meter traveled. If an individual cannot, or is not willing to, increase the rate of energy expenditure, he or she may choose to walk more slowly. This strategy will decrease the energy expenditure rate, but because of the prolonged time in transit, the energy used per meter will be further increased. Most individuals with a locomotor deficit arrive at a compromise between the rate of energy expenditure and energy efficiency. This compromise is usually reflected in their "preferred" walking speed. Figure 3-2 shows examples of energy expenditure and energy efficiency at various walking speeds in healthy subjects and in individuals requiring orthotic and prosthetic devices.

LOWER LIMB FUNCTIONS DURING AMBULATION

A detailed examination of the normal kinematics and kinetics of the major joints of the lower limbs during ambulation is beyond the focus of this presentation but a graphic summary of important factors is presented in Figure 3-3. Also represented in the figure is the activity of the major muscle groups normally responsible for producing and controlling these movements. Of direct relevance to orthotic and prosthetic applications is a consideration of the functions that are provided as a result of these controlled motions. With a sound understanding of normal gait functions, the clinician is in a position to intelligently select and provide devices to substitute for those functions. The following sections will consider the major gait functions provided by

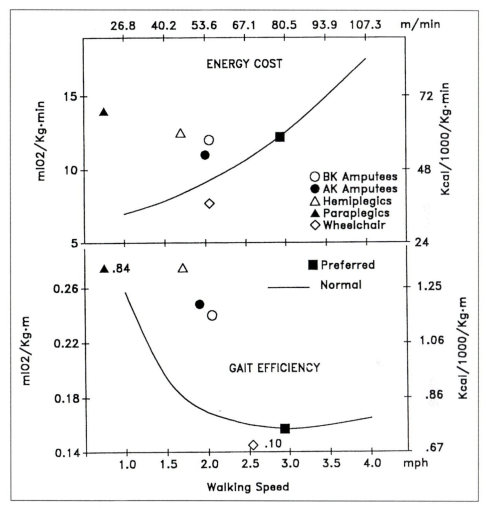

Figure 3-2. Energy expenditure and energy efficiency in individuals requiring orthotic and prosthetic devices.

the foot-ankle, knee, and hip along with a general presentation of the devices and strategies commonly used to externally augment or substitute for those functions. More detailed descriptions of specific components and devices are presented in later chapters.

Foot-Ankle Functions During Gait

From a gait function point of view, five gait functions of the foot-ankle complex can be identified.

Surface Adaptation. The first foot-ankle gait function to be considered occurs in the frontal plane and is the ability of the foot-ankle to adapt to uneven surfaces (Figure 3-4). This is a very important function when walking on other than smooth, flat, straight surfaces. Normally the mobility of the sub-talar and other joints allows the foot to be placed and maintained in a

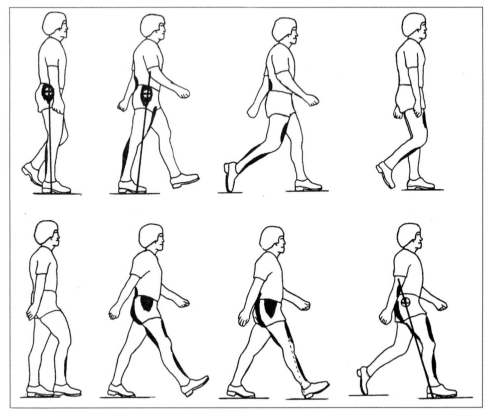

Figure 3-3. Kinematics, kinetics, and muscle activity during normal gait.

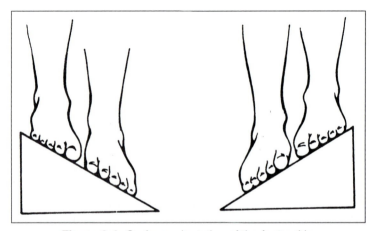

Figure 3-4. Surface adaptation of the foot-ankle.

variety of attitudes throughout the stance phase of gait. Because it requires such intricate and variable muscular control, surface adaptation is a foot-ankle function that is very difficult to substitute for or provide externally. With only a few exceptions, this function is usually sacrificed in lower limb orthotic and prosthetic devices in favor of stability.

Shock Absorption. Immediately following the initial contact of the foot with the floor until the foot is flat, the foot-ankle assists in absorbing the shock of the body weight being loaded on the limb, or more specifically, in decreasing the rate of rise of the ground reaction force. Normally, 15 or so degrees of controlled plantar flexion of the ankle is regulated by the eccentric contraction of the dorsiflexor musculature. Uncontrolled plantar flexion motion following heel-strike produces a classic, usually audible, foot slap.

Two possible prosthetic substitutes for foot-ankle shock absorption are depicted in Figure 3-5; others will be described is later chapters. Figure 3-5d shows the widely used solid-ankle cushion-heel (SACH) prosthetic foot in which no motion occurs at the ankle but the shock absorption function is accomplished by compression of a foam wedge in the heel. In chapter 4, the vertical shock pylon (VSP) by Flex-Foot will introduce a prosthetic option for vertical loading, in addition to a saggital plane motion during stance phase. Figure 3-5e depicts what is referred to as a single axis foot in which the amount and rate of plantar flexion following heel-strike is regulated by the stiffness of a small rubber bumper or pad within the foot. Orthotically, several options are commonly used to achieve the foot-ankle shock absorption function. Metal uprights in an ankle-foot orthosis may contain a joint where the motion into plantar flexion and foot-flat is controlled by a spring (Figure 3-5c) which is incorporated into the joint. In a molded plastic AFO, movement into plantar flexion is regulated by the posterior "leaf spring" portion of the orthosis (Figure 3-5b).

In general, shock absorption is a function in which the force of gravity on the body is absorbed by body tissues, using the elastic properties of metal, plastic, or foam to duplicate this function. It should be noted that reducing the speed of walking generally reduces the magnitude and rate of rise of the ground reaction force or shock imparted to the limb. Chapter 4 also describes the urethane, gel, and silicone socket liners that act to reduce shock or impact on the residual limb during stance.

Center of Mass Motion. The third function of the foot-ankle during ambulation is the effect that this segment has on the movement of the body's center of mass. In the saggital plane, we can consider the center of mass to be approximately one thigh length above the knee joint. Little can be done between the knee and the hip to smooth out the center of mass path. Adjustments in limb length can be done, however, at the ankle. By progressively changing the pivot point of the foot-ankle from the apex of the heel to the ankle axis and then to the metatarsal area of the forefoot, the displacement path of the knee joint, and consequently the approximate center of mass of the body, undergoes a smooth minimal vertical change (Figure 3-6). One reason for, or at least a benefit from, decreased walking speed is that it reduces the vertical motions of the body's center of mass, and therefore, the need for making large limb length adjustment using the foot-ankle. Figure 3-7 illustrates this point.

With an intact neuromusculoskeletal system, limb length adjustments in early stance phase occur as a result of ankle plantar flexion, under the control of the dorsiflexor musculature, from

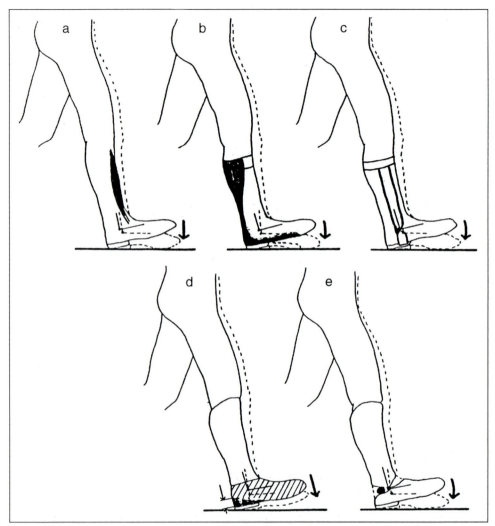

Figure 3-5. Normal shock absorption mechanism of the foot-ankle (a) along with examples of orthotic (b and c)and prosthetic substitutes (d and e).

heel strike until the foot is flat on the floor. The orthotic and prosthetic options that were previously discussed regarding shock absorption usually also produce satisfactory limb length adjustments during this phase of gait. Following foot-flat in an intact limb, gradually increasing activity in the posterior calf muscles controls and then completely limits the rotation of the tibia over the stationary foot, causing the rotation point to shift to the forefoot and the metatarsal heads.

Figure 3-8 illustrates several prosthetic and orthotic mechanisms used to limit continued rotation of the tibia over the foot, preventing a drop off of the center of mass in late stance. By definition, a SACH foot has a solid ankle which allows no movement into dorsiflexion (Figure 3-8b) so that, beginning with the mid-stance phase, the heel rises and weight is born on the

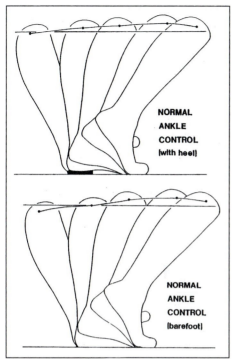

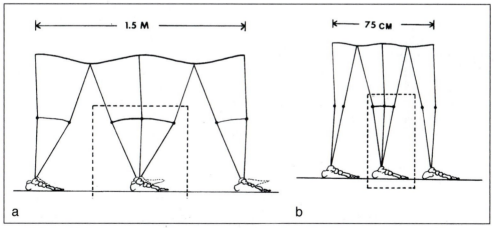

Figure 3-6. Normal foot-ankle control and its effects on the movement of the center of mass.

Figure 3-7. Knee path and approximate center of mass path displacements during (a) normal and (b) reduced walking speeds.

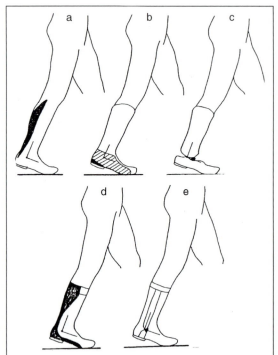

Figure 3-8. Mechanism used to limit tibial rotation over foot during late stance.

forefoot as the body continues to move forward. Another prosthetic option is shown in the single-axis foot in Figure 3-8c in which resistance to motion is provided by an anterior rubber bumper whose compression limits the amount and rate of dorsiflexion motion. In the modern energy-storing prosthetic foot, the design and materials allow a resistance to dorsiflexion in the extreme range of motion (when the amputee is on toe) that then is returned at toe off. A short toe lever will produce drop off. Orthotically, an anterior "stop" or spring used in the joint(s) of a metal upright orthosis (Figure 3-8e) and the posterior "leaf-spring" action of a molded plastic AFO (Figure 3-8d) are examples of ways to externally control center of mass movement in mid and late stance. A weak gastroc in the stance phase can also produce a dropoff.

The normal gait progressive buildup in joint moments to eventually equal a steadily increasing external moment is a difficult function to produce artificially. In many instances, motion into dorsiflexion in late stance is severely limited or simply not allowed by the prosthetic or orthotic mechanism. This concept of a fixed or solid ankle raises the question about what ankle angle should be used to provide optimal gait performance for the user of the prosthesis or orthosis. From the point of view of the influence of the foot-ankle on the center of mass movement, the angle at which the ankle is fixed has predictable effects. As illustrated in Figure 3-9, no resistance to dorsiflexion about the ankle joint results in a compass-like movement pattern on the knee joint center and a severe dropoff of the center of mass. Fixing the ankle in 10 degrees of plantar flexion causes the pivot point to shift to the forefoot relatively early in stance so that the center of mass must "ride up" over the foot during late stance. A foot-ankle fixed in a neutral position has a similar but less dramatic effect than one set in plan-

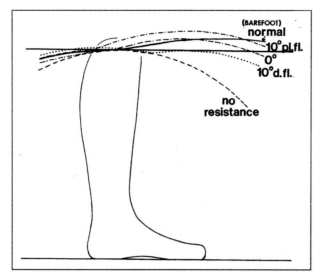

Figure 3-9. Effect of "free" and "fixed" ankle on knee.

tar flexion while an angle of slight dorsiflexion seems to produce a flatter trajectory but one with a slight dropoff.

Answering the question about which fixed ankle angle is ideal is not a simple matter but requires consideration of at least two other foot-ankle functions, namely, knee stability and swing phase shortening, to be discussed later. It is also important to remember that the slower walking speeds selected by many users of prosthetic and orthotic devices are accompanied by reduced requirements for limb length adjustments at the foot-ankle and less energy requirements.

Knee Stability. Support and movement of the mass of the body through space is in response to the ground reaction forces from the supporting surface. As the foot (or an assistive device) pushes against the ground, the reaction force against this push causes the body to move (or remain stationary) in proportion to the magnitude and direction of the force. In the sagittal plane, the line of action of the ground reaction force, on its path from the contact point under the foot to the body center of mass, may pass anteriorly, posteriorly, or directly through the axis of the knee joint. If the ground reaction force passes through or anteriorly to the knee axis, the knee is considered to be mechanically stable, because either no joint moment is required or the opposing moment is provided by passive posterior joint structures. If, however, the force line passes posteriorly to the joint axis, opposing moments must be provided by knee extensor musculature or motion into flexion or knee buckling will occur. In this case, the knee is considered to be mechanically unstable. For example, walking in a crouched position with excessive knee flexion requires a great deal of knee extensor activity and is an exaggeration of a very unstable knee.

For individuals with compromised or absent knee function and reduced ability to control and/or maintain a flexed knee during weightbearing, configuration of an orthotic or prosthetic device to externally enhance knee stability may be very important. The factors that can affect the relationship of the supporting force line to the knee axis, and therefore, its mechanical stability, are the location of the body's center of mass, the contact point (or center of pressure) under the foot, and the ankle angle. Using information from Cook and Cozzens, Figure 3-10 illustrates how knee moments during quiet standing can be affected by an ankle-foot orthosis that fixes the ankle at a particular angle. In the normal, unconstrained condition (Figure 3-10a), the supporting ground reaction force line passes very close to the knee joint center so that minimal muscular control is required. Maintaining an attitude of dorsiflexion (Figure 3-10b) shifts the knee joint center forward and results in a knee flexion moment that must be counteracted by appropriate activity in the knee extensor muscles. Maintaining a plantar flexed ankle angle (Figure 3-10d) produces the opposite effect, shifting the knee center posteriorly behind the supporting force line so that the equal and opposite moment is provided by the posterior joint structures. The same principles apply to configuration of a prosthesis and are especially important in the case of an amputation above the knee where there is no attachment of the knee extensor muscles across the knee joint.

During gait, foot-ankle configuration becomes even more important to knee stability because the ground reaction force is constantly changing in terms of both magnitude and direction throughout stance phase. By maintaining the foot-ankle in either plantar flexion or dorsiflexion, it is possible to make the knee either more or less stable. Figure 3-11 illustrates these effects. The more extreme the angle in which the foot-ankle is maintained, the more dramatic the effect on knee stability. In patients who have difficulty maintaining the knee in extension during weightbearing, the prosthetic or orthotic foot-ankle can be fixed in a plantar flexion position so that the contact point tends to be anterior under the foot with the force line located near or anterior to the knee joint center. Conversely, for patients with increased exten-

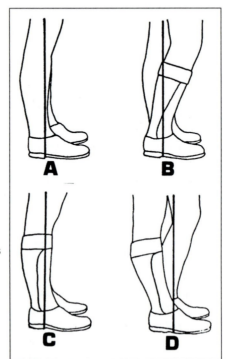

Figure 3-10. Knee moments ala fixed ankles.
(Source: Cook T, Cozzens B. The effects of heel height and ankle-foot orthosis alignment on weight line location: a demonstration of principles. Orthot Prosthet. 1976; 30(4):43–46.)

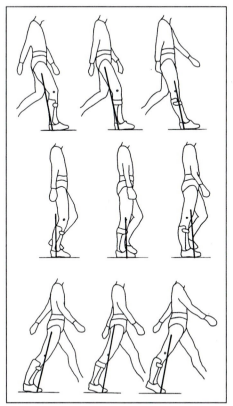

Figure 3-11. Knee moments via solid ankle.

sor tone or a tendency to severely hyperextend the knee, the foot-ankle can be maintained in dorsiflexion tending to keep the contact point more posterior under the foot and the ground reaction force line closer to the knee joint center.

It must be remembered from the discussion in the previous section, however, that fixing the ankle in a particular attitude also has consequences for the movement path of the body's center of mass. A compromise must be reached to achieve adequate knee stability without excessively increasing the energy requirements associated with the center of gravity riding up or dropping off during late stance. The situation is further compounded by the need to control the foot-ankle during the swing phase.

Swing-Phase Control. In normal gait, the ankle is in a posture of approximately 20 degrees of plantar flexion when the toe leaves the supporting surface (Figure 3-12). The ankle is returned to a neutral or near-neutral position by the time of midswing phase by contraction of the ankle dorsiflexors. Inability or failure to accomplish this motion results in an elongated limb requiring that other compensatory motions must occur elsewhere to prevent or to minimize the dragging of the foot as it is brought forward.

Orthotically and prosthetically maintaining the foot-ankle in a near-neutral position often is not difficult, although there are exceptions. A near-neutral position usually provides adequate

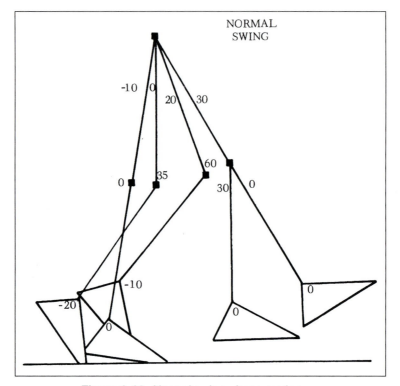

Figure 3-12. Normal swing-phase motion.

swing-phase control, but some compromises in selecting an optimal ankle angle often need to be made to also provide adequate knee stability and optimal center-of-mass movement during stance.

The dragging of the foot or toe during the swing phase does not necessarily indicate that a problem exists at the foot-ankle. As will be discussed shortly, adequate and coordinated motions of the knee and hip are also essential for clearance of the limb during the swing phase.

Knee Functions During Gait

From a functional viewpoint, three major functions of the knee during gait will be discussed: shock absorption, support, and limb shortening. The knee has motion in all three planes. This helps to explain why orthotic and prosthetic devices never approach normal functions.

Shock Absorption. Concurrently with the shock absorption function of the ankle immediately following foot contact, the knee normally allows 15 degrees of controlled knee flexion to also absorb the shock of loading the limb. The quadriceps musculature eccentrically controls the rate of flexion and then concentrically returns the knee to nearly full extension by the time of midstance (see Figure 3-3). This slight knee motion also assists in smoothing the movement path of the center of mass, which is at its lowest point during the double-support period and is changing direction from a downward motion to an upward motion at this time. Without this "yielding" of the knee, the limb is loaded more abruptly, causing a greater impact to the body tissues. Just as with most gait functions, reducing walking speed reduces the rate at which the limb is loaded, and consequently, the demand for controlled knee flexion in early stance.

Orthotically and prosthetically, shock absorption at the knee is difficult to provide with a mechanical device. Controlling the variable resistance needed to maintain a partially flexed, loaded knee, yet still provide adequate support and rapid swing-phase flexion, requires a sophisticated mechanism. Such components are likely to be complex, heavy, bulky, and expensive and are used only in a limited number of prosthetic applications. This function usually falls on the hydraulic units to provide.

Support. An important function provided by the knee during stance is support of body weight. As discussed earlier with regard to the influence of the ankle on knee stability, the line of action of the ground reaction force is of key importance. If that line is maintained anterior to the knee-joint axis, passive posterior structures provide the counteracting moment to prevent motion. If the force line is posterior, active knee extensors usually regulate the tendency for the knee to flex from body weight.

If active control of knee extension is compromised or absent, as is often the case in orthotic and prosthetic applications, the supporting force line must be maintained anterior to the knee to prevent knee buckling. A crucial time for establishing and maintaining knee stability is during early stance, when the ground reaction force tends to originate posteriorly under the foot and to pass posterior to the knee center. The relationship of the force line to the knee joint can be affected in three ways. The first method is to change the alignment of the device to affect the relationships among the origin of the force line under the foot, the knee axis, and the body's center of mass. Changing the foot-ankle posture, as previously discussed, is one option (see Figure 3-11). Locating the knee axis more posteriorly and allowing hyperextension in a prosthetic system is another example (Figure 3-13a). A second method for achieving greater knee stability is for the patient to locate the body's center of mass more anteriorly by leaning forward or using some other similar strategy to reconfigure the body segments (Figure 3-13b). A third method is to produce an increased extension moment at the hip, causing the heel to "dig in" so that the force line tends to be angled more vertically than usual. Figure 3-13c illustrates this last technique.

The preswing phase is a period that may be particularly difficult with regard to support and knee stability for some users of prosthetic and orthotic devices. During this phase of "normal" gait, the knee joint begins to flex while still partially loaded (Figure 3-14). As is discussed later, this preswing knee flexion is an important element in achieving a normal swing phase but may be very difficult or impossible for an individual with limited or absent control of the knee. Many times an individual with a prosthesis or orthosis will delay knee flexion in this phase of gait until the contralateral limb has been securely placed and loaded. Such delays result in a less smooth, usually slower, and less efficient gait pattern. Some sophisticated prosthetic knee units can successfully duplicate controlled yielding of the knee in preswing. In most prosthetic and orthotic applications, however, the point at which the knee begins to flex is determined by a combination of the three factors already mentioned: device alignment, center-of-mass location, and hip moments.

Normally, mediolateral control of joint moments at the knee is provided by the intrinsic structural integrity of the joint. When the knee joint has been affected by pathology or by

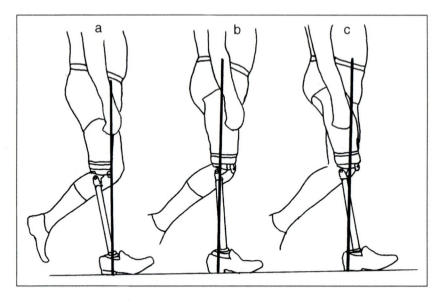

Figure 3-13. Techniques for knee stability.

trauma, structural deformities may result, and an external device may be needed to limit malalignment and pain and to improve function. Figure 3-15 shows an example of inadequate mediolateral support at the knee.

Limb Shortening. The most obvious function provided by the knee joint during normal gait is 60 to 65 degrees of flexion during initial swing phase to shorten the limb (see Figure 3-3). It should be noted that approximately one half of this motion occurs before the toe leaves the supporting surface (see Figure 3-14). If an individual, for whatever reason, does not get this

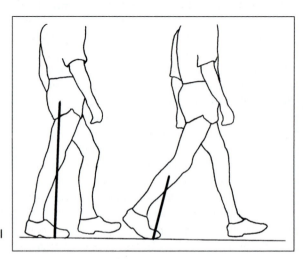

Figure 3-14. Normal terminal stance.

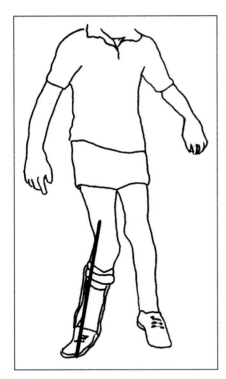

Figure 3-15. Inadequate mediolateral control.

start on knee flexion, it is virtually impossible to obtain the full knee flexion necessary for a normal swing. Consequently flexion during preswing is a necessary precursor to adequate limb shortening during swing. In some individuals and at faster walking speeds, the knee flexors may assist knee flexion in preswing. During preswing and initial swing, again depending on walking speed, the knee extensors normally contribute to limiting knee flexion and to initiating knee extension. In prosthetic and orthotic applications, the challenge is to provide swing-phase control of the knee to replicate normal knee flexion and extension as closely as possible. Too much knee flexion in early swing results in excessive heel rise, while too rapid knee extension in late swing may result in a terminal swing impact as the knee reaches the limits of its extension motion. Clearly an external device that can accomplish normal control and adjust to various walking speeds is likely to be rather sophisticated. Some devices of this kind are available, especially for TF amputees. However, simpler devices, which are adjusted to a particular walking speed, are used in most cases. Such a sophisticated unit is the "C" leg from Otto Bock. This computer controlled unit embodies a microprocessor to assist the amputee with both swing and stance phases. The unit is programmable, using a laptop computer.

Frequently, because of concerns for knee stability and patient safety, an orthotic or prosthetic device may use a locking mechanism that allows no motion at the knee. Sometimes, too, because of increased tone associated with neurologic deficits, some individuals maintain a rigid, fully extended knee during ambulation. The resulting "stiff-knee" gait poses some real problems during swing phase (Figure 3-16). When preswing and swing phase knee flexion are absent, the individual is faced with the difficult task of advancing a relatively elongated limb

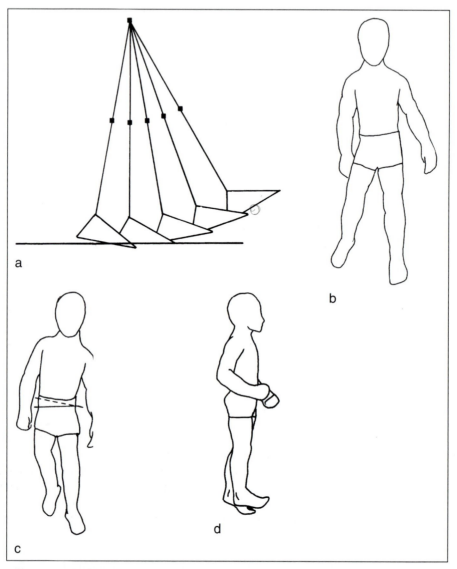

Figure 3-16. Stiff knee swing. a = the problem b = circumduction c = hip hiking and d = vaulting.

during a relatively brief period. Temporal and distance asymmetries are very likely to result, and energy cost increases.

Because the vertical distance between the pelvis and the floor is less than the length of a stiff-knee limb, compensation of some kind must occur. Four common gait deviations often result from absent or inadequate knee flexion during the preswing and swing phases. They are entirely compensatory and may be present in different amounts and various combinations depending on the patient's status and abilities. Circumduction (Figure 3-16b) involves using hip abduction during hip flexion to advance the limb in a semicircular path, and then returning the limb to the line of progression. This strategy increases energy requirements because of the added muscular power used for the additional lateral motion. Hip hiking (Figure 3-16c) is a lateral tilting or relative abduction of the pelvis on the contralateral stance limb to provide a greater distance between the hip joint and the floor for the stiff limb to swing forward. This gait deviation is somewhat more energy consuming than circumduction, because it requires at least a slight vertical displacement of all the body segments except the contralateral stance limb. Vaulting (Figure 3-16d) is the use of active plantar flexion during stance on the contralateral limb to elevate the entire body, thereby increasing the hip joint-to-floor distance for the swing limb. Vaulting is likely to be the most energy consuming of these three gait deviations. (A shoe buildup on one side can be used to prevent/simulate vaulting.) Contralateral side bending of the trunk can allow swing phase and foot clearance for a stiff knee gait.

Hip Functions During Gait

Hip functions during gait are somewhat simpler but are just as important as those of the foot-ankle and knee. In general, however, there are few prosthetic and orthotic devices that can adequately substitute for these functions.

Stance-Phase Extension. At the time of initial contact, the hip is normally in a position of approximately 30 degrees of flexion and progresses to a position of approximately 10 degrees of extension in terminal stance (see Figure 3-3). Because the ground-reaction force line tends to be anterior to the hip-joint axis in early stance, hip extensors are active to control the tendency of the trunk to rotate forward over the newly placed limb and to actively assist in hip extension. By midstance, the force line tends to move behind the hip joint so that the hip flexors become active to control the amount and rate of hip extension and then to initiate the advance of the limb during swing.

Because hip extension during stance is principally an active, relatively powerful function, prosthetic and orthotic substitutes are difficult to devise and generally are not very successful, although there are exceptions to this statement. Compensatory gait deviations used by individuals with inadequate hip control may include backward leaning and lumbar lordosis (Figure 3-17) in early stance (to keep the reaction force line closer to the hip joint center) and forward leaning and anterior pelvic tilting in late stance (to assist in the initiation of flexion during swing).

Swing-Phase Flexion. Beginning with preswing, the hip flexes to advance the limb through swing phase until initial contact and the next stance phase. As was mentioned previously, active flexion of the hip is required to attain adequate knee flexion. Additionally, the timing of hip flexion is important, because the hip must pass the neutral position before the knee begins extending, or clearance will be insufficient (see Figure 3-12). As with hip extension, swing-phase hip flexion is a difficult function to produce with an external artificial device. Individuals with hip flexion control problems often compensate with exaggerated motions of the pelvis and/or lower spine.

Mediolateral Stability. In the frontal plane, the supporting force line is always medial to the hip joint throughout the stance phase of normal gait (Figure 3-18a). The hip abductor group

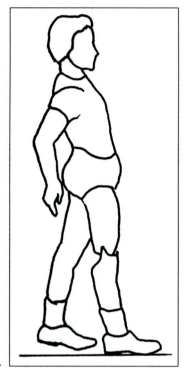

Figure 3-17. Lordosis.

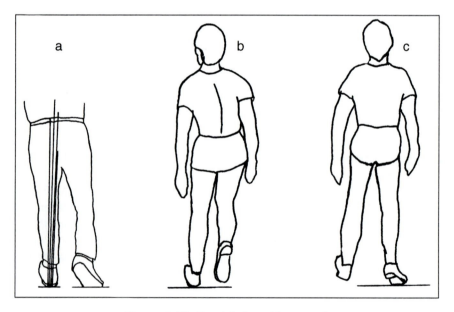

Figure 3-18. Frontal plane hip control.

is active during initial contact, foot flat, and midstance, allowing the pelvis to go through a slight (approximately 5 degrees) relative adduction on the femur. The hip abductors control the lateral shift of the center of gravity over the single limb, at first decelerating and then reversing lateral motion. In some applications, particularly with transfemoral prostheses and hip-knee-ankle-foot orthoses using pelvic bands and hip joints, it is possible to provide mediolateral stability of the hip joint(s) using these external devices.

Lateral leaning of the trunk toward the affected side is a common gait strategy for moving the force line closer to or through the joint so as to minimize the hip abductor requirements (Figure 3-18b). The result is the classic Trendelenburg gait pattern. Another strategy adopted by some individuals is to use an abducted gait pattern to achieve a wider base of support (Figure 3-18c). The advantage of such a pattern is that if control is lost, gravity will cause the body mass to move medially, a much safer situation than to get the body weight too far over the limb laterally and to fall away from the midline.

Other Causes of Gait Deviations

The preceding sections have discussed the principal functions accomplished by the lower limb during gait along with some common biomechanical causes of gait patterns that deviate from normal. There are certainly other reasons why a particular individual may choose to adopt a specific way of ambulating. Many of these will be presented in greater detail in chapters 4 through 6 and 8. These reasons may include discomfort, feelings of insecurity, cosmesis, and a host of other physiologic, psychologic, and sociologic factors. It is the role of the health care provider to evaluate these factors as thoroughly as he or she can and to positively affect as many as possible.

REFERENCES

Stauffer S, Hoffer M, Nickel V. Ambulation in thoracic paraplegia. *J Bone Joint Surg.* 1978; 60A(6):823–824.

CHAPTER 4

Transtibial Amputations and Prostheses

The Custer National Cemetery reminds us of the cost in morbidity and mortality, and the impact wars have had on our society. Injuries from wars also heighten the need for research and development in order to provide better care for the survivors. The field of prosthetics and orthotics benefited greatly over the years from grants awarded by the U.S. government and from our Veterans Administration to advance the state of the art and offer surviving veterans more functional lives.

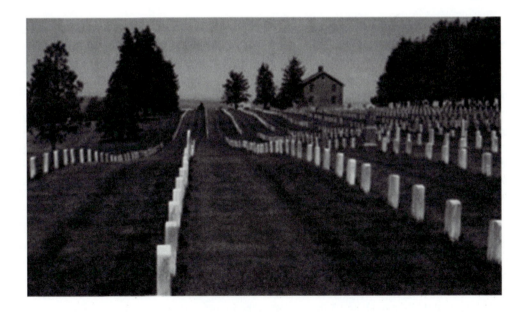

Following completion of reading this chapter, the student will be able to:

1. Describe the major levels of amputation of the foot and leg and the advantages of each to the amputee.

2. Discuss the causes and respective components available to the amputees, specific to age, functionality level, and level.
3. Describe the role of the physical therapist in the preoperative discussions with the amputee.
4. Compare and contrast the major types of feet available and describe their effect on energy efficiency to the amputee.

As was mentioned in chapter 1, lower limb amputations are 11 times more common than upper limb amputations. Leg amputations are divided into two general categories, transtibial (TT) and transfemoral (TF). Amputations below the knee joint are the most common level of lower limb amputation encountered today. In this chapter, we will discuss different anatomical levels of TT amputation, the components commonly used in TT prostheses, how TT prostheses are suspended and aligned, and postoperative management of individuals who have experienced an amputation of the lower limb at the transtibial level. The chapter concludes with a consideration of energy expenditure and gait in transtibial amputees.

LEVELS OF TRANSTIBIAL AMPUTATION

Transtibial amputations can occur within the foot (referred to as a partial foot amputation), at the ankle (referred to as an ankle disarticulation or Syme amputation), or at any location through the tibia and fibula (usually simply referred to as a transtibial amputation).

Partial Foot Amputation

Various levels of partial foot amputation are depicted in Figure 4-1. Amputations of the toes are a common form of partial foot amputation. Toe amputations may be performed for a variety of reasons including vascular disease, trauma, or secondary to a congenital deficiency. Except when the great toe is involved, little, if any, residual effect is usually noted and the need for prosthetic restoration is small. Prosthetic restoration for cosmetic purposes is possible with the advent of modern plastics technology although these prostheses are usually covered by a shoe.

An amputation at the transmetatarsal level creates a weight-bearing stump while minimizing the need for a prosthetic device. Transmetatarsal amputations are done for vascular as well as traumatic reasons. In either case, a long plantar flap, using the skin from the bottom of the foot, provides a good, weight tolerant residuum. Although the length of the foot lever is shortened following the amputation, it creates a limited functional impairment as shown by Garbalosa et al, Hobon et al, and Sanders. Often the incorporation of a piece of spring steel or a graphite insole in the shoe is sufficient to achieve good walking function. The gait of patients with a transmetatarsal amputation typically looks like they "fall off" at heel off due to the shortened anterior foot lever. Functionally, this presents little difficulty unless there is a need for forceful push off, as in walking quickly or uphill, or in running. Gait studies by Garbalosa et al resulted in distal weight-bearing pressures increasing compared to the longer, normal side.

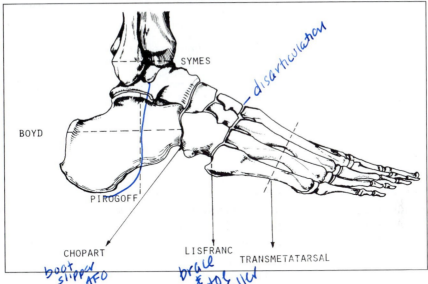

Figure 4-1. Partial foot amputation levels.

The tarsal-metatarsal or Lisfranc amputation is named after the French surgeon Jacques Lisfranc and describes a disarticulation done at the junction of the three cuneiforms and the cuboid. The anterior foot lever is further shortened compared to the transmetatarsal amputation. Because the extensor mechanism is still intact, muscular balance about the ankle is maintained. The shorter the dorsum of the foot, the more difficult it becomes to keep a shoe on the remaining residuum. The Lisfranc level of amputation is the most proximal ankle sparing level that may be used without complications in young children. Studies have shown that the potential for ankle flexion contracture increases when the amputation occurs above the insertion of the foot extensor musculature making functional use of a prosthetic device difficult.

Amputation at the mid-tarsal or Chopart level is named after the French surgeon Francois Chopart and leaves only the talus and calcaneus. Chopart amputation is not usually a level of choice because the extensor mechanism will be absent and an unbalanced foot and deformity may occur.

Figure 4-2 shows an example of a partial foot prosthesis or shoe filler. The exact configuration will vary depending on the level of partial foot amputation.

Functional outcome studies have been published on several levels and etiologies. Garbalosa et al studied 10 unilateral, diabetic, transmetatarsal (TMA) amputees, comparing the peak plantar pressures with their "normal" or remaining foot. Results showed a significantly greater mean peak plantar pressure on the TMA side. The heels of the TMA foot also had significantly lower mean peak pressures and a significantly reduced dynamic dorsiflexion range of motion, even though static dorsiflexion range of motion between both feet was similar. The authors concluded that because the TMA foot did not use all available range of motion and had greater peak plantar pressures, foot wear management of this group of patients is critical. Millstein concluded that with traumatic, partial feet, Lisfranc and Chopart levels did better than transmetatarsal or digital levels. Eighty-one percent rated their long-term (16 years) results as either good (43 percent) or fair (38 percent).

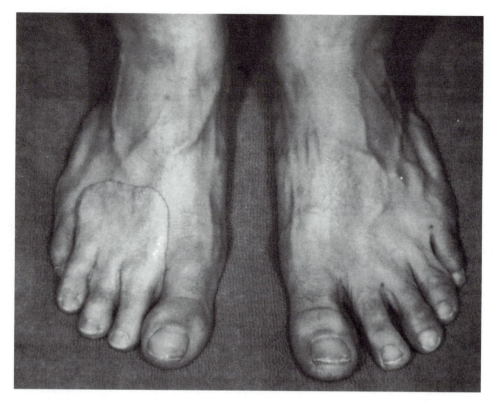

Figure 4-2. Partial foot prosthesis. (Courtesy of Horst Buckner, Life-Like, Dallas, TX)

Ankle Disarticulation (Syme Amputation)

The Syme amputation is named for the famous surgeon Dr. James Syme, a Scot who practiced in Edinburgh between 1833 and 1869. Because he operated in the pre-Listerian and pre-anesthesia era, Syme needed a procedure that would allow him quick and sure amputation of the foot in cases of nonunion fracture or life-threatening infection. Syme wrote that he could disarticulate the ankle in less than 1 minute and was successful in saving patients while retaining a stump that tolerates full weight bearing on the end (end bearing).

Syme amputation is currently used for traumatic, congenital, and sometimes for vascular reasons. Wagner reported up to 95 percent success rate using Doppler noninvasive testing prior to two-stage Syme amputations in dysvascular patients. Two-stage Syme procedures disarticulate the foot in the first stage and close the wound using the plantar skin 6 weeks later. Among the indications for a Syme amputation is that the patient must be a potential prosthesis user.

There are basically three types of Syme prostheses: the medial opening type, designed by the Veterans Administration; the posterior opening type, designed by Colin McLaurin in Canada; and the closed panel or hidden wall design first described by LeBlanc (Figure 4-3). Hornby, in Toronto, has questioned the long-term use of the Syme level. In reviewing 68 patients with Syme level amputations, he found that the majority of patients required proximal

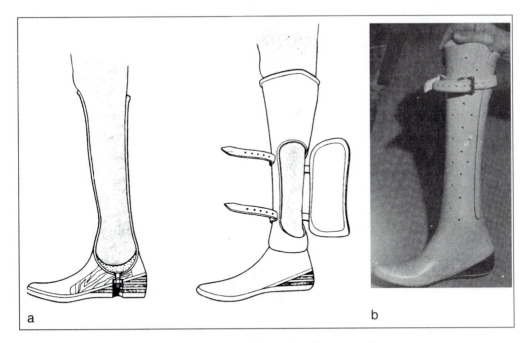

Figure 4-3. Medial (a) and posterior (b) opening Syme prostheses.

unloading of weight and distal relief from weight bearing. He concludes that a lacer-type socket is most efficient in relieving distal weight bearing.

The Syme or ankle disarticulation level is also used in children secondary to trauma, congenital anomalies, or tumors. The Syme offers a long, end-bearing residual limb, free from the problems of bony overgrowth often seen in pediatric amputations that transect long bones. The lower leg, particularly the fibula, tends to overgrow following transection. The fact that a patient may end bear and ambulate indoors without a prosthesis is often considered the advantages of the Syme level. Davidson and Bohne reported positive results using the Syme procedure in 23 children with a myriad of congenital problems. All patients walked within 3 months of their operations, using standard Syme prostheses. This group included patients with fibular dysplasia, proximal femoral focal deficiency (PFFD), and other problems. Leg length discrepancies and foot/ankle deformities were the most common indications for Syme amputation in children. Eilert and Jayakumar compared the Boyd and Syme level amputation outcomes in 34 children. The Boyd amputation transects the calcaneus and fuses it to the distal tibia, thus preserving length. Although good results were found using both techniques, the best results occurred when the heel pad was plantigrade (neutral), occurring more often using the Boyd technique. All 34 patients were excellent prosthetic users and all were fitted within 3 months of their operations. Most could bear full weight on the end of the stump with or without the prosthesis.

In 1967, Sarmiento, Gilmer, and Finneston reported on a new approach to the large, bulbous, uncosmetic Syme amputation. Their modified approach is based on the premise that weight bearing can occur on the patellar ligament and on the medial flare of the tibia, thus eliminating the need for total end bearing in the prosthesis. By surgically shaving the malleoli, the overall stump circumference is reduced by one-third. The same posterior flap and heel pad is used to cover the stump and close the wound. By making the end of the stump smaller, the need for a trap door in the prosthesis is eliminated. The resulting hidden-panel Syme prosthesis looks smaller and is, therefore, more acceptable to many patients, particularly females.

In his classic energy cost study published in 1976, Waters reported a longer residual limb increased gait efficiency while wearing a prosthesis. Recently, a single subject, longitudinal, comparison of both Syme and transtibial level indicated that while using a Flex-Foot, the gait efficiency (6 to 10 percent) and walking speed (8.3 percent) both improved at the TT level. According to Lin et al, this finding calls into question the long-standing thoughts about Syme level and perhaps demonstrates the value of energy storing prosthetic feet to the amputee.

Birch et al reported on the physical and psychological results of 10 young adults with Syme amputation done for fibular deficiency. All used Syme prostheses and none reported difficulty walking or running. Psychological testing, done at a mean age of 21.7 years, revealed normal satisfaction with occupation, personal growth, relationship, and recreation. Quality of life and self-esteem were also normal. This amputation study begins to establish outcomes for comparison with multistaged lengthening procedures.

McCarthy and Eilert reported on outcomes of Syme or Boyd amputation compared with limb lengthening for the same group of patients with fibular hemimelia. Thirty patients with either procedure done at least 2 years previous were studied. Mean age at amputation was 1.2 years and 9.7 years for lengthening. Patients having amputation had fewer complications (0.37 versus 1.0), fewer procedures (1.9 versus 7.0), at a lower cost ($7,016 versus $26,900) than the lengthening group. The amputation group also had less pain (0.2 versus 1.2), were able to perform more functional activities (0 versus 1.2), and were more satisfied (100 percent versus 50 percent) when compared with the lengthening group.

Cottrell-Ikerd reviewed the Syme surgical procedure as well as indications and contraindications. In reviewing the biomechanics of the Syme prosthesis, the authors stress the need for a more perfect prosthetic solution, which they believe is partly responsible for the poor outcomes seen in Syme prosthetic wearers.

Fowler et al compared gait kinematics and kinetics in adults with PFFD who underwent Syme amputation versus Van Nes rotational osteotomy. The patients having the Van Nes procedure were able to support a flexed-knee posture at both SSWV and fast walking producing greater knee extensor moments, compared with the Syme group. The authors believe that the improved gait should be considered in planning for PFFD children with excessive limb length discrepancy.

The Syme level remains controversial but will continue to offer options to children and adults. Further prosthetic studies and research will hopefully help clarify this interesting issue.

Transtibial

Most authors and surgeons agree that the majority of lower limb amputations in North America are largely related to severe vascular disease. The exact percentage is not known, but most agree that the percentage falls between 80 and 90 percent. Some authors such as Reiber et al suggest that the number of vascular-related lower extremity amputations exceeds 130,000 per year in the United States. According to the American Diabetes Association, 56,000 amputations are performed annually on diabetics. Most vascular amputations occur as elective procedures; that is, amputations performed by surgeons at an "elected" level, often at the TT level. Kay and Newman reported that nationwide, the TT is more popular than the TF. This fact represents a turnaround from the TF level; historically the more commonly done procedure. This change may be related to two phenomena: the advent of noninvasive Doppler blood flow detection equipment, and efforts by the American Academy of Orthopaedic Surgery following published studies demonstrating more successful rehabilitation when the amputation was done at the transtibial level. According to Reiber, from 1989 to 1992, there were still more amputations done at the TF level than TT, 28,640 to 24,527. These data include both diabetic and nondiabetic patients. Diabetes affects only 3 percent of the population, but is the primary diagnosis for 51 percent of all diagnoses for which limb amputation was done. Kay and Newman data presented only amputees fitted with prostheses thus describing a younger and probably healthier overall population.

McCollough states that 75 percent of patients with TT amputations related to vascular disease can become satisfactory users of a prosthesis, compared to less than 50 percent for the TF. He cites the increased energy cost associated with the use of the transfemoral prosthesis as the primary cause. He further states that many transfemoral amputees prefer wheelchair locomotion because it may be safer as well as less energy consuming. Moore reviewed the literature and reported that between 48 and 77 percent of all TF amputees may be prosthetically rehabilitated. In his series of 18 cases, all healed primarily and all were rehabilitated with a permanent prosthesis. Information from Linds et al shows cigarette smoking causes not only an increased chance of limb amputation, but it also contributes to a greater risk of infection and reamputation.

The TT amputation is a transmedullary amputation, resulting in a surgical ablation of the limb through the bone. This process creates the need for a prosthetic device designed to unload the weight proximal to the cut bone. Through-bone amputations do not tolerate end weight bearing nearly as well as disarticulations, such as those performed at the level of the ankle or knee. Persson and Liedberg investigated the ability of 69 amputees to tolerate end bearing. The average maximal weight bearing was 13 Kg. TF amputees tolerated 13.7 Kg, compared to 11 Kg for the TT amputees. Vascular TT amputees averaged 10.7 Kg. The ability of a residual limb to tolerate end bearing apparently does not change with time. Figure 4-4 illustrates different levels of below the knee amputation and the terms generally used to describe them.

Long Transtibial Amputation. Most authors agree that saving all possible length is advantageous, often resulting in greater prosthetic function. Charles Truax, in a classic article written in 1899, described the virtues of saving all possible length. Although not a surgeon, he wrote very enlightened surgical philosophy, as a strong proponent of saving all length possible. Shea reports that saving all possible length consistent with good circulation and wound healing is often difficult due to vascular compromise. Many authors prefer a mid-tibial length or longer, and the use of the long posterior flap or closure. This is thought to be a better approach than either an equal length flap or a long anterior flap. Not placing the suture line on the very end of the residual limb makes prosthetic fitting easier.

Some authors report success using a side-to-side flap approach. Tracy described a side-to-side, saggital flap approach. Persson demonstrated the superiority of this procedure when compared to anterior and posterior flaps. Termensen randomly compared this approach to the conventional long posterior flap described by Burgess. Results indicated nearly equal rates of

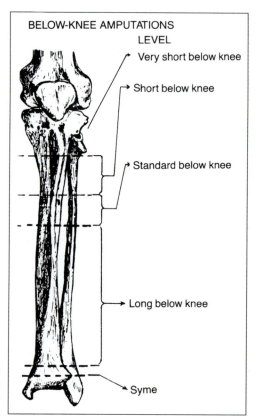

BELOW-KNEE AMPUTATIONS
LEVEL

→ Very short below knee

→ Short below knee

→ Standard below knee

→ Long below knee

→ Syme

Figure 4-4. TT amputation levels. (*Source:* Northwestern University Prosthetic Orthotic Center, 1987, with permission.)

primary healing, although these rates were low when compared to other similar published works. There were no reported differences in outcome relative to limb fitting, occupation, or ambulation. More recently Robinson described the "skew flap." The skew flaps use antero-medial and posterolateral cutaneous flaps based on blood-flow studies that indicate a richer blood supply. Robinson reported on use of a side-to-side flap, and reducing the amount of muscle side to side, thus making the fresh residual limb more conical. This skew flap uses an anteromedial and posterolateral fasciocutaneous flap, based on basic research involving cutaneous perfusion studies.

Medium Transtibial Amputation. The length of a TT residual limb, usually thought to be "medium" or standard in length, is 5 to 6 inches. This length was recommended by Burgess for the elective TT amputation. A 3-to-5 inch flap is left in order to cover the end of the stump. This skin flap, with continuous nerve and blood supply, is thought to assist the amputee with proprioceptive feedback and a sense of position of the residual limb within the socket. This standard length residual limb allows for easy fitting of the patellar tendon bearing (PTB) socket and any number of standard types of suspension, which will be discussed later in this chapter.

Short Transtibial Amputation. The term short is usually used to describe a TT residual limb that is 4 cm or less in total length, when measured from the medial joint line of the knee. Residual limbs of this length may present the prosthetist with great challenges. Considering the overall length and the small area of anterior skin upon which to unload the complete body weight, it is often necessary to use the distal end of the stump for weight bearing. As was mentioned earlier, end bearing is not well tolerated, and is usually not done. In the case of the very short TT residual limb, however, there is often no other choice. Flexion contractures may add to the difficulties encountered in the prosthetic fitting of the very short TT amputation. There is a greater risk of developing a flexion contracture when the residual limb is quite short, due in part to the imbalance created by the knee flexors, and the tendency of patients with very short residual limbs to want to flex their knees while sitting or lying. Great care must be taken to prevent such a deformity from occurring.

COMPONENTS OF TRANSTIBIAL PROSTHESES

The basic configuration in a TT prosthesis includes a socket, a spacer, and a foot. In addition, some form of suspension is necessary in order to maintain the device in place on the residual limb. The pylon or spacer, between the socket and foot, may be made of wood, plastic, foam, or metal, depending on the type of system used or the special needs of the patient. A so-called conventional prosthesis is one that is often prescribed and fitted within a certain geographic area, and often is specific to a given level of amputation. An example might be if a PTB socket with thigh corset and knee hinges were always prescribed for TT amputees in spite of specific patient criteria or needs. A conventional fitting is usually not wrong, but does not always consider and include the patient's thoughts or needs in the prescription process. There is no universally accepted "conventional" prosthesis used equally in all areas of the country. Often the so-called conventional prosthesis is dictated by the preferences or skills of the prosthetist or physician in the area.

Prosthetic Feet

As presented in chapter 3, the prosthetic foot should—ideally—substitute for the functions of the normal foot-ankle. These functions include adaptation to uneven surfaces, shock absorption following heel strike, limb length adjustments to smooth out the path of the body's center of gravity, stabilization of the knee, and limb shortening during swing. Clearly, the prospect of substituting for all these function with a simple, mechanical prosthetic foot is unrealistic. Several configurations present workable compromises and are commonly used in lower limb prosthetics, both transtibial and transfemoral.

A commonly prescribed prosthetic foot used in the United States is the solid ankle cushion heel (SACH) foot (Figure 4-5). The SACH foot has a wooden keel and a polyurethane foam heel wedge. The remainder of the foot is a poured polyurethane foam, which will turn dark when exposed to direct ultraviolet light. For that reason, many prosthetists will coat the foot with a plastic dip to prevent the foot from changing color. A survey by Fishman et al of practices in the 1970s revealed that the SACH foot was used 81 percent of the time on TT amputations and 74 percent of the time on transfemorals. A later study by Lehneis revealed that the SACH foot was used on 82 percent of all prostheses. Mechanically, the SACH foot has no moving parts, but simulates plantar flexion as the heel wedge compresses at heel strike and into early foot flat. Because there are no moving parts on the SACH foot, very little maintenance is required. However, occasionally a new heel wedge is needed if the compression becomes too easy. Heel wedge density is selected by the prosthetist based on the weight and gait characteristics of the patient. If the heel wedge is too stiff, foot flat is delayed and a knee flexion moment may be created. Conversely, in the case of weak knee extensors, a soft heel cushion or wedge is important to ensure that early and quick foot flat is achieved to maintain the floor reaction line in front of the knee axis, ensuring knee stability. Skinner et al evaluated static load response of the heels of 30 standard SACH feet and found no difference between the medium and regular heel cushions. Consistency between feet of the same heel density rating was quite high. Skinner et al concluded that all grades of heels of SACH feet were too stiff. SACH feet vary in weight from 445 to 490 grams.

Studies done using the SACH foot seem to indicate that the SACH foot does not assist in push off. According to Murray, this may be seen in reports that amputees walk using asymmetrical step lengths, with the longer step that from push off using the remaining limb and foot. Information from Nielsen states it is only after the introduction of the Flex-Foot that studies began to show symmetrical step lengths, and faster self-selected walking velocities.

If one does not choose a SACH foot, a single axis foot may be used. A single axis foot allows limited motion in plantarflexion and dorsiflexion. It does so with the assistance of a plantar flexion bumper made of rubber or hard plastic. A single axis foot may also contain an anterior dorsiflexion bumper as shown in Figure 4-6. As the amputee places weight on the prosthetic foot at heel strike, the bumper allows plantar flexion of the foot, stopping it at the end of the allowable range. Generally, the motion of the foot into plantarflexion is more rapid than the simulated motion with a SACH foot. Indications for the single axis foot are thought to be an old prosthetic user who is accustomed to such a foot, or the TF amputee who relies on the rapid plantar flexion of the foot to assist in knee stabilization. This concept will be further discussed in chapter 5 dealing with TF amputations and prostheses. Doane and Holt compared the differences between SACH and single axis feet on eight male unilateral transtibial amputees. The results indicated that the single axis foot permitted more plantar flexion and dorsiflexion than the SACH foot but the time spent in each phase of gait was approximately equal.

In addition to the SACH and single axis foot, a multiaxis foot is also commercially available. The multiaxis foot allows motion in dorsiflexion and plantarflexion as well as inversion

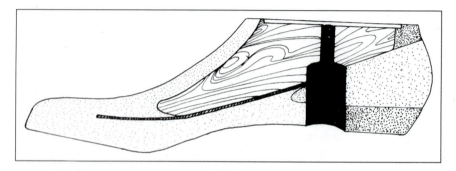

Figure 4-5. SACH foot.

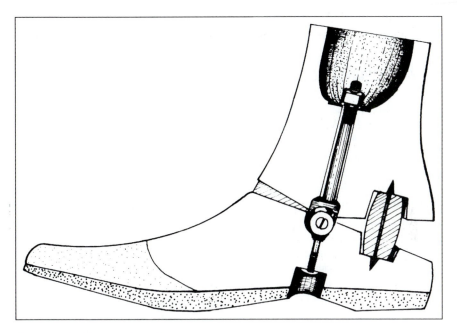

Figure 4-6. Single axis foot.

and eversion. All motions are controlled by a system of bumpers similar to the bumpers previously described with the single axis foot. The addition of inversion and eversion at the ankle allows for a small amount of movement of the foot for changes relative to the walking surface. Stability is afforded the amputee only at the extremes of motion in inversion and eversion, thus any movement in between those extremes is relatively uncontrolled. Otto Bock added a torque rotator to the ankle components of the multiaxis foot and the assembly is known as the Greisinger Foot. The concept of torque rotation or conversion will be further discussed in chapter 5 in the section dealing with TF prosthetic components.

Intuitively, amputees are thought to profit from other than SACH feet and much effort has gone into the research and development of multiaxis feet. However, little clinical evidence exists to compare the benefits derived from a multiaxis foot with the increase in cost to the amputee. There is also increased weight at the end of the prosthesis, and because multiaxis feet have a number of moving parts, there is an increase in the need for maintenance or replacement.

A number of new prosthetic feet have become available for use in TT prostheses. No attempt will be made to discuss all feet as there are many. Feet with referenced literature are cited, as well as information useful to team members. One change in prosthetic feet is the availability of sculptured toes. Because many amputees prefer to wear sandals or open toed shoes, the presence of the sculptured toe makes the acceptance of the prosthetic foot easier.

Studies by Burgess of amputees indicate that running requires some pronation and supination of the foot to allow the foot to bear weight on the lateral border following contact with the ground. To assist the amputee in this activity, the Seattle Foot incorporates a leaf spring made of Delrin, which aids in the push-off phase of running. The foot incorporates a rubber bumper angled at 22 degrees and an extension limitation cable that does not allow the foot to extend. Subjectively, the foot allows more comfortable running and jumping. It weighs 595 grams.

ENERGY-STORING FEET

Another prosthetic foot is the Flex-Foot (Figure 4-7), which actually looks more like a ski than a foot. Developed by Van Phillips, the Flex-Foot is made from graphite laminate heel and forefoot components. Early biomechanical studies by Wagner and Supan suggest that using this foot provides a mechanical advantage to the amputee, even the geriatric amputee. Biomechanically, once the amputee has loaded the toe of the foot, the stored energy is returned at push off, thus assisting in propelling the amputee forward. Energy consumption studies by Nielsen suggest that there is as much as a 20 percent energy savings by using the Flex-Foot compared to a SACH foot, depending on the speed of the amputee's gait.

Recently, Flex-Foot has introduced a foot with pylon-loading capabilities. Known as the VSP (Figure 4-8), (vertical shock pylon), this foot allows the amputee to not only load the toe during stance phase in the sagittal plane, but also to load the pylon as if it were a shock absorber. Once the weight has progressed forward and at toe off, both the pylon and the toe of the foot propel the amputee forward. Studies done on small numbers of TT amputees indicate that the VSP is more efficient than the original Flex-Foot, particularly at higher walking speeds.

When comparing weights of various feet, the Carbon Copy is the lightest, weighing only 415 grams. By comparison, the Seattle Foot weighs 595 grams, and Otto Bock's SACH foot weighs 445 grams.

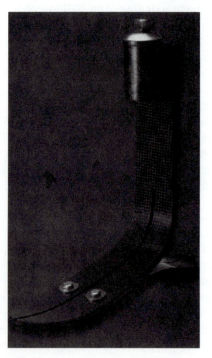

Figure 4-7. Flex-Foot®. (*Source:* Flex-Foot, Laguna Hills, CA, with permission.)

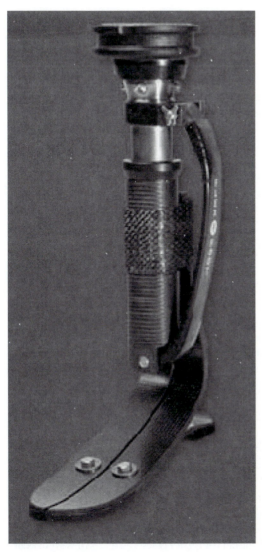

Figure 4-8. VSP

Prosthetic Feet

The need for and use of sensory feedback from prosthetic feet has not received the same attention that upper extremity terminal device feedback has received. Twenty-four amputees, 12 transfemoral and 12 transtibial, were fitted with a "sense-of-feel" device coupling a heel sensor and the metatarsal sensor to the corresponding front and back of the residual limb. Pre- and post-testing procedures measured symmetry of weight distribution, duration of single limb standing balance over the involved limb, and symmetry of step length and of stance phase times. Weight distribution symmetry scores increased by 7 percent. TF subgroup demonstrated a 24 percent increase in standing balance duration. Step symmetry increased 11 percent overall, despite a relatively short acclimation period.

Whether the prosthetist utilizes the SACH, single axis, multiaxis, or an energy-storing foot in the components of the transtibial prosthesis, all foot/ankles are either glued, laminated and/or bolted to an ankle block in the prosthesis. In an exoskeletal system, the plastic laminate is added to the outside of the prosthesis in order to produce a cosmetically acceptable foot/ankle assembly. Endoskeletal systems, which have an aluminum pylon attached to the foot/ankle assembly, utilize a foam cover and stocking to provide cosmesis. This foam cover for the endoskeletal prosthetic system will be described in chapter 5 dealing with TF prosthetic components, because a large number of endoskeletal systems are fitted to amputees at the TF level.

The Patellar Tendon Bearing (PTB) Socket

Prior to the 1950s, most TT prostheses contained a plug socket, which consisted of a wooden, leather-lined ring, generally shaped in the form of a circle, into which the amputee placed the residual limb. Because the volume of a residual limb may change frequently, it was not uncommon for plug sockets to fit differently day to day, or even hour to hour. The plug socket may be conceptualized as a cork in a bottle and the distance that the cork is forced into the bottle depends on the size and shape of the cork as well as the force pushing the cork downward.

In contrast to the plug socket, the PTB socket, developed in the 1950s by James Foort and Charles Radcliffe, utilizes total contact, a concept to be distinguished from end bearing. Total contact, in regard to the PTB socket, denotes a firm, but gentle force exerted by the socket over the entire area of the residual limb, in order to contain the volume of the residual limb, not allowing the distal portion to swell. Because many TT amputees have serious vascular disease, it is essential that the prosthetist match the total contact socket to the amputee's anatomy, in order to minimize distal oedema problems. End bearing, on the other hand, connotes that the amputee is able to actually bear weight on the end of the residual limb. As was mentioned, most through bone amputations do not accept end weight bearing without pain.

The PTB socket is designed to have specific areas of weight bearing and specific areas of relief, where very little or no weight is borne (see Figure 4-9). Areas that are intended to accept weight are the patellar tendon (ligament), the medial flare of the anterior tibia, the lateral aspect of the residual limb, the pre-tibial muscle mass between the tibial crest and fibula, the lateral surface of the fibula distal to the head and proximal to the cut end, and the popliteal fossa. The pressure sensitive areas of the TT limb include the patella, tibial tubercle, crest of the tibia, anterodistal tibia, anterolateral tibial condyle, distal end of the tibia, fibular head, hamstring tendons, lateral distal fibula, common peroneal nerve, and saphenous nerve.

When the prosthetist prepares the positive model for the PTB socket, areas of weight bearing and relief are developed by modification to the model. If weight bearing is desired, plaster is removed from the positive model. Areas of relief receive extra plaster (buildup) in order to develop recesses in the final socket. In order to assess the socket fit, a standing X-ray of the amputee in the socket may sometimes be used.

The PTB socket has essentially four sides or walls. Although the anterior wall is thought to be the primary weight-bearing wall, the other three walls play very important roles in the overall utilization of the PTB socket.

The top of the anterior wall is referred to as the anterior trim line. Generally, the anterior trim line is finished in such a manner that the top bisects the patella. This bisection may be important as an anatomical landmark for evaluating proper socket fit. In some prosthetic designs, the anterior trim line may exceed the proximal edge (or pole) of the patella as part of a supracondylar-suprapatellar suspension system as will be discussed in a subsequent section. The

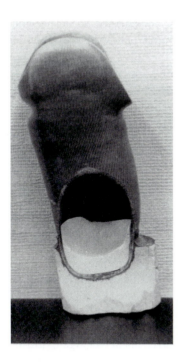

Figure 4-9. Patellar tendon bearing socket, medial view, with exposure to demonstrate total contact on bottom.

medial and lateral walls are rounded in shape and rise above the proximal pole of the patella. These walls can be used to control the knee mediolaterally in stance phase.

The posterior wall functions to produce a counterpressure to maintain the anterior residual limb against the anterior wall for the purpose of weight bearing. Too great a distance between the front and back walls will not properly load the anterior wall. The height of the posterior wall depends on the overall length of the residual limb. The longer the limb, the lower the posterior wall can be in order to allow for full knee flexion without the wall forcing the limb out of the socket. The shorter the residual limb, the higher the posterior wall, in order to retain the soft tissue in the socket. Generally, the height of the posterior wall is equal or just distal to the mid patellar tendon. The posterior wall may be level or slanted downward from lateral to medial to clear the hamstring tendons. Usually the prosthetist attempts to enclose as much soft tissue as possible within the posterior wall in order that these structures are not strangulated.

In addition to the features just described, the PTB socket is usually pre-flexed 8 to 10 degrees by the prosthetist as it is incorporated into the prosthetic limb. The purposes of pre-flexing the socket are to allow greater exposure to the anterior aspect of the residual limb for weight bearing; to maintain the knee joint in at least a neutral position, discouraging knee hyperextension; and to assist in the suspension of the prosthesis. Flexion of the socket is usually accompanied by slight dorsiflexion of the foot. This alignment assumes the use of a SACH foot.

Using a PTB and SACH foot, new amputees often need to be taught to walk in some knee flexion throughout the stance phase, due to the alignment of the socket. Therefore a slightly shorter step may need to be taken, and a shorter initial contact period can be anticipated. It is important to keep in mind that TT prostheses may incorporate a SACH foot, and that slight dorsiflexion of the solid foot will cause the knee to remain slightly flexed during weight-bearing, discouraging hyperextension. The greater the amount of flexion (dorsiflexion) of the foot, the earlier in stance phase knee flexion will occur.

Special anatomical circumstances may dictate modifications to the typical prosthesis previously described. An amputee with a 35 or 40 degree flexion deformity of the knee can still be fitted with a functional prosthesis. However, the prosthesis would need to be flexed to 40 or 45 degrees, making the step lengths even shorter.

PTB sockets may be of two basic types: hard sockets or sockets made with liners. Liners provide an interface between the residual limb sock and the socket and are preferred by some prosthetists and many amputees. Liners are thought to provide somewhat of a cushion, thus offering the amputee a more comfortable fitting. Indications for the use of a socket liner are often a very bony residual limb and one where weight bearing may place undue force on the tibia, usually on the crest. In children, liners are often used to offer greater flexibility of socket fitting as the child grows. As growth occurs, stump socks are removed. When no more socks can be removed, the liner is removed, making the socket larger, and allowing the amputee more time between socket fabrications. Socket liners may be fabricated from many different materials ranging from leather to plastic. Materials used for socket liners include Pelite, Plastazote, and various combinations of foamed plastic materials. In 1970, Koepke, Giacinto, and McCumber described a silicone gel socket liner covered with horsehide. This gel socket liner was intended for amputees with skin problems such as skin grafts, extensive scars, and limbs without sensation. This silicone gel insert, developed at the University of Michigan, distributes pressure evenly and is thought to lessen shear forces that can contribute to skin breakdown and ulceration. Usually when a socket liner is worn, the amputee first dons the liner and then inserts the liner into the socket (Figure 4-10). Today, prefabricated gel liners, often termed comfort liners, are commercially available and widely utilized.

In the PTB hard socket, stump socks are nearly always used as an interface between socket and skin. They may be wool or synthetic and serve to add volume within the socket as limb volume decreases. The smaller the limb, the more plies of sock necessary. Socks come in many sizes and thickness from 1 to 6 ply.

Total Surface-Bearing Socket Design

Previous research and development produced the PTB socket, and the notion that areas of the residual limb were either pressure tolerant or pressure sensitive. Great care was taken by the Certified Prosthetist (CP) to relieve the positive impression to load only those areas that accepted loading.

Total surface-bearing socket designs suggest that forces may be applied over the entire residual limb, with the magnitude varying according to the type of tissue. There are no areas of relief because all surfaces are tolerant, using the older vernacular. The new design still does not propose end bearing on the cut end of the bones, but rather to transfer as much force as can be comfortably borne. It eliminates the focused pressure of the PTB "bar" across the anterior surface, and relies on the use of the new comfort liner technology to allow the force to be applied evenly through gel materials such as silicone, elastomers impregnated with mineral oil, and urethane. Although such total contact propositions are used in other areas of orthotics, such as total contact casts for diabetic plantar ulcers, the difference lies in the problems created by shearing and friction, which at least for now appear to be answered by the newer comfort liner materials.

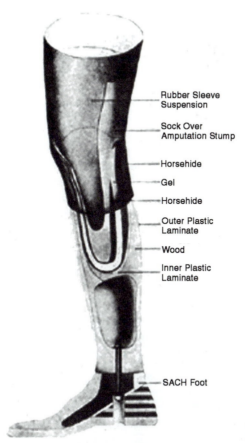

Rubber Sleeve
Suspension

Sock Over
Amputation Stump

Horsehide

Gel

Horsehide

Outer Plastic
Laminate

Wood

Inner Plastic
Laminate

SACH Foot

Figure 4-10. Michigan silicone insert

Liners: Silicone, Viscoelastic, and/or Urethane

As has been previously identified elsewhere, sockets were originally unlined, using the so-called "hard socket" concept. Amputees requiring more cushioning used whatever materials were available at the time. Socks are often used to soften the interface/skin junction, with patients choosing to vary thickness by ply of sock. As newer materials became available, they eventually found their way into prosthetic practice. An example of a material used in the 1950s and 1960s was Kemblo, a rubber-like material used in the early socket liners. The material cushioned the residual limb to reduce painful forces and rubbing often experienced by bony residual limbs, and ushered in the liner concept.

In 1970, Koepke from the University of Michigan published a paper detailing the advantages of medical grade silicone, which was covered with leather and used as a socket liner. The application was designed for use by TT amputees with myelomenningocele (spina bifida) to help reduce ulceration over bony prominences due to lack of sensation. Also note that these sockets were suspended using a latex rubber sleeve, an obvious precursor to the suspension sleeves now commonly used for prosthetic suspension (see Figure 4-10).

During the mid 1980s, reports began appearing about new silicone socket liners being produced in Iceland by Össur Kristinsson in Reykjavik. Known as ICEROSS, an acronym for Icelandic Roll on Silicone Socket, the system offered prosthetic users an alternative to rubber, foam, or sock interfaces. The system was available in many sizes and introduced the added feature of inherent suspension by way of a pin. With the pin attached to the distal plastic or metal stabilizer, suspension is accomplished by inserting it into a catch or shuttle lock located in the distal socket (Figure 4-11). This eliminated any additional need for straps, belts, or wedges, and completed a self-suspending socket.

Because early sizing was limited some prosthetists began providing custom-molded so-called (3S) *silicone suction suspension* liners. Pritham and Fillauer pioneered this technology for patients whose limbs were of odd size or configuration. As the quality and range of pre-fabricated liners has improved, the need for custom-made solutions has diminished.

Currently, liners are made from medical-grade silicone, urethane, or thermoplastic elastomers, sometimes infused with mineral oil, vitamins, or aloe vera. They may be covered on the outside with nylon or textile in an effort to increase useable lifetime and decrease wear relative to socket forces on the anterior limb.

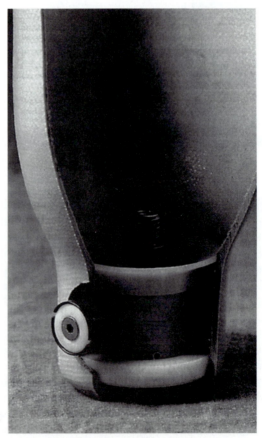

Figure 4-11. Shuttle lock system.

Examples of currently available systems include:

- ICEROSS: Clear and two-color silicone, covered with fabric, 19 sizes, multiple thicknesses, with or without shuttle lock (Figure 4-12).
- Alpha: From Ohio Willow Wood, made from mineral oil-impregnated gel, covered with a spandex-like material, available in three sizes, three gel thicknesses, and three configurations of gel distribution. Available with or without locking pins, these also may be heated over modified casts to provide custom sizing (Figure 4-13).
- TEC: Total Environmental Control, developed by Carl Caspers, offers a custom-molded or off-the-shelf urethane liner with nylon proximal enhancement. A bit thicker than

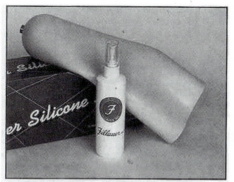

Fillauer's flesh-colored Silicone
Suspension Liner

Figure 4-12. ICEROSS.

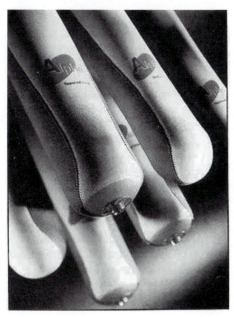

Figure 4-13. Alpha.

many others, the TEC provides shock-absorbing functions and is preferred by many runners and/or jumpers (Figure 4-14).

- Otto Bock: 6Y10 silicone liner offers distal attachment suspension and a pneumatic bladder. It differs from the rest by the addition of an inflatable bladder to produce total contact on the bottom of the liner (Figure 4-15).

- Aegis: Combines a tapered and preflexed transtibial shape allowing for popliteal relief in a clear silicone liner (Figure 4-16).

- Silipos: Offers a hybrid between conventional stump socks and a silicone liner, using a mineral oil gel. They are available with both single and double nylon sheaths to wick perspiration from the limb and in standard thicknesses of conventional stump socks (Figure 4-17).

Liners offer distinct purported advantages via skin/socket pressure reduction and the ability to self-suspend. They do require some degree of maintenance and demand regular cleaning on the inside. They are more fragile than foams or rubber materials and require moderate to good dexterity in order to don and doff.

Some caution and judgment must be used when attempting to fit large patients with large thighs. Due to the extreme size and quickly increasing circumferences moving proximally, suspension may be compromised and difficult.

Lake surveyed 56 amputees using silicone suspension sleeves to determine the incidence of dermatological problems presumably related to the use of the sleeves. He discusses the subject thoroughly and reports the results of the survey. Also of interest is the publication of the opinions of several ABC-Certified Prosthetists as to criteria for the use of silicone sleeves: superior suspension, management of unstable limb volume, secure feeling, decreased perceived

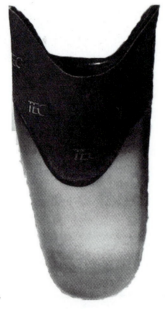

Figure 4-14. TEC.

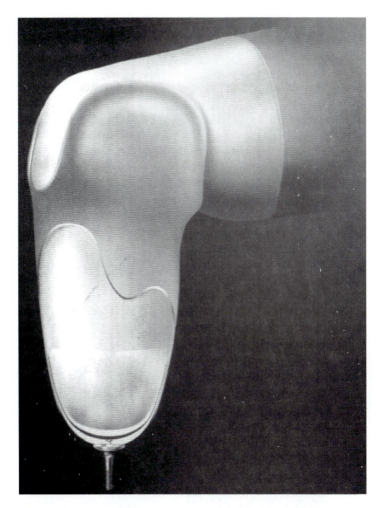

Figure 4-15. Otto Bock.

weight, flexible interface, and improved cosmesis. Other points of interest were reasons that silicone sleeves might be avoided: known sensitivity to silicone, poor cognitive capacity, poor skin (invaginations), adherent scars, and compromised hand function. Their conclusion about skin problems related to the use of silicone sleeves was guarded, and was expressed as a by-product of age, pathology, physiology, and activity level.

Comfort liners have been reportedly used at other prosthetic levels including trans-femoral, transradial, and transhumeral. Caution is needed when fitting sleeves at the TF level. Because of the increased mobility of the distal residual limb, carefully selected patients can benefit assuming good hands and a willingness to learn.

Trieb, of Vienna, Austria, presented his work at the 1990 American Academy of Ortho-paedic Surgeons meeting. He reported on 61 TF amputees wearing silicone suspension sys-tems. He contrasted them with 18 amputees wearing ischial containment sockets without

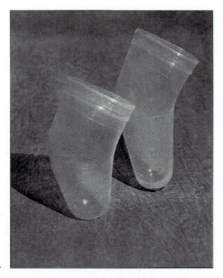

Figure 4-16. Aegis.

silicone sleeve systems. No differences were observed for satisfaction, average daily use, or the use of assistive devices. Although data about gait was presented, no causative affect was established.

Boonstra, van Duin, and Eisma, of the Netherlands, evaluated the preference of TT amputees for the 3S compared to the supracondylar PTB socket with pelite liner. Eight amputees wore both for 10 weeks and completed questionnaires concerning comfort, ambulation, ADL, working conditions, and sports. Of the six that completed the testing, two preferred the 3S, two the PTB with pelite, and two were satisfied using both styles.

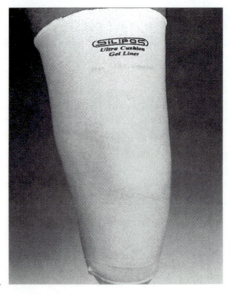

Figure 4-17. Silipos.

Outcome of Fitting an ICEROSS Prosthesis:
Views of Transtibial Amputees

The ICEROSS prefabricated liner has been available since 1986 (see Figure 4-12), although custom liners had been described by Kristinsson and Fillauer. Kristinsson reported that the main advantages of the new liner were improved suspension and greater weight-bearing capabilities at the interface of the socket and residual limb. Follow up reports on ICEROSS use have been slow in coming.

The views of the amputees who wore the new silicone system were solicited between April 1993 and October 1994. A total of 69 unilateral TT amputees were provided ICEROSS systems on Endolite pylons and multi-flex ankle joints. All had been previous PTB wearers.

A composite questionnaire was devised to evaluate the amputees' views of the new system. Fifty-four of the 69 questionnaires were returned. The etiology of the group was interesting; 27 were traumatic; 11 to diabetes or peripheral vascular disease; 6 were congenital; and 10 were miscellaneous. Ages ranged from 22 to 80 years. Follow up took place at an average of 22 weeks post fitting. The results were as follows:

- Wearing time per day was not significantly different.
- Distance walked per day was not significantly different.
- Walking on uneven ground was not reported to be easier.
- Amputees did not use walking aids any less frequently.
- Stump sweating was greater in the first 3 weeks, then diminished.
- Skin breakdown was less, and walking up and down stairs was easier.

Fifteen of the 54 patients ultimately rejected the ICEROSS completely. Ten of the 15 reported skin rash as the reason, along with irritation and severe sweating. Two of the 15 found the distal compression too tight to tolerate. Of further interest is that the overall rating favored the ICEROSS. However, this must be taken with caution because the pre-selection process tended to place patients with skin problems in these sockets in the first place.

The results of this study clearly indicate why the use of outcomes is only of value when parallel clinical research with measurable criteria are also collected and scientifically analyzed. Without the science, the notion that 36 percent of these patients had an unsatisfactory outcome tells us little of what we did wrong and, more importantly, what we need to change to make the outcomes better.

A review of a recent database reveals 26 articles dealing with some phase of this new technology. Most of these articles deal with anecdotal looks at the use of the new materials. None of the articles used the scientific method to compare these systems with others or even with current technology, such as foam liners. Until this is done, it is impossible to report the effect of using these new products with amputees who have peripheral vascular disease, diabetes, scars secondary to burns or frostbite, or infection from trauma.

The Prosthetic Skin

The external covering, or prosthetic skin, of the prosthesis may be plastic laminate, a heavy cotton stocking over soft foam, or a water and stain-resistant coating. The function of the prosthetic skin is to cover the device in a cosmetically acceptable manner and to protect the mechanism from contamination. With an exoskeletal type, a combination of fiberglass stockinette and thermal setting plastic combine to provide the amputee with a hard plastic shell, similar to the shell of a turtle. This prosthetic skin provides the structural stability for the prosthesis, as well as protection for the residual limb and component parts. With an endoskeletal system (Figure 4-18) the actual structure of the device is provided by an aluminum or titanium pipe and connectors, with the cosmetic restoration produced by a foam cover and a heavy sock or water-resistant covering. The polyurethane foam cover is shaped by the prosthetist based on circumferential measurements of the amputee's remaining limb. It should be understood that the exoskeletal type of hard plastic shell is far more durable and acceptable to amputees who work or play in rugged environments or otherwise damage the foam cover of an endoskeletal limb.

Preparatory Prostheses

A preparatory prosthesis is any prosthesis that is not "definitive," or intended for long-term use and one that allows ample opportunity for modifications. The purpose of any preparatory prosthesis is to allow early ambulation at an efficient and safe level, and yet allow for the rapid changes in volume that often occur in the days and weeks post operatively. Preparatory prostheses may be made of many materials, including plaster, wood, plastic, and metal. Preparatory prostheses cost less than a finished limb, but allow the patient to walk safely in a custom fabricated socket (Figure 4-19). Preparatory prostheses will be discussed further in the section on rigid dressings.

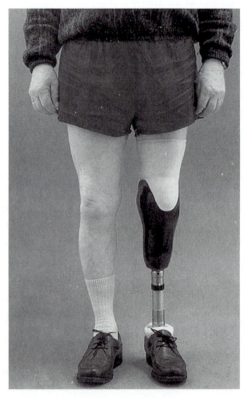

Figure 4-18. ENDO.

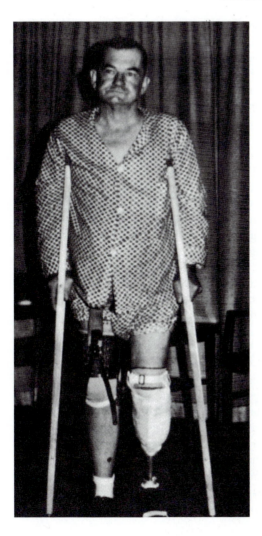

Figure 4-19. TT preparatory prosthesis, with removable pylon and SACH foot.

When using modular prosthetic component systems, the endoskeletal tube may also serve as the temporary prosthesis. This allows the care team to begin training with the prosthetic device and to withhold final cosmetic restoration pending the results of the training. In this case, the temporary is also the permanent limb, with the difference being the completion of the cosmetic cover. A socket replacement for volume or configuration changes may be done and added to the endoskeletal pylon system.

SUSPENSION OF THE TRANSTIBIAL PROSTHESIS

Suspension refers to the components and design features used to hold a prosthesis in place while the amputee ambulates and performs other functional activities. Suspension of the TT prosthesis may take many forms. It is desirable to use the easiest and simplest possible form of suspension because most amputees resist the addition of straps, belts, and the like, particularly if they are functionally unnecessary. The anatomy of the knee and thigh often determine the ease with which the prosthesis may be suspended. Normal anatomy of the thigh allows many suspension applications that center around the fact that the femoral condyles provide a useful attachment location. Amputees who are overweight or have excessive soft tissue around the thigh and knee, make the suspension of TT prostheses more difficult. Figure 4-20 shows examples of different types of suspension as discussed in the following sections.

The Supracondylar Cuff

A frequently used means of suspension in the TT prosthesis is the supracondylar cuff (Figure 4-20a). The supracondylar cuff is usually made of leather, vinyl, or other plastic, and is riveted to the medial and lateral walls of the socket and closes circumferentially around the lower thigh. The supracondylar cuff classically either buckles or closes using Velcro, so that only one hand is required to fasten it. In some cases, the supracondylar cuff may not be sufficient to completely suspend the prosthesis in all circumstances and an auxiliary waist belt may be added to ensure adequate suspension. An additional feature of the supracondylar cuff is that it may act to limit hyperextension of the knee during stance phase. A disadvantage to the supracondylar cuff is that it may present a high amount of force in the popliteal space, particularly while the amputee is sitting, or when the knee is flexed to 90 degrees, and using many thicknesses of sock.

The Medial Wedge

Another means of suspending the PTB prosthesis is the removable medial wedge. Medial wedging is the technique that involves a soft, pliable, often leather or plastic wedge, inserted by the amputee inside the medial wall of the prosthesis by the spuracondylar fossa. Once the residual limb and wedge are in place in the socket, no further straps are necessary. The lateral wall must be rigid and not yield so that the medial wedge pressure pushes the residual limb against the lateral wall. This compression may cause some discomfort in the early wearing periods, often necessitating gradual periods of wearing in order to accustom the medial aspects of the leg to the wedge and its pressure. Sometimes the medial wedge is incorporated into the medial side of a socket liner (Figure 4-20c) so that no other removable wedge is necessary, providing the amputee with a very cosmetic PTB prosthesis that is self-suspending.

The Removable Medial Wall

When the medial wedge used for suspension is the medial wall itself, one has a PTB suspension variant known as the removable medial wall or removable medial brim. This type of suspension allows the amputee to remove the entire medial wall, insert the leg, and then insert the medial wall into a steel channel laminated into the side of the prosthesis. The removable wall has a wedge-shaped protrusion formed on it, which conforms to the medial musculature of the knee. Through both swing and stance phase, the wedge in the medial wall maintains the limb in place (Figure 4-20b).

Sleeve Suspension

A relatively new form of suspension for the PTB prosthesis is sleeve suspension. Sleeves may be made of many different materials such as neoprene rubber, knitted cotton, elastic, or a cotton-polyester blend. Koepke, Giacinto, and McCumber in 1970 described the silicone gel

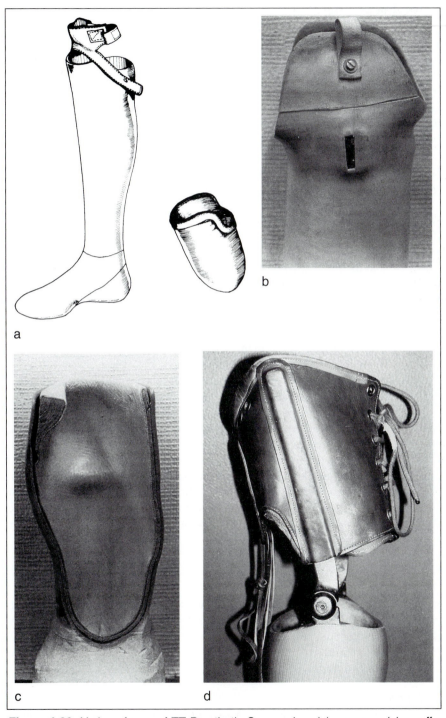

Figure 4-20. Various forms of TT Prosthetic Suspension: (a) suparcondylar cuff (b) removable medial wall or brim (c) removable med. wedge linear (d) thigh corset with knee joints.

socket used for problematic residual limbs, or ones with difficulties in pressure distribution (see Figure 4-10). Part of that "Michigan leg" was a latex rubber sleeve that was used for suspension. The rubber sleeve attached to the socket of the prosthesis, and was pulled over the knee by the amputee following insertion of the leg into the socket. Other suspension sleeves made of many materials are commercially available and function in ways similar to the Michigan sleeve. Although the rubber sleeve may not be used in all climates, it is a viable form of suspension when heat and humidity are not a problem.

Thigh Corset and Knee Hinges

Another form of suspension for the TT prosthesis is the thigh corset and knee hinge (Figure 4-20d). This form of suspension is quite bulky and is used only when necessary. Usually, the amputee using this form of suspension has some instability of the knee, and therefore uses the knee hinges as an orthosis (see chapter 7). The instability may be either medial-lateral or anterior-posterior. Other candidates for thigh corset and knee hinge suspension are amputees whose skin on the residual limb is unable to tolerate the applied forces and who need an additional area over which to distribute the forces. This situation occurs in amputees doing heavy lifting and in juvenile diabetics, patients with systemic lupus erythematosis (SLE), and rheumatoid arthritis. Knee hinges used with PTB sockets may be either single axis or polycentric. Polycentric hinges have a moving center of rotation and are thought to act more like the normal anatomy of the knee joint. For this reason, many amputees prefer polycentric hinges since undue pressure from socket binding can be avoided.

Thigh lacer and knee joints (joints and corset) reduce the interface pressure between skin and socket. Textbooks estimate that these systems may reduce interface pressure between 25 and 60 percent. Shem reported on this topic by measuring these pressures using the Rincoe Socket Fitting System (SFS). Percentage increase in the interface pressures without the thigh lacer ranged from 3.4 to 39.8 percent, with an average of 19 percent. Although Bowker and Michael reported that only 1 percent of all TT amputees use the thigh lacer, it has been verified and quantified that the reduction in residual limb pressure is real.

According to Foort, criteria for the use of a thigh lacer include stabilizing the prosthesis against rotation with the knee flexed, heavy lifting, knee instabilities, inability to stand without pain or skin breakdown, donning and doffing, and preference or history of wearing thigh lacer.

MANAGEMENT OF THE RESIDUAL LIMB

An important part of postsurgical care of the amputee is devoted to managing the residual limb. This management consists of simultaneously attending to wound healing and to shaping and conditioning the residual limb for its new function of weightbearing. Two techniques have developed as important aspects of residual limb management, application of a rigid postsurgical dressing and compression wrapping.

Rigid Dressings

The concept of early prosthetic fitting dates back to the early eighteenth century, and probably long before. During World Wars I and II, early temporary prostheses were made from plaster and broom handles. These prostheses were used successfully throughout Europe. In the 1950s interest in the United States in active mobilization of the residual limb and the development of the elastic bandage sparked a renewed interest in early prosthetic fitting. In 1957, surgeons first used plaster and pylons to serve as provisional or temporary prostheses. Early experience with this system confirmed what had been written years before: that walking on an immature residual limb had positive effects on residual limb maturation. In 1958, Berlemont recorded the first immediate postoperative prosthetic fitting while the patient was on the operating table. The technique was soon refined and popularized in this country by Dr. Burgess of Seattle.

The components of the rigid dressing as described by Burgess include Lycra Spandex stump sock, scived relief pads for tibia and patella, elastic plaster, regular plaster, waist belt and suspension strap, and pylon and SACH foot assembly. The stump sock is pulled over the wound, covering the distal residual limb with sterile lamb's wool to allow for wound drainage. Beveled felt pads are placed on the patella and on both medial and lateral sides of the crest of the tibia. Elastic plaster is wrapped over the residual limb followed by regular plaster. A suspension strap is encased in the plaster near the end of the procedure and a waist belt is placed on the patient. The patella covering is removed and any extra plaster cut away. Drying time is 12 to 24 hours, depending on temperature and humidity. The pylon and SACH foot are added and the final pylon adjustment is done with the patient standing.

The results attributed to the use of the rigid dressing in the middle to late 1960s included better wound healing, need for fewer postoperative narcotics, earlier ambulation, less oedema, and the psychological advantage of never being without a limb. Through the 1960s and early 1970s, there were many reports concerning the use of new surgical techniques that benefited the dysvascular amputee. Few, if any, studies were sufficiently controlled to allow fair evaluation of the influence of any one aspect of new treatment procedures. Many of these new procedures improved patient care simply by emphasizing the saving of the knee joint, particularly in the elderly. It was not until Mooney published his work in 1971 that the use of immediate postoperative rigid dressings in the dysvascular amputee was questioned. In 182 cases of TT amputation on dysvascular patients, he concluded that rigid dressing and ambulation were good and probably contributed to the overall well-being of the patients. However, he also concluded that ambulation within the first 2 to 4 weeks may deter wound healing. In 1977, Baker et al, in a prospective study, reported evidence that the use of the rigid dressing procedure did not result in a higher percentage of wound healing in vascular diseased patients with TT amputations. Wound healing was reported as 85 percent using the rigid dressing, and 83 percent using soft dressings. However, patients with rigid dressing were discharged on postoperative Day 7.3 on the average, whereas patients in soft dressings were discharged in an average of 14.7 days. Patients with rigid dressings began ambulation using a prosthesis at postoperative Day 29.6, whereas patients with soft dressings began at postoperative Day 35.5.

Rigid dressings with pylons are intended for partial weight bearing. Slight dorsiflexion of the prosthetic foot usually allows the patient to have a smoother advance through stance phase during early ambulation because the knee is stiff. The pylon is often shortened to permit swing phase without circumduction, vaulting, or hip hiking. The pylon/foot assembly may be removed while the patient is in bed. This avoids the tendency for the hip to passively externally rotate secondary to the round heel of the foot. The combination of a rigid dressing and pylon is one form of a temporary prosthesis. Generally, temporary prostheses are used in cases where large volume reductions in the residual limb are anticipated. So long as the distal residual limb has a larger circumferential measurement than the proximal measurement, a plaster dressing may well be the treatment of choice.

Rigid dressings, with or without pylon, are generally in use throughout the United States today and the technique may be learned by anyone. The rigid dressing is generally applied by a prosthetist or surgeon although, in some facilities, it may be applied by a physical therapist or orthopaedic physician assistant.

Semirigid Dressings

Swanson reported on his version of the use of a semirigid dressing using a custom-molded PTB socket made of polyethylene. He recommends the use of a stump shrinker and sock under the socket for fluid resorption in the early postoperative days until the wound heals. The stated goals for use include protection and volume reduction. Swanson concludes that CAD-CAM could expedite the use of this technique and allow data collection about limb shrinkage, allowing studies to evaluate these effects for purposes of payment justification by third parties. Vigiers et al reported on residual limb wound healing after vascular, TT amputation: They compared, randomly, the time to healing of open wounds treated with a plaster cast, supracondylar type, with a silicone sleeve liner and with an elastic compression wrap. The cast and silicone interface group healed in 71.2 days whereas the elastic bandage group required 96.8 days.

Compression Wrapping

Compression wrapping is a procedure that assists in the shrinking and maturation of the residual limb or stump. It is often done using rubber or synthetic elastic wraps, and is usually taught to the patient or significant other so that it may be carried out in the patient's home. Compression wrapping is a part of a system often referred to as a soft dressing. Soft dressings usually consist of cotton mesh gauze, wrapped over the stump, followed by a compression wrapping often referred to as an "Ace" wrap. Compression wraps are commercially available in many sizes, and in a number of different materials. Generally, wraps are 2, 3, 4, and 6 inches wide. The length may vary and it is often necessary to sew two wraps together to produce one longer wrap. Generally, compression wraps are applied in order to create pressure gradients, with more pressure being applied distally, and less pressure as the wrap proceeds proximally. Wrapping continues indefinitely, as the maturation process frequently takes 6 to 12 months, and often longer.

There are two basic techniques of application for the compression wrap. One is called the recurrent, and the other a figure eight (Figure 4-21). The figure eight style requires only two hands and is very simple to learn. Pressure should be applied on the oblique turns, and not on the circular turns. The result of applying too much pressure on the circular turns is a tourniquet, which may compromise the viability of the residual limb, as well as delay prosthetic fitting, due to large amounts of "boggy" oedema. The wrap should extend above the knee and above the proximal pole of the patella. This allows for a consistent shrinking of the entire residual limb, as well as affording some degree of suspension for the wrap. Wrinkles in the wrap can cause skin problems and care should be taken to avoid them. Patients should be discouraged from active knee flexion exercise while the wrap is in place. This will serve to increase the pressure over the patella and tibial tubercle, and will also lead to an ultimate loss of

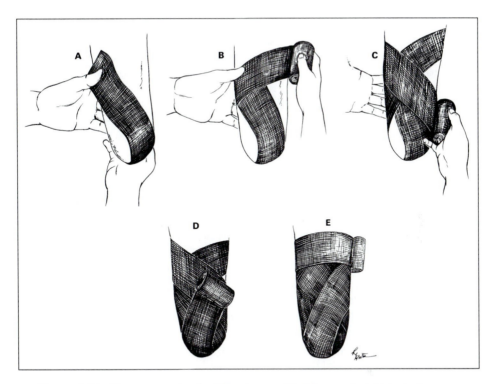

Figure 4-21. Stump wrapping for TT using modified figure-of-eight technique.

suspension of the wrap. Isherwood et al studied the pressure associated with the use of soft dressings and particularly elastic compression dressings. Results of their work indicate that the greatest pressure on the TT residual limb occurs over the tibial tubercle. In fact, the mean pressure for both skilled and unskilled bandagers was greater by 28 mm Hg over the tibial tubercle, from 39 to 67mm Hg.

An alternative to a rolled compression wrap is a shrinker sock which is typically an elastic sleeve with one end tapered and sewn shut. The sock is pulled over the residual limb and held in place using tape or Velcro. Shrinker socks are available in many sizes, thicknesses, lengths, and knittings. The advantages cited for using the shrinker socks compared to compression wraps are ease of application and no need for understanding or learning wrapping techniques. The cost of the device is more than most compression wraps, but may be worth the investment when dealing with home bound patients who have difficulties with stump wrapping. Varghese reported comparisons of compression wraps, shrinker socks, and a modified shrinker sock. The modification was done based on measured pressure readings taken from the stump. Results indicated that patients had excessive pressures when regular compression wraps were used. The best results came from the modified shrinker sock that showed increased venous return in the residual limb. The sock maintained pressure longer and was easier to apply. Single knit shrinker socks delivered less than ideal pressure and deteriorated following several washings.

Lilja studied TT, vascular amputees from amputation to 120 days postamputation to evaluate the changes in volume and to determine if a proper time exists in which to fit the definitive prosthesis. Other researchers have studied this phenomenaon to identify factors affecting the process. This study utilized a CAD-CAM scanner to test one of the oftmentioned advantages of this new technology. The range of volume reduction over the 120 days measured 17 to 35 percent. Body weight during the study remained stable. Based on these results, the authors recommend an early preparatory prosthesis and the definitive to follow 4 months later. This agrees with the Scandinavian prosthetists, Liga and Oberg, who believe an acceptable fitting includes no more than two, presumably five-ply, socks

Other Stump Maturation Options

Wu and Krick reported on an alternative to either conventional rigid dressings or compression wraps. The removable rigid dressing (RRD) involves the use of a plaster shell, socks, a stockinette sleeve, and a thermoplastic supracondylar cuff. Tube socks are used under the plaster shell to accommodate volume loss. Additionally, the cast may be safely used while standing, with the assistance of a simple car jack. The RRD is usually applied following the removal of the first thigh-length rigid dressing. It may, however, be used with both recent and long-term amputees. The removable rigid dressing reportedly saved 90 days of hospital stay by eliminating many breakdowns of the skin often seen in TT amputees using compression wraps.

In addition to the postoperative dressings or systems previously discussed, other options exist. These options may be generally referred to as soft, or semirigid. Although soft dressings of gauze and cotton are commonly used with a more delayed prosthetic fitting, 80 percent healing success was reported by Gay and Heard when the soft dressing was used in conjunction with surgical techniques that left a long posterior skin flap. The two principal types of semirigid dressings are the unna paste boot and the air splint. Unna boot is the term used to describe a zinc oxide impregnated gauze, which is commercially available like plaster. The boot never hardens but provides some external pressure to the stump, while giving it some shape. The procedure for application has been described by Ghiulamila. Felt relief pads are used along the crest of the tibia, in a way similar to a plaster rigid dressing. Unna boots do not allow for any swelling and may be applied by anyone knowledgeable in the technique.

Writing primarily in British publications, Little reported on the postoperative use of an air splint. The use of the air splint is said to facilitate early ambulation and balance training and to allow partial weight bearing on the recently amputated limb. Little's article, published in 1970, described the use of air splints on five patients, all dysvascular, and all having long posterior flaps. Following closure of the wound, the air splint was applied and inflated to a pressure of 25 mm Hg. Sweating under the splint was noted as a nuisance and the addition of a walking pylon was reported to be difficult, if not impossible. Little doesn't claim that the air splint system is better or even equal to the rigid dressing system. He does, however, believe it to be easier to apply and use. In the United States, use of the air splint was reported by Kerstein and Sher. Both cite the same advantages as Little, plus the ability to see the wound and to inspect it at any time without the problems of removing and reapplying a plaster cast. The technique of Kerstein involves a stump sock and felt relief pads, similar to a plaster rigid dressing. Kerstein reported results on 11 patients indicating, as did Little, that no pylon attachment was possible with the air splint. Sher first used the air splint when no prosthetist or early prosthetic program was available.

Other Factors Affecting the Residual Limb

It is not possible to describe, in detail, all the possible stump conditions that might be encountered in an active prosthetics/orthotics clinic. However, this section will describe some general considerations that may affect the course of treatment or the indications for specific components or modifications.

The presence of a break in the skin or a sore does not, in and of itself, contraindicate the use of a prosthesis while the sore is open or even draining. Although physician preference may dictate some situations, it is imperative to understand why the sore or ulcer first appeared. Appropriate steps may then be taken to relieve the area and the patient may return to limited ambulation, always being careful not to increase the size or severity of the sore. This approach may be difficult for some patients and families to grasp because many equate skin sores with potential trouble and with the series of events that may have led to the amputation in the first place.

Burns, either thermal or electrical, can result in limb amputations and often leave scars that can be difficult to manage. If the scarring occurs on the lower extremity, the need to bear weight on that extremity may make the prosthetic fitting fraught with skin breakdown, particularly in the early weeks and months following the amputation. As the skin contracts, the chance of ulceration increases. Careful and watchful follow up and well-educated family members are very important.

Perhaps the most common problem dealt with in the follow up of patients with amputations is oedema. No other problem is seen so frequently and is such a source of frustration for amputees and their families. Because the great majority of amputations are done for vascular reasons, it should not be surprising that the postoperative problem list includes oedema. As was mentioned in the section describing the PTB socket, oedema can affect socket fit and lead to ulceration when bony prominences are not resting in their designated places within the socket. It also can confuse the amputee regarding the correct number of plies of stump socks to wear.

In cases of severe diabetes or other vascular conditions, as well as any of a group of peripheral neuropathies, normal feeling in the stump is diminished or lost altogether. When this occurs, skin breakdown is often persistent. The important factors involved in evaluating these situations are the type and fit of the socket as well as the adherence to recommended amounts of ambulation and the use of proper numbers of plies of stump socks. In some instances, nothing can prevent ulceration, and patient management is from one episode to another. In other situations, more proximal unloading of weight is helpful. This may take the form of a thigh lacer, which is reported to relieve as much as 40 percent of the patient's weight from the PTB socket. In extreme cases, patients are placed in a quadrilateral socket, similar to the sockets used with TF amputations, as described in the next chapter. Additionally, special liners, such as the comfort liners, used inside the socket can help to distribute the weight more evenly. Adequate length of the residual limb can be important in the prevention of ulceration by affording a large surface area for weight bearing, resulting in less force per unit area.

In those cases where a marked flexion contracture exists, and conservative measures fail to improve the clinical picture, a bent knee prosthesis may be fitted. Such a device usually incorporates thigh corset and knee-hinge suspension and allows the patient to walk with the knee in a bent or flexed position, taking all the weight on the anterior tibial aspects of the stump. A cosmetic problem exists when the bent knee prosthesis is used. However, in those few cases where no other device will function, this option should be considered. Clinical experience dictates that the patient should be fully informed beforehand as to exactly what the device will look like.

ALIGNMENT OF THE TRANSTIBIAL PROSTHESIS

The term alignment refers to the physical relationship between the socket and the prosthetic foot. Much attention is paid to alignment in order to attain the optimal function for the amputee, particularly during stance phase when the amputee is in a position of full weight bearing. Proper alignment will provide the amputee with the opportunity to comfortably bear all weight on the limb without undue forces causing either pain or ulceration.

Static Alignment of the Transtibial Prosthesis

As was discussed in chapter 2, alignment occurs in two phases: static (bench) and dynamic. Static or bench alignment is the configuration in which the prosthetist places the prosthesis prior to the initial limb fitting. This usually occurs in the office of the prosthetist and prior to any visit to the physician or physical therapist. The bench alignment will usually allow most amputees to begin ambulation. Bench alignment allows the amputee to proceed to static alignment. Static alignment starts the patient weight bearing. Changes necessitated during walking begin dynamic alignment. Changes may be made while the amputee walks in order to provide the most comfortable and efficient gait possible.

One of the primary devices used by the prosthetist in bench aligning a prosthesis is a plumb bob, a pointed weight on the end of a string, providing a true vertical reference. The prosthetist initially aligns the prosthesis so that a plumb line hung from the center of the posterior wall will fall about 1/2 inch lateral to the center of the heel of the shoe of the prosthesis as seen in Figure 4-22. Thus, the foot will be 1/2 inch inset from true vertical. This insetting of the foot in bench alignment accommodates for the bowing of the tibia, helps load pressure tolerant areas, and allows for a reasonable distance between the heels during gait. As was discussed in chapter 3, the narrower the base of support, the less energy consuming the gait.

In the anterior-posterior plane, the prosthesis is initially aligned so that a plumb line from the center of the lateral wall will fall just anterior to the foremost edge of the heel, a location sometimes referred to in prosthetics as the breast of the heel. Although there is no ankle axis in a SACH foot, the plumb line would pass just anterior to it if there were one.

Dynamic Alignment of the Transtibial Prosthesis

Following acceptable bench alignment, dynamic alignment occurs while the amputee is walking and in full weight bearing on the involved side. The guiding principle in dynamic alignment is that the sole of the shoe must be perfectly flat on the floor when the amputee is full weight bearing at midstance. This determination must be made both from the front and back, as well as from the side. The prosthetist adjusts the alignment, attempting to optimize the amputee's gait pattern. Experience is necessary to perform this alignment and can be learned through the eyes and assistance of an experienced prosthetist. It is important to remember that any changes made are likely to alter the forces on the limb, so a thorough understanding of the process should precede any attempted changes in alignment.

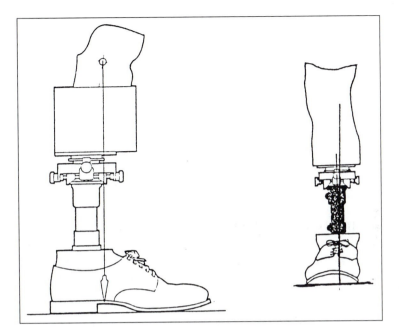

Figure 4-22. Bench alignment for a PTB prosthesis.

Heel Height

Changes to the heel height of the shoe, or the absence of a shoe, can alter prosthetic alignment. The amputee must decide on a heel height and remain very close to that height throughout. Early education about the problems of changing shoe/heel heights will prevent many later problems.

FUNCTIONAL TRAINING OF THE TRANSTIBIAL AMPUTEE

Individuals who undergo amputation for vascular insufficiency are generally deconditioned, often diabetic, and have been hospitalized or at home attempting to heal a long-standing foot or lower leg ulcer. Silbert reported that 41 percent of the diabetic amputees he studied lived longer than 3 years postoperatively, but that 51 percent of those surviving the surgery lost their remaining limb within 5 years. Mazet reported similar results, stating that a second amputation occurred 33 percent of the time within 5 years of the first. Whitehouse stated that the dysvascular amputee is more likely to die than to lose the remaining limb. McCollough reported that in 27 cases of bilateral TT amputations, 20 lost the second limb within 2 years, and 7 before 6 years. In view of this data, amputees should have well-fitting, protective, and sometimes custom-made insoles or entire shoes in order to make every effort to preserve the contralateral extremity. A well-fitted, large toebox shoe may be helpful in this regard.

Ng, Berbrayer, and Hunter studied 59 TT amputees and evaluated ambulatory status over time. Using the scale of Volpicelli, follow up was obtained at least for 6 months, or the last chart entry. Ambulatory status demonstrated 42 percent to be community ambulators, 46 percent to be household ambulators, and the rest more limited.

The authors concluded that the prognosis was determined by a number of factors, including the age and general health, along with the etiology of the amputation and the status of the remaining limb.

Pre-Prosthetic Care

The postoperative care following amputation surgery is a team effort, conducted jointly by all parties concerned. It is important for the success of the patient that the care be consistent with what was promised preoperatively, and that all parties continue to communicate. In large general hospitals, it is convenient to house amputees close together, if possible, for consistent nursing care, and to allow each patient to talk with and watch the others, and to share their successes. Generally, the postsurgical care of an amputee may also be thought of as the pre-prosthetic time when care goals by all team members focus on wound healing, limb and/or joint preparation, and early exercise, including ambulation. The specifics of each case may differ due to etiology, concomitant disease or trauma, age, motivation, and philosophy of the managing team.

The involvement of the physical therapist in the postoperative management of the TT amputee starts as early as the amputee has been discontinued from any strong pain medication. The program can be much the same for all TT amputees, irrespective of the type of postoperative dressing used. Amputees usually come to the department twice daily and are involved with an overall exercise program graded to each amputee's tolerance. Short periods of standing can reacquaint the amputee with balancing in the upright position. Mirrors are very helpful in providing visual feedback. Standing often occurs in a graded sequence, starting with bedside activity prior to coming to the physical therapy department. Initial standing may start on a tilt table, to better control the body as well as blood pressure.

In addition to standing, amputees can begin doing quadriceps-setting exercises, done every hour they are awake. This exercise increases strength and control of the quadriceps mechanism and can easily be done irrespective of the type of postoperative dressing applied. Progressive resistive exercise is usually discouraged, due to the potential danger to the antero-distal tibial skin closure. Skin problems are the primary reason for not wearing a prosthesis in TT amputees, and for that reason great care should be exercised in order to keep the antero-distal tibia and tibial tubercular skin free of ulceration. Attention must also be given to the upper extremities and progressive resistive exercise, using either diagonal patterns or conventional shoulder and elbow extension.

Soon after the amputee is able to stand comfortably and safely, transfer training can begin. This enables the amputee to begin independent self care. Bed-to-chair, chair-to-commode, and chair-to-mat transfers are all important. During transfer and ambulation training, amputees often fall. Amputees who fall with a rigid dressing properly in place are less likely to injure the residual limb than with a soft dressing.

Once standing is safe, and transfers are possible, one-legged hopping can be started. Hopping usually begins in the parallel bars and moves on to a walker and eventually crutches. Amputees usually do quite well with this phase, but may expect too much from themselves too early. Very often amputees need to be told to rest, because they are eager to perform. If the amputee has been fitted with a plaster postsurgical dressing, it is imperative that the waist belt suspension strap remains tight. Once the amputee is able to handle both the plaster and the walker, he or she is free to walk with assistance on the hospital unit, to encourage bed-to-toilet independence.

Sutures may be removed at Day 14. However, many surgeons desire to leave sutures in much longer, particularly if wire has been used, because wire tends not to cause problems with suture line infections. On or around the postoperative Day 14, the sutures may be evaluated following removal of the first rigid dressing. Whether the sutures come out or not, another rigid dressing is applied and a pylon may be added if the wound is healing satisfactorily.

If the amputee is placed in a soft dressing, stump wrapping begins in an effort to start shrinking and shaping the residual limb. If possible, another member of the family is asked to share in the responsibility for stump wrapping. Diagrams illustrating the modified figure eight method can be given to the amputee to act as a guide once the amputee leaves the hospital (see Figure 4-20).

Gait Training with a Preparatory Prosthesis

The goals associated with the use of preparatory prostheses include independent ambulation, independent donning and doffing, understanding of socket fit, understanding potential excessive pressure areas, and learning who to call if problems arise. Most preparatory prosthetic systems at the TT level allow the amputee to ambulate well independently, while using cane, crutch, or walker. Amputees should learn to walk with little assistance from others, unless balance or other problems precludes safe ambulation. The preparatory prosthetic device functions mostly as the definitive limb; it just does not have the cosmetic appearance of the finished limb.

Gait training begins in the parallel bars and progresses to whatever type of assistive device is mutually acceptable. Many amputees remain with a walker for some time. This is done to allow the residual limb to become conditioned by remaining in a partial weight-bearing situation. Amputees may be moved to forearm crutches, by choice, to enable them to load the prosthesis and not lean on the axillae. In time, and in appropriate cases, amputees are encouraged to walk without any assistive devices. Typically, amputees may take a long prosthetic step with the involved side, which makes equal step lengths difficult. A force plate can be used to make certain that the amputee is not overloading the new device.

Applying and removing the prosthesis, or donning and doffing, are goals of the new amputee. Most amputees are able and should be encouraged and instructed in proper technique, because proper fit begins with donning.

Depending on whether socks or comfort liners are used, amputees are instructed in the proper methods of application of each. Care should be taken to pull the socks or liner on straight, and to leave no wrinkles, because wrinkles may add to skin problems and breakdown. Socks are made in thicknesses or plies, and liners are available in different thicknesses, sometimes with weight-bearing thicknesses being different than nonweight bearing locations. For those liners, front and back identification is a critical lesson.

Vascular disease may include venous disease making volume swings common. Instruction in proper fitting following donning includes a lesson about anatomical landmarks and where these points match up with the socket. Instruction must include regular socket fit checks, particularly in the early phases, because volume swings necessitate changes in thickness of socks to produce the desired fit.

Walking may reduce socket volume necessitating addition of socks. Phased walking early on will help teach the new amputee about the effects of distance walking on socket volume.

Amputees should always take a sock along on the walk in case socket loosening occurs. Socks may be added over comfort liners to offset loss of limb volume. If a pin suspension is used, a hole must be made in the sock to allow the pin to engage.

The changes in volume during gait represent a potential danger to the amputee if skin problems arise. Because many amputees do not sense pressure or pain normally, patient education should include frequent checks of residual limb skin for signs of pressure, redness, or ulceration. The new amputee should be instructed to check the skin each and every time volume checks are made, either before or after socks are added or removed. This habit will help assure that no patient walks any long distance on a limb that has begun ulcerating due to either too many socks or too few. Too many socks may produce an unstable gait that may seem as if the limb is too long. Skin breakdown occurs when bony prominences do not match up with socket relief areas, and increased pressure over these bony prominences produces ulceration during dynamic ambulation. Often ulceration can be prevented if volume changes are neutralized prior to ambulation.

Time must be spent teaching the amputee and family members about evaluating correct socket fit. Powder can be dusted into the socket and then examined after the residual limb is removed to determine if there has been total contact with the distal portions. Plastic temporary devices are often fabricated over at least one three-ply sock, which means that the chances of adding socks over the next 3 to 6 months are quite high. Care should be taken to instruct the patient in the correct socket fit. Circumferential changes and the relative sock thickness changes should be recorded at each follow-up visit, thus yielding an objective means to determine when the limb volume has stabilized and when it is time to fabricate the definitive device.

Progression to independent ambulation includes the progression to full weight bearing on the new prosthetic limb. This process involves strength in the hip and knee and balance, with or without assistive devices. Early gait training requires an accurate assessment of dynamic alignment to assure that the alignment in both saggittal and frontal planes allows optimal gait.

Often limbs may be set up in a safer configuration. This includes a slightly outset foot and a slightly posterior set socket. This combination produces a wide base gait and a longer toe lever. It requires less work of the hip abductors and the knee extensors. As the gait improves, these changes may be reduced or softened to allow a more normal, energy-efficient gait. These changes need to be monitored in conjunction with skin condition because alignment changes can and do produce loading differences on the skin of the residual limb.

The goals for the TT amputee should include a safe, flowing gait, with step lengths and widths equal. A slight knee varus moment at midstance on the prosthesis should help place the prosthetic foot directly under the trunk. The hip abductors should minimize any lateral trunk lean over the foot. Speed will vary but should progress between 50 and 80 m/min for most adults, slightly slower for severe vascular patients.

The Definitive Prosthesis

When the amputee is ready for the definitive fitting, another plaster impression or cast is taken. The socket is then mounted on the pylon and gait resumes. Following successful fitting and alignment, the device returns to the prosthetist for definitive finishing. The use of adjustable endoskeletal components that can be readily realigned throughout the lifetime of the prosthesis. This allows the prosthetist to incrementally improve the alignment as the gait training progresses, over the life of the prothesis.

Amputees should learn to put on and take off the prosthesis with little assistance from others. The acceptance of any prosthesis depends a great deal on the ease with which the patient independently applies the device. It is the job of the physical therapist to teach the patient about the fit of the socket prior to discharge from the prosthetic training program. The understanding of the pressure and relief areas of the socket design will allow the amputee to continuously check the fit and know when a stump sock must be added or removed. If the amputee is taught where excessive pressure areas are likely to develop, it is possible to trouble shoot problems at home. It is also important to discuss the difference between end bearing and total contact. Often it is beneficial to teach this same information to a significant other so that the amputee has another person to discuss these matters with in times of question. The last item necessary for the amputee is the name and phone number of someone to call if problems arise. In many cases this person is a member of the prosthetic/orthotic clinic team and is likely to be the physical therapist. This gives the care a specialized touch and allows the amputee exact knowledge of who to contact if a question or problem arises.

ENERGY EXPENDITURE AND GAIT IN TRANSTIBIAL AMPUTEES

As was presented in chapter 3, any abnormal gait pattern, whether associated with TT amputation or not, results in an increased energy requirement. Energy efficiency is also related to walking speed, body weight, and the disease states present, particularly vascular diseases which affect the heart, lungs, and the peripheral vessels, both arterial and venous. The presence of a major limb amputation represents yet another confounding variable. Although the literature is difficult to evaluate because of inconsistent methods and terms, certain conclusions can be drawn. Waters et al is probably the most quoted article dealing withTT amputation and energy expenditure. Ambulation with a transtibial prosthesis increases energy requirements by 30 percent. Waters reported on a comparative study of the energy expenditure of normal subjects and TT amputees. Results indicated that the speed of walking of the vascular TT amputee was 41 percent less than normal, and that those vascular amputees expended 55 percent more energy at that speed, when compared to normal. For comparison, traumatic TT amputees walked 13 percent slower than normal, using 25 percent more energy than normal. The average TT amputee walked 36 percent slower than normal, expending 41 percent more Kcal/m/min. Gonzalez reported that the TT amputees in his study walked at 64.4m/min or 22 percent slower than normal, but that the energy to walk at that speed was equal to normal. Ganguli reported a speed of 50 m/min and an increase of 33 percent in energy expenditure. Reitemeyer reported that unilateral TT amputees walked 60 m/min, using 28 percent more energy per unit of distance walked. Ralston reported a TT walking speed of 48.8 m/min compared to normal non-amputees at 73.2 m/min. Ralston also reported that energy expenditure per minute was equal for TTs and normals when self-selected velocities were used. From these various studies there appears to be a consensus that TT amputees walk slower than normal and expend more energy than non-amputees. No study quantifies the specific contributions of length of residual limb, height, or the severity of the underlying peripheral vascular disease.

DuBow et al reported on six bilateral, dysvascular, transtibial amputees compared to eight non-amputee, age-matched controls. Both groups walked 40 meters at a self-selected rate and exercised on a stationary ergometer. Results indicated that the controls walked 63 m/min, compared with 40 m/min for the amputees. The controls walked 48 percent faster than they propelled the ergometer. Oxygen consumption was 157 percent more walking than using a wheelchair. Bilateral TTs walked 39.9 m/min or 1.5 mph, using 7.84 ml O_2/kg.min and 0.232 ml O_2/kg.m. Given the 39.9 m/min waking speed, this represents about half normal walking speed, with equal consumption and efficiency. Because energy to propel a wheelchair was 157 percent less than ambulation, it is easy to understand why bilateral amputees often choose a wheelchair.

Volpicelli, Chambers, and Wagner reviewed 44 cases of bilateral, transtibial amputation, fitted with prostheses. Results indicated that 35 were rehabilitated, while 9 were wheelchair ambulators. Twenty-three of 35 were defined as community ambulators, while 12 were house-hold ambulators. Eighteen of 19, aged 59 years or less, were rehabilitated, while only 17 of 25, aged 60 or more, were rehabilitated. TTs from trauma did better than those with dysvascular diagnoses, and those not having major organic complications of diabetes did better than those who did. The data appeared to support the conclusion that bilateral Syme or one TT and one Syme did better than bilateral TT amputees. Although these numbers are quite small, several failures existed in these groups. However, the group with bilateral TTs was greater than 70 years of age and had major organ complications from diabetes. The results emphasize the importance of saving the knee joint, but caution about the ultimate predictable success of re-habilitation with bilateral TT amputation and vascular disease. From these studies and others, it has generally been concluded that the shorter the length of the TT stump, the more energy consuming the gait.

Nielsen, Shurr, Meier, and Goldman reported on seven traumatic TTs, comparing the energy cost using a conventional foot (SACH) and the Flex-Foot. Prior to this study, research centered on the length of limb, age, or medical condition of the amputee, with little, if any emphasis focused on 41 prosthetic components. Seven amputees walked on a level treadmill at speeds ranging from 1.0 to 4.0 mph (80m/min = 3 mph). Although the number of subjects was small, several conclusions were warranted. Ambulation using the Flex-Foot facilitated a more normal walking speed (77.8 m/min), when amputees were allowed to select their own walking speed. Ambulation using the Flex-Foot at walking speeds greater than 2.5 mph (69 m/min) tended to conserve energy, on the average about 20 percent (ml/kg.M), resulting in lower relative levels of exercise intensity and enhanced gait efficiency.

Macfarlane reported using high-speed photography to evaluate the vertical rise and fall of the center of mass during gait using a Flex-Foot and a SACH or conventional foot. Results indicated that the total rise and fall was less with the Flex-Foot partially identifying a reason for the lower energy cost with that foot.

Nielsen et al compared physiological gait with those who had suffered a type IIIC tibial fracture and other patients who proceeded to amputation following a IIIC fracture. Results indicated that the amputees, wearing a Flex-Foot, walked faster (15%). Although the IIIC patients walked slower, less efficiently, and with more energy consumption, when compared with transtibial amputees wearing a Flex-Foot, further studies of larger samples are necessary to achieve statistical significance.

Lehman et al studied the metabolic requirements of transtibial amputees during running and found no energy savings comparing FF with SACH. Torburn et al compared FF with SACH feet at self-selected-walking-velocity and found no differences.

Testing has revealed that the VSP produces greater movement vertically during running or as the speed increases. This is consistent with the findings of Nielsen and may begin to explain the findings of the VSP where the greatest energy saving in gait efficiency comes at the higher ends of speed including jogging and slow running.

Because many studies now have compared amputees at similar ages, sexes, and levels, the interest has focused on a comparison of prosthetic feet, holding other variables constant. Results of studies appear inconsistent, but may be partially explained due to the inconsistencies in methods, patient groups, speeds walked, and levels of physical activity and motor adeptness.

Future studies must center on new component technology, but must also include alignment, suspension, and changes in socket design.

REFERENCES

1. Amputee Clinics Newsletter. "A Matter Of Dressings." April 1975; 8(2).
2. Baker WH, Barnes R, Shurr DG. The healing of transtibial amputations: A comparison of soft and plaster dressings. *Am J Surg,* 1977; 133:716.
3. Berlemont M, Weber R, Willot JP. Ten years of experience with the immediate application of prosthetic devices to amputees of the lower extremities on the operating table. *Prosthetics International.* 1969; 3:8–18.
4. Birch JG, Walsh SJ, Small JM et al. Syme amputation for the treatment of fibular deficiency. An evaluation of long-term physical and psychological functional status. *J Bone Joint Surg Am.* 1999; 81(11):1511–1518.
5. Blessey RL, Hislop HJ, Waters RL, Antonelli D. Metabolic energy cost of unrestrained walking. *Physical Therapy.* 1976; 56(9):1019–1024.
6. Bobbert AC. Physiological comparison of three types of ergometry. *Journal of Applied Physiology.* 1960; 15(6):1007–1014.
7. Borsch P. Energy expenditure during ambulation with the Seattle foot, SACH foot, and Flex-foot: An amputee case study. Unpublished report, 1988.
8. Bowker JH, Michael JE, ed. Atlas of Limb Prosthetics: Surgical, Prosthetic and Rehabilitation Principles. St. Louis: Mosby Year Book, 1992:461–462.
9. Burgess EM, Zettl JH. Amputations below the knee. *Art Limbs.* Spring 1969; 13(1): 1–12.
10. Burgess, EM et al. Amputations of the Leg for Peripheral Vascular Insufficiency. *J. Bone and Joint Surg.* July 1971; 53A(5);874–890.
11. Burgess EM et al. The Seattle foot—a design for active sports: 42 preliminary studies. *Orthotics and Prosthetics,* 37. Spring 1983; 25–31.
12. Corcoran PJ., Brengelmann GL. Oxygen uptake in normal and handicapped subjects in relation to speed of walking beside velocity controlled cart. *Archives of Physical Medicine and Rehabilitation.* 1970; 51:78–87.
13. Cottrell-Ikerd V, Ikerdd F, Jenkins DW. The Syme's amputation: A correlation of surgical technique and prosthetic management with an historical perspective. *J Foot Ankle Surg.* 1994; 33(4):355–364.
14. Datta D, Gopalan L. Outcome of fitting an ICEROSS prothesis: Views of trans-tibial amputees. *Prosthetics and Orthotics International.* 1996; 20: 111–115.
15. Davidson WH, Bohne WHO: The Syme amputation in children. 1974; 56A: 1312.
16. DeLisa JA (ed). Rehabilitation medicine—Principles and Practice. 2nd ed. Philadelphia: J.B. Lippincott Company: 1993; 516–525.
17. Doane N, Holt LE. A comparison of the SACH and single axis foot in the gait of unilateral transtibial amputees. *Prosthetics and Orthotics International.* 7: April 1983; 33–36.

18. DuBow LL, Witt PL, Kadaba MP, Reyes R, Cochran, GVB. Oxygen consumption of elderly persons with bilateral below knee amputations: Ambulation vs. wheelchair propulsion. *Arch Phys Med Rehabil.* 1983; 64:255–259.

19. Durnin JVGA, Passmore R. Energy, Work and Leisure. London: Heinemann; 1967.

20. Eilert RE, Jayakumar SS. Boyd and Syme amputations in children. 1976; 58A: 1138.

21. Fishman S, Berger N, Watkins D. A survey of prosthetic practice–1973–74. *Orthotics and Prosthetics.* September 1975; 29(3) 15–20.

22. Fowler EG, Hester DM, Oppenheim WL, et al. Contrasts in gait mechanics of individuals with proximal femoral focal deficiency: Syme amputation vs Van Nes rotational osteotomy. *J Pediatr Orthop.* 1999; 19(6):720–731.

23. Ganguli S, Datta SR, Chatterjee BB et al. Performance evaluation of amputee-prosthesis system in transtibial amputees. Ergonomics 1973; 16:797–810, 1973.

24. Garbalosa JC, Cavanagh PR, Wu G et al. Foot function in diabethc patients after partial amputation. *Foot Ankle* 1996; 17:43–48.

25. Gay R, Heard G. Long Posterior Flap Transtibial Amputation for Obliterative Vascular Disease of the Lower Limb. *I. J. Med. Science.* January-February, March 1972; 141(1–3):141–143.

26. Ghiulamila, RI. Semirigid dressing for postoperative fitting of transtibial prosthesis. *Arch. Phys. Med. and Rehab.* April 1972; 186–190.

27. Gonzalez EG, Corcoran PJ, Reyes RL. Energy expenditure in below knee amputees: Correlation with stump length. *Arch Phys Med Rehabil.* 1974; 55:111–119.

28. Hobson MI, Stonebridge PA, Clason AE. Place of transmetatarsal amputations: A five-year experience and review of the literature. *J R Coll Surg Edinb.* 1990; 35:113–115.

29. Hornby R, Harris WR. Symes' amputation: Follow-up study of weight-bearing in 68 patients. *J Bone Joint Surg.* 1975; 57A:346–349.

30. Isherwood PA, Robertson JC, Rossi A. Pressure measurements beneath below knee amputation stump bandages: Elastic bandaging the puddifoot dressing and a pneumatic bandaging technique compared. *Br. J. Surg.* 1975; 62:982–986.

31. Kay HW, Newman JD. Relative incidences of new amputations. *Orthotics and Prosthetics.* 1975; 29:3–16.

32. Kerstein, MD. Utilization of an air splint after transtibial amputation. *Amer. J. of Phys. Med.* March 1974; 53(3):119–126.

33. Kihn RB et al. The immediate postoperative prosthesis in lower extremity amputations. *Arch Surg.* July 1970; 101:40–44.

34. Koepke GH, Giacinto JP, McCumber RA. Silicone gel below-knee amputation prostheses. *U Mich Med Ctr Jour.* Oct.-Dec. 1970; 36:188–189.

35. Lake C, Supan TJ. The incidence of dermatologial problems in the silicone suspension sleeve user. *J Prosthetics & Orthotics.* 1997; 9(3):97–106.

36. LeBlanc MA. Elasti-liner type of Syme's prosthesis: Basic procedure and variation. *Artificial Limbs.* 1971; 15:22–26. 44

37. Lehmann JF, Price R, Boswell-Bessette S et al. Comprehensive analysis of dynamic elastic response feet: Seattle Ankle/Lite foot versus SACH foot. *Arch Phy Med Rehabil.* 1993; 74:853–861.

38. Lehneis, HR. Prosthetics update 1980: Foot and knee components. Prosthetics and Orthotics Clinic, spring 1980; 4(1):1–8.

39. Lilja M, Oberg T. Proper time for definitive transtibial prosthetic fitting. *Jour of Prosth and Orth.* Spring 1997; 9(2):90–95.

40. Lin SJ, Nielsen DH, Shurr DG, Saltzman C. Physiological response of multiple speed treadmill walking for Syme versus transtibial amputation. 2000. In press.

41. Linds J, Kramhoft M, Bodtker S. The influence of smoking on complications after primary amputation of the lower extremity. *Clin Orthop.* 1991; 267:211–217.

42. Little JM. A pneumatic weight-bearing tempory prosthesis for transtibial amputees. *The Lancet.* February 6, 1971; 271–273.

43. Macfarlane PA, Nielsen DH, Shurr DG, Meier K. Gait comparisons for below-knee amputees using a flex-foot versus a conventional prosthetic foot. *Jour of Prosth and Orth.* Summer, 1991; 3(4):150–161.

44. Mazet R. The geriatric amputee. *Artificial Limbs.* 1967; 11:33–41.

45. McCarthy JJ, Eilert RE. Fibular hemimelia: Outcome measurements of amputation versus lengthening. Shriners Hospital for Children, Philadelphia, 1999 (unpublished).

46. McCollough NC. The Dysvascular Amputee, *Orthop. Clin. of North America.* July 1972; 3(2):303–321.

47. McCollough NC, Jennings JJ, Sarmiento A. Bilateral below the knee amputations in patients over fifty years of age. *J Bone Joint Surg.* September 1972, 54A(6):1217–1223.

48. Millstein SG, McGowan SA, Hunter GA. Traumatic partial foot amputations in adults. A long-term review. *J Bone Joint Surg (Br).* 1998; 70(2):251–254.

49. Molen NH. Energy/speed relation of transtibial amputees walking on motor- driven treadmill. *Int Z Angew Physiol.* 1973; 31:173–185.

50. Molen MH, Rozendal RH, Energy expenditure in normal test subjects walking on a motor driven treadmill. Nederlandse Akademie von Wetenshappen, Series B Physical Sciences Proceedings, 1967; C70: 192–200.

51. Mooney V et al. Comparison of postoperative stump management: Plaster vs. soft dressings. *J Bone and Joint Surg.* March 1971; 53A(2):241–249.

52. Moore W, Hall AD, Wilie EJ. Below knee amputations for vascular insufficiency. *Arch Surg.* 1968; 97:886.

53. Murray MP et al. Gait patterns of above-knee amputee using constant-friction knee components. *Bull Prosthetic Res.* 1980; 17:35–45.

54. Ng EK, Berbrayer D, Hunter, GA. Transtibial amputation: Preoperative vascular assessment and functional outcome. *Jour of Prosth and Orth.* Fall 1996; 8(4):123–129.

55. Nielsen D. Physiological measurements of walking and running in people with transtibial amputations with 3 different prostheses. *Journal of Orthopaedic and Sports Physical Therapy,* September 1999; 29(9):526–533.

56. Nielsen D. Personal Communication, 2001.

57. Persson BM. Sagittal incision for below knee amputation in ischemic gangrene. *Jour Bone Jt Surg.* January 1974; 56B:110–114.

58. Persson, BM, Liedberg, E. Measurement of Maximal End-Weight Bearing in Lower Limb Amputees. *Pros Orth Int.* December, 1982; 6:147–151.

59. Petersson BM, Sunden G. Amputation at the below knee level for ischemia. *Nord Med.* 1992; 86:1045–1049.

60. Piznur MS, Sage R, Stuck R, Osterman H. Amputations in the diabetic foot and ankle. *Clin Orthop.* 1993; 296:64–67.

61. Pritham C. Suspension of the below knee prosthesis: An overview. *Orthotics and Prosthetics.* 1979; 33:1–19.

62. Ralston HJ. Energy-speed relation and optimal speed during level walking. *Internationale Zeipschrife fuer Angewandte Physiologie. 1958;* 17:277–283.

63. Reiber GE, Boyko EJ, Smith DG. Lower extremity foot ulcers and amputations in diabetes. In: Harris MI, Cowie CC, Stern MP et al, eds. *Diabetes in America,* 2nd ed. Washington, DC: National Institutes of Health Publication. 1995; 95–1468:409–428.

64. Reitemeyer H. Energieumsatz und gangbild beim gehen und radfahren mit einem unterschenkelkunstbein. *Z Orthop.* 1955; 86:571–582.

65. Robinson KP, Hoide R, Coddington T. Skew flap myoplastic below-knee amputation: A preliminary report. *Br J Surg.* 1982; 69:554–557.

66. Sabolich JA, Ortega GM. Sense of feel for lower-limb amputees: A phase-one study. *Jour of Prosth and Ortho.* Spring 1994; 6(2):36–41.

67. Sanders LJ. Transmetatarsal and midfoot amputations. *Clin Podiatr Med Surg.* 1997; 14:741–761.

68. Sarmiento A, Gilmer RE, Finnieston A. A new surgical-prosthetic approach to the Syme's amputation: A preliminary report. *Artificial Limbs.* 1966; 10:52–55.

69. Shea, JD. Surgical techniques for lower extremity amputation. *Orth Clin Nor Amer.* July 1972; 3(2):287–301.

70. Shem KL, Breakey JW, Werner PC. Pressures at the residual limb-socket interface in transtibial amputees with thigh lacer-side joints. *Jour of Prosth and Orth.* Summer 1998;10(3):51–55.

71. Sher, MH. The air splint. *Arch Surg.* May 1974; 108:746–747.

72. Silbert S. Amputation of the lower extremity in diabetes mellitus: Follow-up of 294 cases. *Diabetes.* 1952; 1:297–299.

73. Skinner HB et al. Static load response of the heels of SACH feet. *Orthopedics.* February 1985; 8(2):225–228.

74. Swanson VM. Transtibial polyethylene semi-rigid dressing. *Jour Prosth and Ortho.* January 1993; 5(1):30–35.

75. Termansen, WB. Below knee amputation for ischemic gangrene. *ACTA Orth Scand.* 1977; 48:311–316.

76. Torburn L, Perry J, Ayyappa E, Shanfield SL. Below-knee amputee gait with dynamic elastic response prosthetic feet: A pilot study. *J Rehab Res Dev.* 1990; 27:369–384.

77. Tracy, GD. Below knee amputation for ischemic gangrene. *Pac Med Surg.* September-October 1966; 74:251–253.

78. Truax, C. Prosthetic Surgery. The Mechanics of Surgery. San Francisco: Norman Publishing, 1988.

79. Varghese G. Pressure applied by elastic prosthetic bandages: A comparative study. *Orthotics and Prosthetics.* December 1981; 35:30–36.

80. Vigiers S, Casillas JM, Dulieu V et al. Healing of open stump wounds after vascular below-knee amputation: Plaster cast socket with silicone sleeve versus elastic compression. *Arch Phys Med Rehabil.* 1999; 80(10):1327–1330.

81. Villaret M, Roederer C. Prosthesis, functional retraining and occupational readaptation of individuals with wounds or in accidents. 1923; Paris: Library of J. B. Bailliere et Fils.

82. Volpicelli LJ, Chambers RB, Wagner FW. Ambulation levels of bilateral lower-extremity amputees. *J Bone Joint Surg.* 1983; 65A(5):599–605.

83. Wagner FW. Amputations of the foot and ankle. *Clin Orthop.* 1977; 122:62–69.

84. Wagner J, Supan T, Sienko S, Barth D. Motion analysis of SACH vs. Flex-foot™ in moderately active transtibial amputees. *Clin Prosth Orth.* 1987; 11(1):55–62.

85. Warren, R et al. The Boston interhospital amputation study. *Arch Surg.* December 1973; 107:861–865.

86. Waters RL, Perry J, Antonelli D, Hislop H. Energy cost of walking of amputees: Influence of level of amputation. *J Bone Joint Surg.* 1976; 58A:42–51.

87. Whitehouse FW, Jurgensen C, Block MA. The later life of the diabetic amputee: Another look at the fate of the second leg. *Diabetes.* 1968; 17:520.

88. Wu Y, and Krick H. Removable rigid dressing for transtibial amputees. *Clin Prosth and Orthotics.* 1987; II(1):33–44.

89. Wyndham CH, van der Walt WH, van Rensburg AJ, Rogers GG, Strydom NB. The influence of body weight on energy expenditure during walking on a road and on a treadmill. *Internationale Zeipschrife fuer Angewandte Physiologie.* 1971; 29:285–292.

CHAPTER 5

Knee Disarticulation and Transfemoral Amputation and Prostheses

No one symbolizes the plight of the TF amputee better than Terry Fox. Fox, following amputation due to cancer, stunned the world when he announced that he would run 5,300 miles across Canada to raise money for research to find a cure for this disease, which remains the cause of many amputations today. Starting at St. John's, Newfoundland, Fox ran across Canada in a very primitive preparatory prosthesis at the pace of 26 miles per day. He completed 3,339 miles before progression of his disease forced him to stop near Thunder Bay, Ontario.

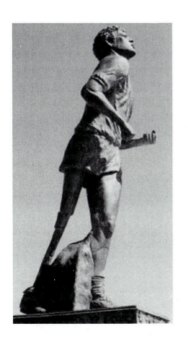
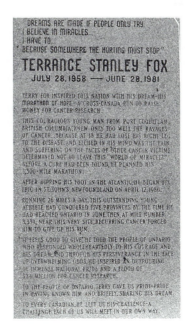

Following completion of reading this chapter, the student will be able to:

1. Describe the major muscle groups necessary to succeed with a TF amputation, and the pre-prosthetic exercises used to prepare the amputee for prosthetic wear.
2. Describe the importance of the knee component and the design of four different types of prosthetic knees.
3. Describe the relationship between the hip, knee, and foot on standard TF or Knee Disarticulation [KD] prosthesis.
4. Discuss the four major means of TF or Knee Disarticulation [KD] prosthetic suspension and the indications for each.

Amputations at or above the level of the knee joint are performed for the same reasons as transtibial and lower level ablations: trauma, tumor, disease, and congenital malformations. In North America, many of the traumatic losses at these levels are due to vehicular accidents. Regrettably, Aitken reports primary bone tumors often affect the proximal thigh and necessitate high level amputation, often in relatively young individuals.

In developed countries such as the United States, the average age of amputation has been gradually increasing over the past 50 years due to improvements in safety regulations and medical treatment. It has been reported by Kay that approximately 85 percent of all TF amputations in the United States occur between the ages of 50 and 80 years of age. Data from Kald published in the late 1980s demonstrated that at that time, 47 percent of Swedish amputees were more than 80 years old. According to Torres, TF amputation is less common than TT ablation, but appears to have increased in recent years perhaps due to a larger percentage of bilateral lower limb amputations being performed.

It is now very clear that the biomechanical loss is much higher for these individuals than for amputees who have an intact biological knee joint, and that rehabilitation is much more challenging as a result. The situation is further complicated because the majority of all TF amputations are performed due to dysvascularity and its sequelae, which means that cardiopulmonary limitations are common in this population. This double disability of dysvascularity plus loss of the biological knee is the primary reason that only selected elderly TF amputees can successfully use a prosthetic limb. McCullough et al reported in the 1970s that 45 percent of TF amputees over 50 years of age could be expected to walk with a prosthesis. Moore et al reported similar success rates in the late 1980s, and suggested that a screening method should be developed for elderly, dysvascular amputees to determine when prosthetic rehabilitation was feasible.

Unfortunately, no practical screening techniques have been identified to date. The general consensus remains that those elderly amputees who are motivated to try a prosthesis, and physically capable of doing so, should receive a preparatory limb as soon after amputation as possible. Corcoran and others have shown the importance of prompt fitting and delays have been clearly shown to diminish prosthetic outcomes, presumably due to the well-documented debilitating effect of inactivity. New amputees' experience with the preparatory prosthesis then forms a very clear basis for subsequent prescription of a definitive device. Those who do not show promise with the preparatory prosthesis typically choose wheelchair mobility, because that requires far less effort than walking with an artificial limb, although some prefer to use the prosthesis for selected activities or for limited periods each day.

It should be emphasized that non-dysvascular amputees typically do well with TF prostheses and are almost always good candidates for prosthetic rehabilitation. This is particularly true for children and younger adults, but vigorous elderly amputees can usually also manage transfemoral artificial limbs regardless of their secondary diagnoses.

LEVELS OF AMPUTATION

Figure 5-1 depicts the major levels of amputation at or above the knee joint. The most common level is in the mid-transfemoral region.

Knee Disarticulation

The knee disarticulation, or through-knee amputation, is a level not often seen in North America. Most support for this level comes from European and, particularly British, literature. In the older population, the through-knee level is said to offer an advantage, because side-to-side flaps are thought to enhance wound healing. Radcliffe reports that for those individuals who are not likely to be functional ambulators, this level is thought to offer the mechanical advantage of a longer lever arm for greater ease in transfers and related activities.

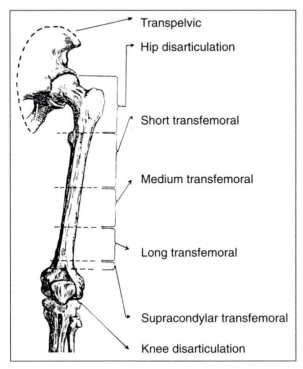

Transpelvic

Hip disarticulation

Short transfemoral

Medium transfemoral

Long transfemoral

Supracondylar transfemoral

Knee disarticulation

Figure 5-1. Levels of upper leg amputation. (*Source:* Adapted from Northwestern University Prosthetic Orthotic Center, with permission, 1987)

Shea states that the through-knee amputation offers an end-bearing residual limb with increased proprioception as compared to other levels. In addition to affording excellent prospects for suspension of the prosthesis, it is a relatively easy surgical procedure to carry out and is quite safe for the patient. However, Shea also believes that a primary knee disarticulation should not occur if the patient has a preexisting hip-flexion contracture.

According to Wiener, knee disarticulation is a level often considered for growing children, because it preserves the distal femoral epiphysis and allows distal femoral growth to continue following the amputation. In children, the level is often end bearing and does not require a socket design that unloads the limb proximally.

Transfemoral Amputation

Because most above-knee amputations are performed for vascular reasons, the procedure can be considered to be elective; that is, done in a nonemergent situation and at an anatomic level of the surgeon's choosing. This situation allows the surgeon to consult with the prosthetist and physical therapist if questions arise as to the ideal functional prosthetic level.

Although the surgical procedure involved in performing a transfemoral level amputation may not require a great deal of technical skill, Mooney cautions that several important considerations must be taken into account before making the decision to operate. If the amputee is a likely candidate for a prosthesis, a more technical procedure must be accomplished to allow the amputee the best chance of prosthetic and rehabilitative success.

Primary wound healing is usually not a problem at this level. In fact, amputation at this level is prevalent in many developing countries precisely because there is little risk that a revision will be needed.

Gottschalk has proposed that the abductor muscles be preserved and sutured to the distal femur to provide better muscular control of the residual limb. This technique has been endorsed by the International Society for Prosthetics and Orthotics as the preferred method for TF amputation.

Long Transfemoral Amputation. The long TF amputation may be thought of as being supracondylar; that is, the length of the femur extends down as far as the condyles. The supracondylar level produces a long and effective lever arm with which to control the prosthesis. All hip musculature is left intact and available to control the prosthesis. As long as the hip extensors and abductors are not altered, the prosthetic gait should be excellent. A long residual limb with all normal motion and musculature allows both the patient and the prosthetist the freedom to use a variety of components.

Medium Transfemoral Amputation. The medium length, or "standard," TF amputation may be considered as mid-thigh in length, bisecting the femur. In many cases, this level allows the use of standard transfemoral components and results in good gait. At this level, a long anterior flap is often used to avoid having the suture line on the bottom of the socket.

Short Transfemoral Amputation. The short TF level is generally thought to be 5 to 7 cm in length. At this level, the short length of the residual limb makes stabilization in stance phase using hip extension quite difficult. The shorter the residuum, the more difficult it becomes to suspend the prosthesis, because there is less tissue to grasp. Because some weight bearing occurs on the posterior soft tissue of the thigh, the shorter the thigh, the less available surface area. With a short TF stump, the ability of the thigh to generate forces to control the knee during both swing and stance is reduced and provides limitations on the type of knee unit that can be used in the prosthesis. Amputation at the short TF level also increases the chances of muscle imbalance, where the hip flexors overpower the hip extensors, resulting in a hip-flexion contracture. Abduction and external rotation contractures may also be present.

A very short TF amputation may occur at the level of the lesser trochanter of the femur or more proximally. The potential problems that were just discussed become even more pronounced with a very short stump. Mechanically, the very small lever is quite ineffective in controlling a standard TF prosthesis. Much pressure is taken on the lateral distal femur in an attempt to stabilize the hip mediolaterally in the stance phase. Suspension at this level can also be difficult. It may not be possible to use certain suspension techniques, and the amputee needs to be cautioned that the limb may lose suspension at inopportune times.

KNEE DISARTICULATION AND TRANSFEMORAL COMPONENTS

The major components of these prostheses are the ankle-foot mechanism, shin, prosthetic knee, and socket.

Ankle-Foot Mechanisms

Prosthetic ankle-foot mechanisms are selected according to the biomechanical needs and functional capabilities of the individual, as noted in the previous chapter. The primary difference at these levels is that a softer plantarflexion resistance is often appropriate because this allows the foot to reach the ground more quickly and aids in stabilizing the prosthetic knee. Articulated feet are more common in these prostheses for just that reason.

Shin Options

The same basic options are available at these levels as were discussed in the previous chapter on TT prostheses: endoskeletal or exoskeletal construction. Endoskeletal designs predominate because most allow the prosthesis to be realigned and adjusted at any time, as the amputee's abilities or needs change. Exoskeletal configurations are more durable in hazardous environments and are therefore more commonly used for children's prostheses.

Recently, vertical shock-absorbing shin mechanisms have become commercially available. Although Hsu and Yack have shown that clinical acceptance has been encouraging, biomechanical studies verifying the functional characteristics of these new components are just starting to emerge.

Prosthetic Knees

Ideally, a prosthetic knee unit substitutes for the normal knee functions of shock absorption and support during stance phase and swing-phase flexion during gait. Realistically, as with prosthetic feet, compromises in function must be accepted. Numerous knee units are available for TF and KD prostheses and may be thought of as occurring in a functional continuum from a simple locked knee to a relatively sophisticated, hydraulically controlled unit designed to provide control during both swing and stance phase of gait.

Manually Locked Knee.
A locked knee allows no swing-phase knee flexion and provides complete stability in the stance phase. Typical examples of locked-knee prostheses are shown in Figure 5-2 and range from a peg leg having a wooden or metal pipe with no articulation to standard locked-knee units made by Otto Bock and others to ensure knee stability primarily for the geriatric amputee.

Clinically the prosthetic team needs to make a decision based on the individual needs of the amputee as to whether or not to recommend a locked knee. Very often, in the early phases of gait training with the dysvascular amputee, particularly one who the team is not certain will be a successful prosthetic user, a simple locked-knee pipe or pylon may be used. This allows quick evaluation of the amputee's abilities and still allows the amputee to unlock and bend the knee while sitting. It is not uncommon for a definitive TF prosthesis for a geriatric patient to contain a locked knee. Typically these prostheses use knee units that have spring assists that lock when the amputee straightens the knee in extension. For sitting, flexion of the knee is produced by pulling a cord attached to the proximal socket. It is important to remember that the absence of knee flexion in the swing phase will necessitate some other changes in the prosthesis, often shortening of the overall length. Such shortening will allow for the swing phase on the prosthetic side without marked circumduction, hip hiking, or vaulting, all energy-consuming gait deviations. Using a simple locked-knee unit, a definitive TF prosthesis may be made completely from plastic, so the overall weight of the device may be less than 5 lb.

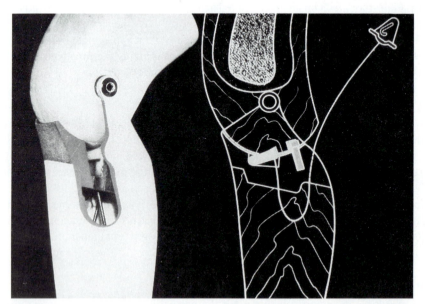

Figure 5-2. Locked knee, also called a positive locked knee. Amputee pulls cord to unlock knee, an internal spring locks knee when knee is initally extended. (*Source:* From Otto Bock, Orthopedic Industry, Inc. Minneapolis, MN, with permission)

Single Axis (Constant Friction) Knee

The single axis knee is the most basic design available, and it is therefore both reliable and inexpensive. This simple hinge allows knee flexion during the swing phase but must be stabilized by ground reaction forces during the stance phase. Radcliffe has described the biomechanics of this knee in detail, noting that the amputee must provide voluntary control using the residual hip musculature to hold the knee in full extension throughout stance phase in order to walk safely.

For many of today's relatively feeble elderly amputees, consistent control of the prosthetic knee under all conditions is an unrealistic expectation. For this reason, use of single axis knees is more common for children than for adults. The exception to this trend is that individuals who live or work in remote areas and find follow-up visits difficult may prefer single axis knees due to their mechanical reliability.

Another limitation is that mechanical constant friction adjustments only permit the amputee to walk smoothly at one fixed cadence. That makes such swing control an inappropriate choice for any individuals who can vary their walking speeds. In a study by Fishman et al, the single axis knee was prescribed less than 20 percent of the time.

Stance Control (Friction Brake) Knee

Given the preponderance of elderly, dysvascular TF amputees, many of whom have limited strength and balance, it should not be surprising that knees that add stance phase stability are among the most commonly prescribed alternatives. Figure 5-3 illustrates one of the most common designs, sometimes termed a friction-brake knee.

When the amputee bears weight on the prosthesis, the knee compresses the spring and contacts a cylindrical brake bushing. The rapidly increasing friction stabilizes the knee and prevents further motion. This allows the novice or feeble amputee to walk safely, even if the prosthetic knee is not always held in extension during weight bearing.

Unfortunately, the same friction-brake mechanism also makes it impossible to flex the knee during preswing until it is fully unloaded and the spring opens the knee, releasing the brake device. This means that such knees are only appropriate for limited ambulators, particularly

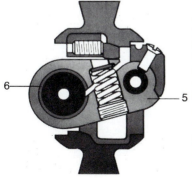

Figure 5-3. This cutaway illustrates a typical design for stance control prosthetic knees. Weightbearing compresses the spring [5] causing the knee to clamp against the cylindrical brake bushing [6]. The resulting increase in friction allows the amputee to safely load the prosthesis even if the knee is not fully extended. When the knee is unweighted, the spring releases the brake pressure and the knee can be flexed for swing phase or to sit down. (Courtesy of Otto Bock Orthopedic Industries, Inc.)

those who walk very slowly. This knee is probably most suitable for amputees who require the use of a walker for balance, and therefore have a slow but steady gait and take small steps.

It is also important to teach the amputee how to shift weight laterally while standing, to fully unload the prosthesis, so the stance control knee can be flexed for sitting. The amount of "braking" can be adjusted by the prosthetist according to the individual's needs. As the amputee's voluntary control improves, the braking feature can be reduced thereby allowing a more normal gait.

Polycentric Knee

Polycentric knees can be recognized by their multiple centers of rotation. The most common designs have four articulations and four connection links or "bars," and are sometimes referred to as "four-bar" knees.

The instantaneous center of rotation (ICOR) may be determined geometrically by drawing a straight line through the anterior and posterior links. The point at which these lines intersect is the functional rotation point for the knee. Interestingly, as the knee is flexed, the functional ICOR moves in a characteristic pattern called the centrode, as shown in Figure 5-4.

Greene has noted that polycentric knees can have three biomechanical advantages over single axis designs. The more posterior the ICOR is located, the greater the alignment stability. The more proximal the ICOR, the easier it is for the amputee to control the knee. Depending upon the design specifics, polycentric knees also increase toe clearance at mid-swing. Gard et al recently quantified the toe clearance for several commonly prescribed knees and noted that it can be as much as 1.5 centimeters.

From a clinical standpoint, polycentric knees are increasingly popular because they offer good stance stability and yet can be flexed under weightbearing load in preswing. The added toe clearance reduces the risk of stumbling. Some have adjustable extension stops that allow

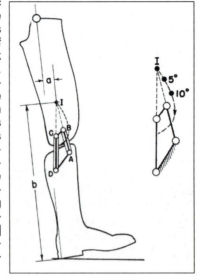

Figure 5-4. The geometric point where a polycentric knee seems to bend functionally is located at the intersection of the posterior and anterior link bars, shown here as point "I". This Intstant Center of Rotation [ICOR] varies as the knee flexes in a characteristic pattern called the Centrode. In this typical example, the knee is relatively stable in full extension but the ICOR moves anteriorly quickly as the knee begins to flex, making it biomechanically less stable during preswing. (Reprinted with permission from Murdock G [Ed] *Prosthetic and Orthotic Practice;* Edward Arnold Ltd, London, 1970.)

the prosthetist to vary the stability according to the amputee's needs. These latter types are often prescribed for bilateral cases.

There is also a group of specialized polycentric knees designed primarily to minimize the protrusion beyond the socket when the amputee is seated. These knees are intended primarily for use in sockets for very long TF amputations or for knee disarticulations (Figure 5-5).

Fluid-Controlled Knees

Staros has shown that fluid-controlled knees provide more normal kinematics than mechanical designs and Gage reports they also are cadence-responsive, allowing the amputee to speed up or slow down at will. Hydraulic units, filled with oil, are most commonly provided but pneumatic knees using air to provide swing-phase control are also available.

Durability of these knees has improved significantly in recent years. However, all fluid-filled mechanisms will need servicing sooner or later, and this must be considered when prescribing these devices. In general, fluid control is indicated whenever the amputee is capable of walking at different speeds.

Although fluid control was originally developed for swing-phase control only, some hydraulic knees use the incompressibility of liquids to provide added stance stability as well. Often termed "stance and swing" or "SNS" knees, these devices are commonly prescribed for active ambulators who negotiate irregular terrain or participate in recreational or competitive sports. The enhanced stance stability features offered by SNS devices have proven to be effective in bilateral cases.

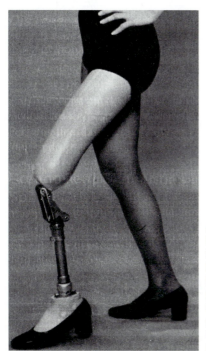

Figure 5-5. Special polycentric knees are available for use with knee disarticulation and similar long residual limbs. Their linkage bars are designed to minimize protrusion of the mechanism when it is flexed beyond 90 degrees, such as when seated. (Courtesy of Otto Bock Orthopedic Industries, Inc.)

Hybrid Knees

According to Michael, most recent knee developments have combined the characteristics of two or more of the noted basic designs, to increase the versatility of the prosthesis and encourage more active use. One common strategy is to combine polycentric construction with hydraulic swing-phase control, resulting in a stable knee that is also easy to flex and cadence responsive, and offers added toe clearance.

Stance Flexion Feature

Historically, amputees have been forced to hold the prosthetic knee in full extension throughout the stance phase to insure proper stability. The stiff-legged gait that results is biomechanically abnormal and requires added vertical displacement of the amputee's center of gravity, which presumably results in a less energy-efficient gait. The lack of knee flexion during stance also eliminates the biological shock absorption inherent in normal gait.

In the past decade, several manufacturers have introduced prosthetic knees that allow a limited amount of knee flexion in early stance but will not collapse. This stance flexion feature has been well accepted clinically, and Blumentritt reports that this capability appears to increase amputee comfort by absorbing some of the impact of weight acceptance on the prosthesis.

Microprocessor Control

Although they are used selectively, fluid controlled knees that incorporate onboard computer controls are becoming more widely available. The most sophisticated design at present is the Otto Bock C Leg, which uses real-time gait analysis based on sensors at the ankle and in the knee to adjust the hydraulic stance and swing control resistances up to 50 times per second. Amputees report greater confidence using such sophisticated knees, and preliminary studies reported by Dietl suggest that the resulting gait may be more energy efficient than with other fluid-controlled devices (Figure 5-6).

SOCKET CONSIDERATIONS

Socket design is one of the most crucial aspects of prosthetic rehabilitation, yet it remains one of the most subjective areas. This section will highlight a few basic principles to provide an overview of this complex topic. Discussion with the ABC-certified prosthetist on the clinic team is recommended for more detailed information regarding specific cases.

Biomechanical Goals

The primary biomechanical goals of the transfemoral or knee disarticulation socket can be summarized as:

- Comfortable skeletal and muscular weightbearing during stance phase
- Triplanar stability of the femur within the socket to provide voluntary control over the socket movements
- Sufficient suspension to minimize swing phase displacement of the prosthesis
- Alignment to permit effective use of the residual musculature

All socket variants must fulfill these criteria in a manner that is comfortable for the amputee.

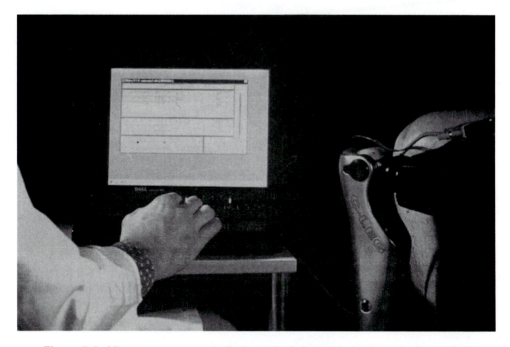

Figure 5-6. Microprocessor-controlled prosthetic knees that automatically readjust themselves to changes in the amputee's gait pattern, offering enhanced swing phase responsiveness and perhaps a more energy-efficient ambulation, represent the present state of the art. The Otto Bock "C-Leg" is shown here temporarily connected to a personal computer so the prosthetist can adjust the parameters. This particular example also offers sophisticated stance stability, changing the hydraulic resistances up to fifty times per second based on data from onboard knee motion and ankle moment sensors. (Courtesy of Otto Bock Orthopedic Industries, Inc.)

Knee Disarticulation Designs

Most knee disarticulation amputations result in a residual limb that can comfortably bear weight through the femoral condyles. Consequently, an end-bearing socket is usually provided.

A small amount of padding is typically incorporated into the distal socket. When full end bearing is comfortable and the patient's muscle tone is good, the socket can terminate inferior to the perineum. When it is necessary to provide some weight bearing or stabilization proximally, the socket brim will be similar to that of a TF prosthesis (Figure 5-7).

Transfemoral Designs

Prior to the 1950s, prosthetic sockets were highly individualized but there were no cohesive design theories for clinicians around the world to follow. Immediately after World War II, Radcliffe and others visited many different countries and studied the local prosthetic fittings. This information was synthesized into what is now known as the quadrilateral or "quad" socket design.

This socket is characterized by its four distinctly differently shaped proximal walls and particularly by a broad, flat posterior shelf that contacts the ischial tuberosity during midstance (Figure 5-8). This ischial bearing concept evolved slightly in the ensuing decades but was gradually accepted worldwide.

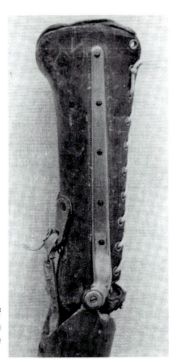

Figure 5-7. A lateral view of a leather knee-disarticulation prosthesis with outside knee hinges.

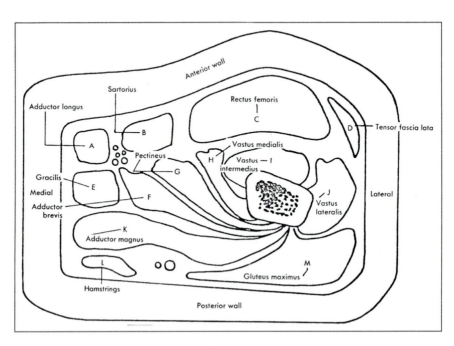

Figure 5-8. Quandrilaterial socket. A cross-section at ischial tuberosity level. (*Source:* From Northwestern University Prosthetic Orthotic Center, with permission, 1987.)

Total Contact. One of the most important contributions of the quad socket concept, which is now considered fundamental to all TF designs, was an appreciation for the importance of total contact: gentle contact of the distal soft tissues of the residual limb with the end of the socket. Without such uniform skin support, there is a tendency for fluids to pool in soft distal tissues and the distal residuum gradually becomes thickened, furrowed, and discolored from small venous hemorrhages that occur over time (Figure 5-9). In severe cases, this verrucous hyperplasia can lead to malignancy and ultimately, death.

It must be noted that such severe consequences do not automatically occur when there is a lack of total contact, but the risk of skin injury increases over time, as the amputee ages, and particularly as their vascular status deteriorates. In view of the preponderance of elderly, dysvascular amputees in the developed world, it is easy to understand why total contact is generally desirable. It should also be noted that the use of suction suspension of various kinds requires total contact in almost every case, as the negative pressure concentrated on the end of the residual limb increases the risk of sequelae.

Socket Alignment. Radcliffe proposed that the TF socket be aligned in a few degrees of adduction and flexion, in part to place the residual hip extensor and abductor muscles in a slightly stretched position and maximize their effectiveness. This also permits the amputee to take a more normal stride length on the contralateral side, and reduces the tendency for a Trendelenberg limp. These recommendations have now become standard practice for all TF

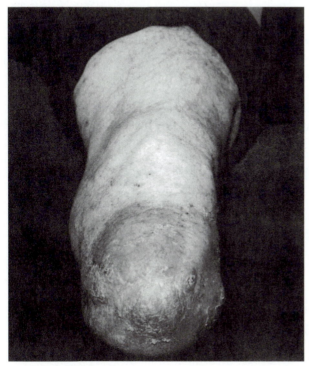

Figure 5-9. Verrucous hyperplasia due to inadequate total contact.

sockets. The specific amount of flexion and adduction must be determined individually for each patient during the fitting process.

Ischial Containment Designs

In the 1970s, Ivan Long began exploring a new socket concept that involved partially encapsulating the tip of the ischium within the socket walls itself. As compared to the quad configuration, this socket had a narrower mediolateral dimension and become known colloquially as a narrow ML or NML socket. Long also advocated increased femoral adduction in an attempt to mimic normal skeletal alignment, and preferred to call his concept a normal shape-normal alignment or NSNA design.

In the 1980s, Sabolich and others refined Long's ideas further by enclosing more and more of the ischiopubic ramus within the socket. Although it is very challenging to fit such an extensive socket in a way that is comfortable for the amputee, clinical experience has shown that the added stability and control that results is well received by many individuals. This is particularly true when the patient has a relatively short residual limb, or one lacking muscle tone. Although Sabolich coined the acronym CATCAM to describe this approach, Michael states the more generic term ischial containment, abbreviated IC, is now more commonly used. (Sabolich obtained a patent in the 1990s on another socket variant that contains a blend of IC and quad features and developed a proprietary training program to promulgate its use.)

The International Society for Prosthetics and Orthotics studied these different TF socket approaches and convened a multinational cadre of prosthetists, physicians, and engineers to report on the efficacy of each design. According to Schuch, the conclusion of this report summarizes the situation succinctly: "There is no contraindication for any particular socket design." The quad, NML, and various IC designs are all well accepted rehabilitation options that have been shown to be clinically effective. The decision as to which specific socket style is preferred for a particular patient is best left to the prosthetist's discretion at this time.

Flexible Sockets

At the same time Long was investigating alternatives to the quadrilateral shape, Ossur Kristinsson of Iceland was investigating socket materials that were more flexible than the ubiquitous hard plastic laminates developed in the quad socket days. Although the early flexible designs were plagued by limited durability, sometimes requiring socket replacements after less than 1 year of use, the development of improved thermoplastics and better fabrication techniques have helped make flexible sockets increasingly popular worldwide.

Pritham reported the advantages of a flexible socket over a rigid, hard socket to be:

- Enhanced suspension
- Increased comfort
- Less heat retention

Figure 5-10 illustrates one example of a flexible thermoplastic socket that is contained within an abbreviated rigid weight-bearing frame that transmits forces to the prosthesis. Many variations in configuration and materials have been reported in the literature and have enjoyed good clinical acceptance. One potential advantage of the socket plus frame approach is that it

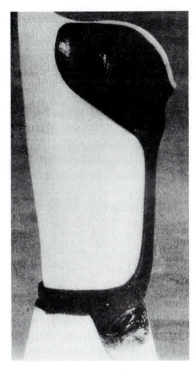

Figure 5-10. The Scandinavian flexible socket; transfemoral example with medial weight bearing frame.

may be feasible to replace only the socket if the patient's residuum volume changes rather than replacing the entire thigh segment of the prosthesis.

Suspension Alternatives

Michael has classified TF and KD socket into four basic groups, each analogous to TT suspensions:

- Vacuum
- Anatomic
- Straps
- Hinge

Vacuum. Vacuum or suction suspension is the most secure option, allowing little or no pistoning or displacement of the socket during the swing phase. This makes the prosthesis feel lighter and gives the amputee the best possible control over the artificial limb.

Traditionally, a suction suspended socket required a very snug, skintight fitting that some amputees found difficult to don consistently. It also required the patient to maintain a constant weight, because volume fluctuations would disrupt either the suspension or comfort. Although many patients found this acceptable, a significant number were unable to use this technique successfully long term.

Ossur Kristinsson of Iceland developed a revolutionary elastomeric suction suspension technique in the mid-1980s in which a custom-made silicone rubber "sock" is applied over the residual limb. Originally, a cord or lanyard at the distal end of the silicone lamination was used to anchor it to the socket. Later researchers developed a variety of mechanical-locking mechanisms that automatically secure the silicone sleeve to the distal end of the socket

The advantages of the 3S technique, as compared to the earlier method, include:

- Ease of donning and doffing the prosthesis
- Ability to accommodate volume reduction by adding textile socks on top of the silicone sleeve
- Increased comfort due to the reduction in shear stresses at the socket brim
- Enhanced suspension, particularly for very short residuums, due to the tendency of the silicone sleeve to remain in contact with the skin

Another option has been termed hypobaric suspension. In this technique, a specially modified limb sock containing a band of silicone that serves as a gasket is used, in combination with a special valve that allows air to be expelled from the socket automatically, to create a vacuum seal in the socket.

It should be noted that all vacuum suspension techniques could be compromised by excessive perspiration, which acts as a lubricant and causes the socket to slide off the limb. For that reason, many clinicians recommend use of an auxiliary suspension in addition to the primary vacuum technique, particularly for very active individuals.

Auxiliary suspension is also necessary if the amputee chooses to wear a thin textile limb sock between the skin and a traditional suction socket, as some do if they have trouble tolerating direct skin-to-socket contact. The resulting partial suction makes the artificial leg feel much lighter and more responsive but is not sufficient to provide full suspension.

Anatomic Suspension. Anatomic suspension may be used when the skeletal contours are such that they can be used to stabilize the socket against displacement in swing phase. In the case of many knee disarticulations, supracondylar suspension is feasible—using a technique similar to that used for TT supracondylar suspension.

Anatomic suspension is also possible with selected congenital malformations. As noted in the previous chapter, the localized pressures inherent in anatomic suspension often require a period of acclimatization before it becomes comfortable for the amputee.

Strap Suspension. The chief advantage of strap suspensions remains that they are amputee adjustable and therefore readily accommodate volume changes. Disadvantages include some inevitable pistoning when this is the sole suspension and objections from some amputees about having anything crossing the abdomen.

The most common TF strap technique uses one or more fabric belts that cross the pelvis. This is sometimes termed a "Silesian bandage" after the European location where this method was first developed (Figure 5-11). There are also a number of commercially available suspension products that can be easily removed by the amputee for laundering, such as the Total Elastic Suspension or TES belt.

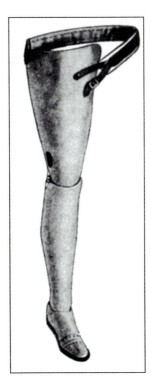

Figure 5-11. Silesian band suspension of above-knee prosthesis. (*Source:* From Wilson AB. Limb prosthetics–1970. *Art Limbs.* 1970; 14:31, with permission.)

Hinge Suspension. The historic metal hip joint and leather belt suspension is increasingly uncommon in today's world (Figure 5-12). Many amputees object to the bulk and restriction to movement inherent in this traditional TT suspension technique. However, it remains a viable alternative when there is a need to provide added mediolateral stability at the hip, as is sometimes the case when the residual limb is very short or if the abductor muscles have been damaged.

PROSTHETIC ALIGNMENT PRINCIPLES

Static Alignment

As was noted in the previous chapter, static alignment is based on the component manufacturers' recommendations. This is the preliminary configuration for the prosthesis, based on the average of a large number of individual alignment results.

The primary distinction from TT static alignment involves positioning the prosthetic knee. An imaginary line running from the greater trochanter near the knee and through the ankle is often used as a reference, and is referred to as the TKA line (Figure 5-13). The more posteriorly the knee center is located, the more stable the prosthesis will be during the stance phase. Conversely, the more anterior the knee placement, the easier it will be for the amputee to flex it for the swing phase. The initial placement is determined by the prosthetist, based on the manufacturer's recommendations and an assessment of the amputee's voluntary control capabilities.

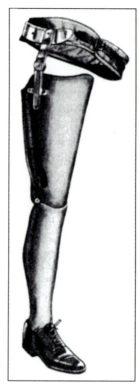

Figure 5-12. Hip joint and pelvic band. (*Source:* From Wilson AB. Limb prosthetics–1970. *Art Limbs.* 1970; 14:31, with permission.)

Socket alignment has been previously discussed. Ankle-foot placement is also typically based on the manufacturer's recommendations.

Dynamic Alignment

Static alignment is only a starting point. The final alignment is determined by iterative walking trials based on visual gait analysis principles.

One of the most critical factors is how readily the amputee can control the prosthetic knee. During dynamic alignment trials, the prosthetist will move the knee more or less posteriorly in small increments and observe the effect on the patient's gait. The goal is to create a prosthesis that is sufficiently stable for the amputee to manage and yet easy to flex during preswing.

Knee rotation is also evaluated, and corrected to eliminate erratic swing phase movements of the shin termed whips. Knee resistance and other parameters are also adjusted to allow the smoothest, most normal gait possible. When stance control elements are present, these are also optimized.

Due to the interaction between the ankle-foot assembly and the knee, it is important that foot flat occur relatively early in the gait cycle, because this allows the ground reaction force to move anteriorly and increases prosthetic knee stability. Careful adjustments to the plantarflexion resistance and the angular and linear position of the foot may be necessary to optimize these variables.

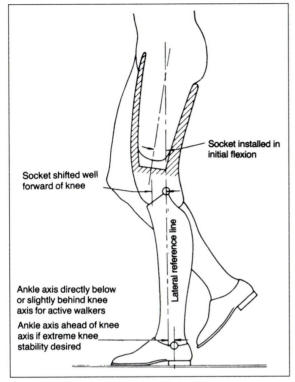

Socket installed in initial flexion

Socket shifted well forward of knee

Lateral reference line

Ankle axis directly below or slightly behind knee axis for active walkers

Ankle axis ahead of knee axis if extreme knee stability desired

Figure 5-13. The preflexed transfemoral socket. (*Source:* From Radcliffe CW. Functional considerations in the fitting of above-knee prostheses. *Art Limbs* 1955; 2:40, with permission.)

Angular socket alignment considerations have been summarized previously. These are varied slightly during dynamic alignment to verify the optimal final position. Two of the more subtle factors are the anteroposterior (AP) and mediolateral [ML] placement of the socket with reference to the knee-shin-foot assembly. Particularly for amputees with a short residual limb or concomitant hip weakness, it can be challenging for the prosthetist to determine the right balance point for these choices.

Many new amputees cannot walk consistently enough in the beginning to allow the prosthetist to refine the alignment fully. As a result, it is often necessary to establish a workable alignment and then refine the details at subsequent visits, as the individual's strength and gait pattern gradually improve.

PERIOPERATIVE MANAGEMENT OF THE NEW AMPUTEE

Preoperative Care

Because most TF and KD amputations are elective procedures performed due to chronic vascular disease, preoperative visits by members of the clinic team may be possible and can do much to allay the patient's fears. In many larger cities, trained peer counselors who are successful prosthetic wearers are available to talk with individuals who have pending amputations.

In some cases, upper limb strengthening exercises can be initiated prior to the amputation. This will make ambulation with parallel bars or external aids easier while the individual is learning to use the prosthesis.

Postoperative Care

Exercise. During the early preprosthetic days following the amputation, care should be taken to prevent any tightness or contracture in the hip joint, because contractures are easily prevented but difficult to treat. The test for hip tightness, the Thomas test, tests for both the presence of hip flexion contracture and the range of hip joint motion. With the amputee supine with pelvis square, a hand is placed under the lumbar spine while flexing the residual limb up toward the trunk. As the hip flexes, the point where the back flattens is the limit of hip flexion. Full hip flexion is 135 degrees and allows the limb to touch the abdomen. With the sound leg resting against the abdomen, any inability of the amputee to bring the residual limb into contact with the examination table without reinitiation of the lumbar lordosis may indicate the presence of a hip flexion contracture. Experience has taught that many geriatric amputees, particularly TF amputees, do not cooperate with the test, because it is physically difficult to do so. It is also necessary to recommend lying prone to stretch the hip flexors and to prevent or retard any hip-flexor tightness.

In addition to evaluating hip flexors and extensors, the hip abductors are also an important muscle group. The hip abductors play a key role in the amputee's ability to stabilize the pelvis in the stance phase of gait. Without the hip abductors, the amputee will lean to the amputated side and produce a cosmetically unacceptable gait as well as expend greater energy. It is important to remember when testing the hip abductors that both hips should remain in a neutral position, because any hip flexion allows the hip flexors to substitute for the abductors and gives the examiner an erroneous impression of the strength of the abductors. Sidelying is another way of testing the strength of the abductors, maintaining the hip in neutral, with the amputated side up.

Rigid Dressings. Rigid dressing for the TF level, as originally described by Burgess, was used in the late 1960s and early 1970s. However, it never gained the overall popularity of the TT system due mainly to the difficulty and complexity of suspending the TF rigid dressing. The system was identical to the TT system, except that the suspension of the cast was accomplished via cables, referred to as Bowden cables, that connected to a waist belt. Suspension was less than ideal, and a great deal of effort and patience were required by both the prosthetist and the amputee.

In 1979, Thorpe et al reported a prospective study on the use of rigid dressings in TF amputees. The rigid dressings were applied by either a physical therapist or prosthetist. Results showed that rigid dressings were beneficial no matter who applied them as long as that person was properly trained in the procedure. Additionally, the study reported that early ambulation usually necessitated greater use of pain medication, suggesting that early ambulation was not advisable. No problems with wound healing could be attributed to the rigid dressing or to the treatment regimen or person applying the device.

Compression Wrapping. Generally the postoperative routine for TF amputees today does not include the use of a rigid dressing. Instead the TF amputee is taught to use a compression wrap for 4 to 6 weeks (Figure 5-14). The spica component of the thigh-wrapping procedure is essential for proper suspension of the wrap. Compression of the medial thigh or adductor region is likewise very important. If wrapping is difficult, a stump shrinker is easily applied.

The short and very short TF amputation levels usually present many problems. Compression wrapping at this level is virtually impossible, because suspension of the wrap is quite difficult, even using proper techniques. There is simply too little residual limb to either wrap or to grasp. Care must be exercised not to overemphasize the importance of stump wrapping, because the amount of edema usually present at this level is not a major problem.

Residual Limb Complications. Factors that may affect the residual limb at the TF and KD level are similar to those at the TT level, as discussed in chapter 4.

In cases where a TF amputation is performed for such reasons as an infected internal fixator or plate, the wound may need to be left open for 5 to 7 days following surgery to allow the wound to clean up and to rid the wound of the infection. Following that period, a secondary closure usually is done. This treatment is most successful in young, otherwise healthy people who heal without delay. When these problems coexist with vascular disease or diabetes, the result may not always be as positive.

In some traumatic cases in which there is denuding of the skin over the residual limb, skin grafts may be required. This makes the surgical procedure difficult, because there is a need to maintain as much length as possible and to surgically close the wound as quickly as possible to prevent further chance of infection. In young children, there is often considerable effort to

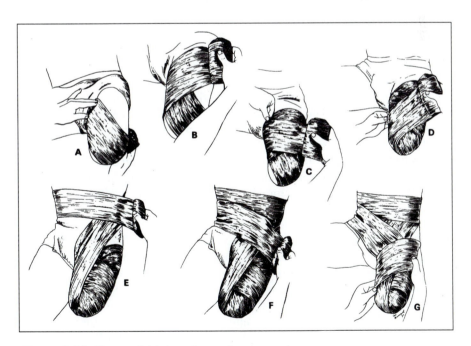

Figure 5-14. Figure-eight, transfemoral compression wrap.

preserve growth plates so as not to create a serious leg-length discrepancy in adulthood. Skin grafting slows down the overall management process and can leave scar tissue that is not very mobile. Tethered or grafted skin without normal mobility makes prosthetic fitting difficult, tending to cause splits or ulcers on the residual limb. Such ulceration should not be misinterpreted as being caused by the prosthesis, when actually the skin simply split due to its inability to stretch. Amputees can walk on prostheses while having splits in grafted skin as long as everyone involved knows what caused the split and the wound itself is kept clean until it heals. Skin grafts from trauma or burns may take a long time to finally heal. Careful observation of such cases can allow the amputee to begin using a TF prosthesis while not bringing further harm to the residual limb.

A major problem associated with management of the TF residual limb is hip-flexion contracture. The more severe the hip flexion contracture, the more difficult the prosthetic fitting, and the more difficult acceptance of the prosthesis will be for the amputee. Severe contractures, in excess of 25 degrees, cause unsightly cosmetic problems for the amputee. The prosthetist can accommodate a relatively large hip flexion contracture by increasing preflexing of the socket within the prosthesis, but there are compromises that have to be made. In sitting, when the prosthesis rests on the chair, a markedly preflexed socket produces an anterior bulge under the pants or dress and does not allow for the even accommodation of a tray or other object placed on the amputee's lap.

Pronounced hip flexion contractures also limit which prosthetic knees are available to the amputee. Because most prosthetic knees require hip extension force to stabilize them in the stance phase, a limitation in hip extension motion often makes the use of such free-swinging knees difficult. It is sometimes necessary to use a locked knee to provide stance phase stability in such cases. The amputee with a severe hip-flexion contracture may also be required to take a shortened step with the sound limb because of his or her inability to extend the prosthetic limb during the late stance phase of gait.

A common complicating factor affecting the postoperative management of the TF amputee is the presence of edema and its associated prosthetic problems. The prosthetic socket is designed for the typical situation, which is that the limb may get smaller due to shrinking or edema absorption but not that the limb will get larger due to increasing edema. When the limb swells, fewer stump socks may be worn, but the socket cannot accommodate gross swelling of the residual limb, even with no stump socks. It is not uncommon to see residual limbs that vary in volume from day to day or hour to hour, making limb fitting difficult. Included in this group are amputees with arteriovenous malformations; their residual limb changes size hourly and they often need two sockets, one for when the residual limb is swollen and one for after it drains and becomes smaller.

Preparatory Prostheses. Originally, the first prosthesis after surgery was termed a temporary limb and it contained only rudimentary components and a primitive socket, often molded directly onto the residuum from plaster (Figure 5-15). The concept was that the amputee could hobble around with this basic prosthesis for several months until the residuum was mature and a definitive quality limb could be prescribed.

Experience showed that although this approach might be feasible for younger, healthy amputees, it was ineffective with the older, often feeble individuals who could not manage such a crude device very well. Contemporary practice is to provide a well-fitted, definitive

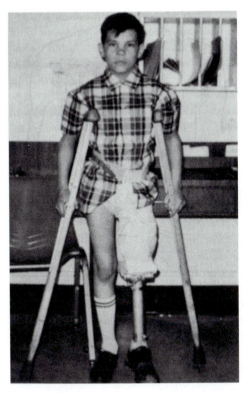

Figure 5-15. Temporary trans-femoral prosthesis.

quality socket and appropriate components in the initial prosthesis, which is now termed a preparatory device. In most cases, endoskeletal construction is used so that the socket portion can be easily replaced due to physical changes in the residuum whenever necessary. This approach has proven to be more effective rehabilitation for today's older amputee population, and the cost of a socket replacement due to residual limb atrophy differs little from the cost of providing a primitive prosthesis that is only used for a few months.

The external protective covering is often omitted from the preparatory limb during gait training to facilitate incremental adjustments to the alignment as the patient's gait matures. Once gait training has concluded, the final covering can be added.

GAIT TRAINING

In chapter 4, results of studies demonstrated that only 4 of 10 TF geriatric amputees are successfully rehabilitated. These findings indicate that the increased physical demands make walking much more difficult for this population than for amputees who retained their own knee joint. The reasons are many and varied and include a loss of muscle strength and limited functional range of motion at the hip, because the frontal plane stability of the prosthesis in the stance phase is controlled by the hip abductors.

The post-operative gait training program for the TF amputee must begin early and pay special attention to the motions and muscle strength of the hip. Flexion of the hip advances the prosthesis; extension of the hip slows the advancement and stabilizes the knee prior to heel strike, and hip abduction stabilizes the socket during single leg stance while the socket is over the foot and the sound limb is advancing in swing phase.

Because all of these motions and muscles are important, pre-prosthetic programs must incororate exercises that include these muscles. Exercises that stress the suture line might wait 2 or 3 weeks until the wounds are completely healed. Mid-range exercises and isometric exercises of the hip extensors and hip abductors may begin as early as Day 2 or 3, as long as they are gentle and are done under supervision. The absolute importance of these muscles for ambulation should be emphasized in order to provide a gentle nudge to work hard.

Once isometric exercise has been mastered, gentle concentric exercise may begin. Eventually, rubber band materials may be used to offer gentle resistance and begin to build strength. These exercises should include the remaining or sound side as well, because the amputee has been relatively inactive prior to the amputation. The sound side muscles need strengthening and stretching as well, particularly because a large number of these TF amputees have diabetes, and elasticity may be compromised.

One-legged ambulation may include the use of walkers, parallel bars, axillary crutches, or forearm crutches. Few, if any, TF amputees can walk on one limb and two canes. For safety reasons, they may also require a wheelchair for long distances, or in situations that include uneven ground, new or unknown territory, or long walks that outstrip the physiological resources available to the geriatric amputee.

Falling on a newly operated limb will slow down the fitting of the prosthesis by causing pain and swelling in the residual limb as well as a potential hip fracture, head injury, or spinal cord problem. As was stated, rigid dressings are not as easily used at the TF level, so the potential injury to the residual limb from a fall is real.

To facilitate gait training, it is customary to align the knee in a very stable manner and often to provide inherently stable knee mechanisms. Every TF amputee is afraid of falling from early on, and it must be the goal of the team to prevent falls. On the other hand, once the amputee has mastered voluntary control of the artificial limb, it is often useful to readjust or realign the knee so that it can be flexed more easily, thereby decreasing the effort required for walking.

Prior to ambulation, the new amputee must understand and be comfortable with the prosthesis. This means that time needs to be spent teaching how the socket goes on and stays on; how the knee works, locks, and bends; how to don and why to add or remove stump socks; and the beginning thoughts about ambulation on level and uneven ground.

Gait training begins with standing in front of a full-length mirror. The goals to be accomplished at this stage include the ability to load both legs equally; the ability to maintain a narrow, yet stable base; and the beginning of weight shifting, first from back to front on the foot of the prosthesis, and later from amputated side to sound side and back. It is critical to master these skills prior to moving into dynamic gait, because socket loading and knee stance phase control cannot be maintained in walking, if they are not mastered statically.

Extrinsicly stabilizing the prosthetic knee, either by using a manual lock or via alignment, may be necessary because many elderly TF amputees are deathly afraid of falling from a buckled knee. Once the fear is gone and the amputee has the skill needed to voluntarily stabilize the knee in stance, the component and/or alignment may be altered to allow more freedom and motion. Endoskeletal designs lend themselves to such realignments and component interchanges, and are increasingly prescribed as a result.

Once static knee motion is understood and easy to accomplish, dynamic ambulation begins. Initially this may be done in the parallel bars and in front of the same, full-length mirror used by the TT amputees. Care must be taken to educate the new amputee about the use of narrow base, short steps in the beginning. Very long strides tend to move the floor reaction force posterior to the knee axis, thus creating a knee flexion moment and making the prosthetic knee unstable.

Once the amputee can ambulate in the parallel bars with full weight bearing and without any loss of knee stability in stance, gait training can move outside the parallel bars and onto a walker, canes, or crutches. At this point, it is important to judge the need for assistive devices to aid stability, and then to proceed, verify that the amputee is standing, first, and then walking with full weight bearing, while using the assistive devices. Once out of the parallel bars, it is quite common for amputees to attempt to transfer body weight to the cane or crutch, which causes their gait to deteriorate. Once the amputee can walk with full weight bearing out of the parallel bars using the cane, crutch, or walker, much practice in order to build up confidence, speed, and the ability to walk on uneven surfaces is in order.

Transfers need to be mastered during every phase, because moving up and down, and in and out of chairs requires much balance, and more strength than simple standing. Most new TF amputees need training to learn getting up from a chair because the prosthetic limb does not participate actively, but can assist in safe standing once the amputee is up. Unless there is a manually locking knee in the prosthesis, the location of the ground reaction force with reference to the knee joint center determines knee stability and amputee safety. Once up, the amputee must learn to position the prosthesis close to the chair and that placing weight on the prosthetic toe will provide knee stability and safety.

Because early gait training has proven to be helpful in fostering long-term prosthetic use, the preparatory prosthesis is generally fitted before the residual limb volume is stable. This demands careful attention to how the the socket is fitting, and the appropriate addition or deletion of socks as the volume changes. Care should be taken to assess how the socket is fitting each and every time the amputee walks to assess any problematic volume changes to assure maximal stability and comfort.

A complete course in TF gait is beyond the scope and purpose of this text. The authors suggest that other references such as Saunders or May be consulted to gain the depth of knowledge necessary to care for the more difficult TF cases. It is also recommended that *prior* to initial gait training with any TF or KD patient, the prosthetist be consulted to determine the exact components and any strengths or weaknesses encountered during the dynamic alignment trials.

ENERGY EXPENDITURE AND TRANSFEMORAL AMPUTEE GAIT

As is the case with the literature on TT amputees, there are few studies of energy expenditure during gait in TF amputees, separating the contributions of vascular disease from the effects of having a TF amputation and prosthesis. Waters studied 13 vascular and 15 traumatic TF amputees and found that the vascular amputees walked 36 m/min, or 65 percent slower than normal speed. The dysvascular TF amputees used 12.6 ml O_2/kg · min to walk 36 m/min. The 12.6 ml O_2/kg · min is approximately equal to the normal predicted rate as described by Corcoran, however, the walking speed is greatly reduced, from 80 m/min to 36 m/min. Traumatic TF amputees fared better using 12.9 ml O_2/kg · min while walking at a rate of 52 m/min. The O_2 use is up a bit from the 12.65 normal value at 80 m/min. The traumatic TF amputees walked 52 m/min or 45 percent slower than normal.

James in his study of 37 TFs aged 21 to 62 years, none of whom were vascular in origin, found that they walked 20 percent slower than normal, using 61 kcal/kg · min. In an article by Otis et al, energy cost during gait was compared between osteosarcoma patients with resection and internal prosthetic replacement versus TF amputation. Results indicate that the patient with resection/internal prosthetic replacement had lower energy costs during gait. Detailed data concerning the components of the TF limbs, however, were not presented. Specifically, free walking speed of resection/replacement patients was 87 percent (54 m/min) of normal, with the TF amputees at 73 percent (45 m/min), with normal measured at 62 m/min. However, 62 m/min is 22 percent less than accepted, normal walking speed. At free-speed walking, the relative energy costs were 160 percent of normal for the resection/replacement group and 209 percent for the amputees. Compared with Waters, this study resulted in a larger net-energy cost for the TF amputees (0.30 +/− 0.05 ml/kg/m to 0.25 +/− 0.05ml/kg/m). MacFarlane compared the energy efficiency and SSWV between SACH feet and Flex Feet. Results indicated a faster SSWV (69 versus 64 m/min) and a more efficient gait with the Flex Foot. Other results of gait speed, reported by Fisher, vary from 20 percent slower to 66 percent slower, from 70 m/min to 28.2 m/min. The associated increase in energy expenditure ranged from 30 percent to 120 percent of normal. As is true of TT amputees, even under the best of circumstances, TF amputees must expend a great deal of additional energy during ambulation. Furthermore, the loss of the biological knee significantly increases the effort needed to walk as compared to the TT levels.

Components at the TF level continue to improve. As was summarized in chapter 4, perhaps these new components may improve the gait and efficiency of walking at the TF level. Nielsen compared five TF amputees, using a repeated measures design, comparing use of the SACH and the Flex-Foot. Sockets, knees, design, and alignment were equal. Only the feet were changed. Results demonstrated a 5 percent increase in walking speed (63–67 m/min) with the use of the Flex-Foot. Future studies with a larger number of subjects are necessary to clarify whether the components are indeed responsible for such gains.

REFERENCES

1. Aitken GT. *Courses on Juvenile Prosthetics.* Northwestern University Medical School, 1974.
2. Blumentritt S, Scherer HW, Wellershaus U et al. Design principles, biomechanical data and clinical experience with a polycentric knee offering controlled stance phase knee flexion: a preliminary report. *J Prosthet Orthot.* 1997; 9:18–24.
3. Burgess EM, Romano RL, Zettl JH, Schrock RD. Amputations of the leg for peripheral vascular insufficiency. *J Bone Joint Surg.* 1971; 53A(5):874–890.
4. Corcoran PJ, Brengelmann GL. Oxygen uptake in normal and handicapped subjects in relation to speed of walking beside velocity controlled cart. *Arch Phys Med Rehabil.* 1970; 51:78–87.

5. Cutson TM, Bongiorni D, Michael JW et al. Early management of elderly dysvascular below-knee amputees. *JRBK J Prosthet Orthot.* 1994; 6:62–66.
6. Dietl H, Kaitan R, Pawlik R et al. C-leg-ein neues system zur versorgung von oberschenkelamputationen (C-leg—a new system for prosthetic management of a/k amputation). *Orthop Tech.* 1998; 49:197–211.
7. Fillauer CE, Pritham CH, Fillauer KD. Evolution and development of the silicone suction socket (3S) for below-knee prostheses. *JRBK J Prosthet Orthot.* 1989; 1:92–103.
8. Fisher SV, Gullickson G. Energy cost of ambulation in health and disability: A literature review. *Arch Phys Med Rehabil.* 1978; 59:124–133.
9. Fishman S, Berger N, Watkins D. A survey of prosthetics practice—1973–74. *JRBK Orthot Prosthet.* 1975; 29(3):15–20.
10. Gage JR, Hicks R. Gait analysis in prosthetics. *JRBK Clin Prosthet Orthot.* 1985; 9(3):17–23.
11. Gard SA, Childress DS, Vellendahl JE. The influence of four-bar linkage knees on prosthetic swing-phase floor clearance. *J Prosthet Orthot.* 1996; 8:34–40.
12. Gottschalk F, Kourosh S, Stills M. The importance of the adductors in the biomechanics of above-knee amputation (abstract). *JRBK Orthop Trans.* 1991; 15:168.
13. Greene MP. Four-bar linkage knee analysis. *Orthot Prosthet.* 1983; 37(1):15–24.
14. Hsu MJ, Nielsen DH, Yack HJ et al. Physiological measurements of gait during walking and running in transtibial amputees with conventional versus energy storing-releasing prosthesis (abstract). *Phys Ther.* 1997; 77, S45.
15. James U. Oxygen uptake and heart rate during prosthetic walking in healthy male unilateral above-knee amputees. *Scand J Rehabil Med.* 1973; 5:71–80.
16. Kald A, Carlsson R, Nilsson E. Major amputation in a defined population: Incidence, mortality and results of treatment. *JRBK Br J Surg.* 1989; 76:308–310.
17. Kay HW, Newman JD. Relative incidences of new amputations. *Orthot Prosthet.* 1975; 29(2):3–16.
18. Kristinsson O. Flexible above knee socket made from low density polyethylene suspended by a weight transmitting frame. *Orthot Prosthet.* 1983; 37(2):25–27.
19. Kristinsson O. The ICEROSS System (abstract). *JRBK Orthot Prosthet.* 1985–86; 39(4): 63–64.
20. Long IA. Normal shape-normal alignment (NSNA) above-knee prosthesis. *JRBK Clin Prosthet Orthot.* 1985; 9(4): 9–14.
21. MacFarlane PA, Nielsen DH, Shurr DG. Mechanical gait analysis of transfemoral amputees walking with the SACH foot versus the Flex-Foot. *J Prosthet Orthot.* 1997; 9(4):144–151.
22. McCollough NC, Jennings JJ, Sarmiento A. Bilateral below the knee amputations in patients over fifty years of age. *J Bone Joint Surg.* 1972; 54A(6):1217–1223.
23. Michael JW Prosthetic knee mechanisms. *Phys Med Rehabil: State Art Rev.* 1994; 8:147–164. JRBK YEAR 1994
24. JW in Spivak et al (eds) Orthopaedics: A Study Guide. McGraw-Hill, 1999; 838.
25. Michael JW. Current concepts in above-knee socket design. *Instr Course Lect.* 1990; 39:373–378.
26. Mooney V. Above knee amputation, surgical procedures. In: *Atlas of Limb Prosthetics.* St. Louis, MO: Mosby; 1981:378–401.
27. Moore TJ, Barron J, Hutchcinson F et al. Prosthetic usage following major lower extremity amputation. *JRBK Clin Orthop.* 1989; 238:219–224.
28. Nielsen DH, MacFarlane PA, Shurr DG, Mechanical gait analysis of transfemoral amputees: SACH foot versus the Flex-Foot. *J Prosthet Orthot.* 1997; 9:144–151.
29. Otis JC, Lane JM, Kroll MA. Energy cost during gait in osteosarcoma patients after resection and knee replacement and after above-the-knee amputation. *J Bone Joint Surg.* 1985; 67A(4):606–611.
30. Pinzur MS, Smith DG, Daluga DJ et al. Selection of patients for through-the-knee amputation. *J Bone Joint Surg.* 1988; 70A:746–750.
31. Pritham CH, Fillauer C, Fillauer K. Experience with the Scandinavian flexible socket. *JRBK Orthot Prosthet.* 1985–86; 39(2):17–32.

32. Radcliffe CW. Above-knee prosthetics. *Prosthet and Orthot Int.* 1977; 1(1):146–160.
33. Radcliffe CW. Alignment of the above-knee artificial leg. In: *Human Limbs and Their Substitutes.* Klopsteg PE, Wilson PP, eds. New York: Hafner Publ; 1954; 676–692.
34. Sabolich J. Contoured adducted trochanteric-controlled alignment method (CAT- CAM): Introduction and basic principles. *Clin Prosthet Orthot.* 1985; 9(4):15–26.
35. Schuch CM. Modern above-knee fitting practice (a report on the ISPO workshop on above-knee fitting and alignment techniques, May 15–19, Miami, FL). *JRBK Prosthet Orthot Int.* 1988; 12:77–90.
36. Shea JD. Surgical techniques for lower extremity amputation. *Orthop Clin North Am.* 1972; 3(2): 287–301.
37. Staros A. The principles of swing-phase control: The advantages of fluid mechanisms. *Prostheses Braces Tech Aids.* 1964; 13:11–16.
38. Thorpe W et al. A prospective study of the rehabilitation of the above knee amputee with rigid dressings. *Clin Orthop.* 1979; 143:133–137.
39. Torres MM. Incidence and causes of limb amputations. *JRBK Phys Med Rehabil: State Art Rev.* 1994; 8:1–8.
40. Waters RL, Perry J, Antonelli D, Hislop H. Energy cost of walking of amputees: Influence of level of amputation. *J Bone Joint Surg.* 1976; 58A:42–46.
41. Wiener DE. Prosthetic stimulation of femoral growth following knee disarticulation. *ICIB.* 1976; 15(11/12):15–16.
42. Yack HJ, Nielsen DH, Shurr DG. Changes in mechanical energy at push-off in transtibial amputees as a function of prosthetic design and walking. *Gait Posture.* 1998; 7:150–151.

CHAPTER 6

Hip Disarticulation, Transpelvic, and Translumbar Amputation

D.B. Marks and A. A. Marks were brothers who opened an artificial limb business in 1853 in New York City. Together they owned many patents, including one for a rubber foot and one for a TT limb, patented in 1854. Following the development of a complete line of prostheses, they published a treatise or catalog that allowed potential clients to see firsthand how prostheses looked and to read about how they functioned. The books also included testimonials from many amputees at all levels from many countries of the world. The hip disarticulation prosthesis seen here was available by mail order for about $100 in the 1902 catalog.

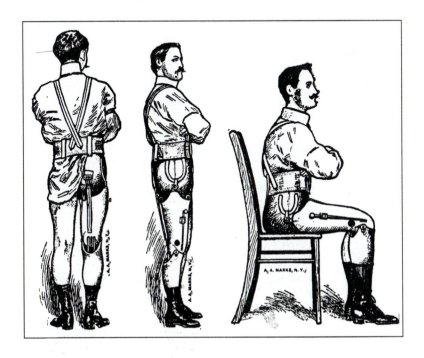

Following completion of reading this chapter, the student will be able to:

1. Discuss the anatomical differences and functional expectations for these high-level amputees.
2. Discuss the common etiologies for these levels of amputation.
3. Discuss the major factors affecting prosthetic use for these levels.

These high-level amputations are only rarely encountered in clinical practice and present obvious challenges to the rehabilitation team. However, with optimal prosthetic design and good gait training, many otherwise healthy individuals with these amputations can ambulate in the community despite the magnitude of their physical loss.

It should be noted that extremely high TF amputation, at or above the trochanteric level, is usually treated prosthetically as if the hip was disarticulated, because it is virtually impossible for most individuals to control a TF prosthesis with such a short residuum. The patient is typically casted with the remnant thigh flexed to 90 degrees and the primary weight-bearing surface is the ischiopubic ramus, as is the case in true disarticulation.

ETIOLOGY

These radical surgical procedures are performed only when there is no other treatment alternative. During the period following World War II, the New York University Medical School noted the presence of metastatic tumor was the primary cause for hip disarticulation and higher level amputations, and many texts from that era imply that cancer is virtually the sole cause.

Due to the steady improvement in cancer treatments in recent decades, amputation is no longer the only effective treatment for pelvic malignancies. Instead, it is increasingly common to resect the limb locally rather than to ablate the entire leg. Shurr reported in 1984 that the etiology in a series of 50 hip disarticulations was 48 percent tumor, 20 percent infection, 20 percent vascular disease, 10 percent trauma, and 2 percent congenital malformation (Table 6-1).

TABLE 6-1. INDICATIONS FOR HIP DISARTICULATION OR TRANSLUMBAR AMPUTATION

Indications	Number of Patients (%)	Number Fitted	Number of Users at Follow-up
Tumor	24 (48%)	9	8*
Infection	10 (20%)	1	0
Trauma	5 (10%)	4	3
Congenital	1 (2%)	1	1
Vascular	10 (20%)	0	0
Total	50	15	12

*Three died following fitting, although prosthetic use was documented prior to death.
(*Source:* From Shurr DG et al. Hip disarticulation. A prosthetic follow-up. *Orthot Prosthet.* 1984; 37:52.)

HISTORICAL PERSPECTIVE

Prior to 1954, the few amputees fitted at these levels received a very heavy, molded leather socket with locked hip, knee, and ankle joints that were released only for sitting. This tilt-table prosthesis (Figure 6-1) was cumbersome to wear, and was propelled by gross pelvic thrust movements. A vaulting gait was common. Not surprisingly, Sneppen reported that the rejection rate for such devices was high.

In 1954, McLaurin described a radical departure that became known as the Canadian design. In the ensuing decades, the clinical superiority of this approach became apparent and it is now the standard treatment worldwide. The Canadian philosophy is based on a thorough understanding of the biomechanics of amputee gait, and uses the ground reaction forces generated during walking to stabilize the free hip, knee, and ankle joints during the stance phase while permitting flexion during the swing phase for a much less abnormal gait than was possible with the tilt table style (Figure 6-2).

Although McLaurin and colleagues described an exoskeletal prosthesis, the same biomechanical principles can be applied to more contemporary endoskeletal devices. Particularly for the high-level amputee, the light weight and adjustability of such modular prostheses has made them the predominant choice of clinicians worldwide (Figure 6-3).

PROSTHETIC DESIGN

Socket Considerations

The anatomical differences among these amputation levels determine the socket design. When the weight bearing structures of the ischiopubic ramus are present, they are encapsulated into the socket (Figure 6-4). Careful contouring immediately above the iliac crests provides suspension and stabilizes the pelvis so the amputee can control the artificial limb.

Rigid laminated sockets are common, but there is a strong trend toward the use of more flexible thermoplastic materials such as polyethylene, advocated by Kempfer. Van der Waarde and others have reported, successful use of very flexible silicone elastomers to accomplish a similar result. In general, the more flexible the overall socket can be, the greater the amputee's comfort and the higher the acceptance rate of the prosthesis, as advocated by Le and other authors.

When the hemi-pelvis is missing in the case of transpelvic amputation, careful contouring of the socket is necessary to contain and support the visceral tissues to provide what has been termed hydrostatic weight bearing. It is sometimes necessary to extend the socket trim lines onto the torso to provide adequate stabilization and sufficient weight bearing surfaces.

For the translumbar amputee, Simon proposed a very special design that includes significant weight bearing on the rib cage, and the use of shoulder straps for suspension is common. Carlson recently described a new socket design for this population that incorporates an adjustable, air-permeable, inner fabric socket within a rigid external frame.

Component Selection

The early literature advocated the use of only the most simplified prosthetic components for this group: a single axis hip joint, knee joint, and ankle joint, or in some cases, the use of a

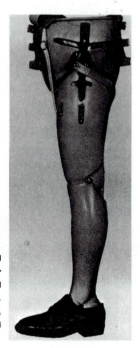

Figure 6-1. Hip disarticulation prothesis with leather bucket-type socket. (*Source:* From *Orthopaedic Appliances Atlas, Artifical Limbs.* Ann Arbor, MI: JW Edwards, 1960; with permission.)

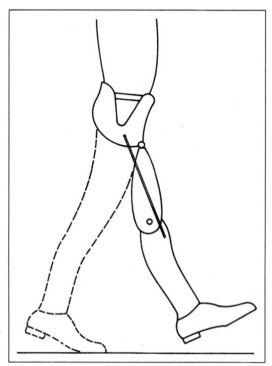

Figure 6-2. CHD prosthesis. (*Source:* From Northern University Prosthetic Orthotic Center, 1987, with permission.)

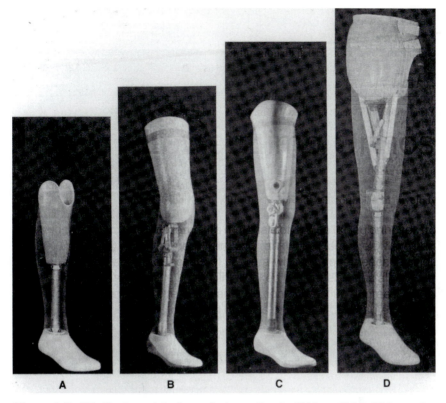

Figure 6-3. Otto Bock modular lower limb prosthesis: (A) transtibial; (B) knee disarticulation; (C) transfemoral; (D) hip disarticulation. (*Source:* From Otto Bock Orthopedic Industry, Inc., Minneapolis, MN, with permission.)

SACH foot. Subsequent experience with more sophisticated socket designs and lighter endoskeletal prostheses has demonstrated that the prescription criteria for these levels are no different than for more common lower limb amputations. It is the individual patient's motivation and functional capabilities that determine the complexity of prosthetic components to be utilized, as noted by Michael.

For example, those high-level amputees who are also somewhat feeble due to age or concomitant disease may benefit from a friction brake stance control knee due to the added stability offered. More active individuals often do very well with a polycentric knee because these designs can offer added toe clearance during swing as well as enhanced stability in early stance. Patients capable of walking at different speeds benefit from a fluid-controlled knee that is cadence responsive. Recent clinical experiences suggest that microprocessor-controlled prosthetic knees are well received by the more active individuals who have sustained these levels of amputation.

In like fashion, although the flexible keel foot is a good basic choice, more active individuals often prefer one of the dynamic response designs. Those who negotiate irregular terrain may prefer a multiaxial ankle although the single axis ankle is best used to aid prosthetic knee stability.

Two specialized components should always be considered for these individuals, because the loss of the entire limb significantly impairs their ability to absorb rotary torque forces while

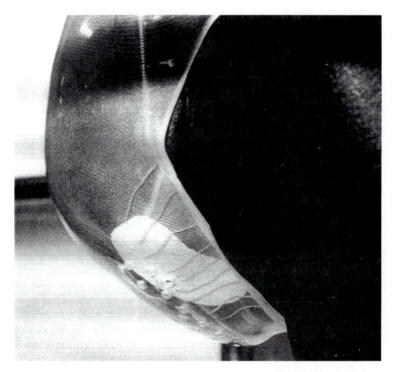

Figure 6-4. Clear test socket demonstrating encapsulation of the ischiopubic ramus, highlighted in white tape, to provide both comfortable weight bearing and control of the prosthetic socket (*Source:* Sabolich J, Guth T. *Clinical Prosthetics & Orthotics.* 1988; 12:112–122. Used by permission.)

walking. The torque absorber is a resilient component usually mounted in the shin segment that allows up to 20 degrees of internal and external rotation with the foot on the ground. This component not only reduces the shear stress on the amputee's skin within the socket, as Lamereaux has noted, but also reduces the stress on the prosthetic joints and enhances their durability.

Moving into confined spaces such as automobiles, classroom desks, and the like is difficult for many amputees. This is particularly true for this group with high-level loss. Van der Waarde and others recommend provision of a locking rotation unit just above the knee to make these tasks much easier and to facilitate dressing and tying shoes (Figure 6-5).

FACTORS AFFECTING PROSTHETIC USE

Basic criteria for fitting a prosthesis at these high levels are:

1. Amputation wound has healed and can tolerate weight bearing.
2. Patient has sufficient cardiopulmonary capacity to walk with a prosthesis.
3. Individual has an interest in using an artificial limb.

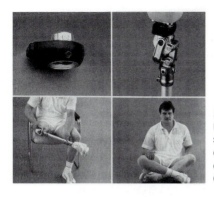

Figure 6-5. Transverse rotation units can be released by pressing a button to permit passive rotation of the shank, making it much easier to enter confined spaces such as desks or automobiles. (*Source:* Otto Bock Orthopedic Industry, Inc.)

In a study by Shurr et al, 15 of a series of 60 patients (25 percent) were fitted with a prosthesis. Most who were fitted had the amputation due to tumor (nine cases) or trauma (four cases). One additional trauma case elected not to be fitted due to severe depression. One toddler with a congenital malformation was fitted uneventfully at 16 months of age.

Only one of those with infections was considered healthy enough to attempt fitting. None of the dysvascular individuals was offered a prosthesis. Several patients with metastatic chest lesions were not fitted. Individuals in this last group lived for 3 months to 5 years after the surgery. Due to improved surgical and therapy techniques, metastatic lesions are no longer considered an absolute contraindication to prosthetic fitting.

As might be expected, those with amputation secondary to trauma who are otherwise healthy can often begin ambulating soon after surgery. In Shurr's study, three of the four traumatic amputees were fitted between 1 and 3 months after the ablation, readily learned to use it, and continued wearing the artificial limb at 15 to 24 months follow up. The fourth individual had sustained triple amputations including shoulder disarticulation and loss of the contralateral leg above the knee. His gait training was understandably difficult, and he concluded at follow up that the energy costs of ambulation were too high for prosthetic use to be practical for him.

All nine of the tumor amputees used prostheses successfully although three expired from their disease within 11 to 60 months. The balance continued wearing the prosthesis long term, with one exception. The one individual whose amputation was due to infection who was fitted rejected the prosthesis after 2 months due to discomfort in the socket.

The percentage of high-level amputees who continue to use a prosthesis long term has varied in the literature from 6 to 80 percent (Table 6-2). The overall trend is for higher usage levels in the more recent reports, presumably due to improvements in the socket designs and components over the years.

GAIT TRAINING

Very little information has been published on gait training of the hip disarticulation or transpelvic amputee. Watkins discussed the number of visits necessary to teach adequate ambulation skills, reporting that they decreased from an average of 20 sessions with the traditional tilt-table prosthesis to 17 sessions with the exoskeletal Canadian to 9 sessions with the endoskeletal modular type.

TABLE 6-2. PERCENTAGE OF FITTED PATIENTS USING HIP DISARTICULATION PROSTHESES

Author(s)	Date	Number of Patients Fitted	Number of Patients Using at F/U
Lewis and Bickel	1957	25	2 (8%)
Miller	1959	32	22 (69%)
Watkins	1962	10	8 (80%)
Higinbothom et al	1966	60	24 (40%)
Douglas et al	1975	50	3 (6%)
Sneppen et al	1978	30	15 (50%)
Shurr et al	1983	15	12 (80%)

Source: From Shurr, DG et al. Hip disarticulation. A prosthetic follow-up. *Orthot Prosthet.* 1984; 37:52.

Regretfully, most physical therapy programs offer little or no instruction in how to train these patients to use their prostheses optimally. Although the images are dated, an excellent training video on this topic is available from the Otto Bock Company at no charge.

As a general rule, the unilateral hip disarticulation or transpelvic amputee should be encouraged to walk without external aids, or to use at most one cane or forearm crutch. If both upper limbs must be encumbered with crutches for the amputee to walk, rejection of the prosthesis is common, because the artificial limb offers little practical advantage in such circumstances.

Studies by Waters and Huang show that it takes approximately the same amount of energy to walk with axillary crutches and one leg as it does to use these high level prostheses, and crutch ambulation is faster. Unless at least one upper limb is freed to carry objects, even though prosthetic use offers an improvement in cosmetic appearance, long-term wearing is doubtful at best.

TRANSLUMBAR AMPUTATION

Translumbar amputation (TLA) has only been technically feasible in recent decades and, according to Friedmann remains an extremely rare procedure. The literature shows, however, that the prognosis for individuals who have lost approximately half of their body mass is surprisingly positive when the individual is highly motivated. Survival rates of more than 20 years post-amputation and return to school or gainful employment have been reported in many cases, including those reviewed by Sneppen.

Lacking a pelvis, the individual with TLA is unable to sit upright and must therefore spend the balance of their lives on a plinth unless they are fitted with some type of prosthetic device. As noted by Smith, most experts advocate fitting with a sitting prosthesis as the first step in rehabilitation. After a carefully monitored "weaning period," many TLA survivors are able to sit upright for several consecutive hours as long as they periodically unweight the torso by "pushing up" with the arms for a minute or so.

Functionally, sustaining TLA is similar to becoming paraplegic in that all volitional movement is above the waist, and special care is required to prevent the development of skin break-

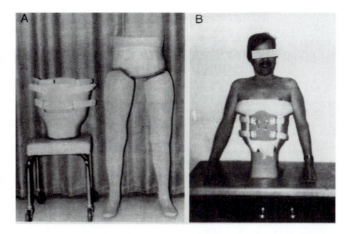

Figure 6-6. Endoskeletal prosthesis described by Dankmeyer and Doshi includes a removable inner socket that can be used independently as a sitting device. (*Source:* Dankmeyer CH Jr, Doshi R. *Orthotics & Prosthetics.* 1981; 35:11–18. Used by permission.)

down. Because the lower limbs have been ablated, the TLA survivor is usually far more mobile than the typical person with paraplegia and some opt to use prosthetic limbs for household or therapeutic ambulation, along with a walker or forearm crutches.

Dankmeyer has described an integrated approach in which he constructs a sitting prosthesis that then nestles inside a limb prosthesis when the client wishes to practice walking (Figure 6-6). When ambulation is not a goal, use of sitting prosthesis alone suffices.

J. Bradlee Aust performed the worlds' first successful TLA in 1961; the individual worked at a nursing home and survived until 1980. Aust summarized his experience with this population:

"Freed of the nonfunctioning lower half, the patient is released from the dead weight holding him down, relieved of his chronic infection and/or cancer, and experiences a new mobility, sense of well-being, and enthusiasm for life."

REFERENCES

1. Aust JB, Page CP. Hemicorporectomy. *J Surg Oncol.* 1985; 30:225–230.
2. Carlson JM, Wood SL. A flexible, air-permeable socket prosthesis for bilateral hip disarticulation and hemicorporectomy amputees. *J Prosthet Orthot.* 1998; 10:110–115.
3. Dankmeyer CH, Doshi R. Prosthetic management of adult hemicorporectomy and bilateral hip. *Orthot Prosthet.* 1981; 35(4):11–18.
4. Friedmann LW, Marin EL, Park YS. Hemicorporectomy for functional rehabilitation. *Arch Phys Med Rehabil.* 1981; 62:83–86.
5. Huang C-T, Jackson JR, Moore NB et al. Amputation: Energy cost of ambulation. *Arch Phys Med Rehabil.* 1979; 60:18–24.
6. Kempfer JJ. Light weight hip disarticulation prosthesis. *J Prosthet Orthot.* 1990; 3:41–42.

7. Lamoreux LW, Radcliffe CW. Functional analysis of the UC-BL shank axial rotation device. *Prosthet Orthot Int.* 1977; 1:114–118.

8. Le N-L, Cribbs DT, Dakpa R et al. The Hugh MacMillan Rehabilitation Centre's experience with the flexible silicone hip-disarticulation socket (FSHDS) (abstract). *J Assoc Child Prosthet Orthot Clin.* 1993; 28:20.

9. Lower-Limb Prosthetics. New York: New York University Medical School; 1975:243.

10. Michael J. Component selection criteria: Lower limb disarticulations. *Clin Prosthet Orthot.* 1988; 12:99–108.

11. Otto Bock *www.ottobock.us.*

12. Shurr DG, Cook TM, Buckwalter JA, Cooper RR. Hip disarticulation: A prosthetic follow-up. *Orthot Prosthet.* 1984; 37(1):50–57.

13. Simons BC, Lehman JF, Taylor N et al. Prosthetic management of hemicorporectomy. *Orthot Prosthet.* 1968; 22(2):63–68.

14. Smith J, Tuel SM, Meythaler JM et al. Prosthetic management of hemicorporectomy patients: New approaches. *Arch Phys Med Rehabil.* 1992; 73:493–497.

15. Sneppen O, Johansen T, Heerfordt J, Dissing I, Peterson O. Hemipelvectomy. *Acta Orthop Scand.* 1978; 49:175–179.

16. Terz JJ, Schaffner MJ, Goodkin R et al. Translumbar amputation. *Cancer.* 1990; 65:2668–2675.

17. Van der Waarde T, Michael JW. Hip disarticulation and transpelvic amputation. In: Atlas of Limb Prosthetics, 3rd ed. Bowker JH, Michael JW, eds. St. Louis, MO: Mosby-Yearbook; 1992.

18. Van der Waarde T. The Ottawa experience with hip disarticulation prostheses. *Orthotics & Prosthetics.* 1984; 38:29–33.

19. Waters RL. Energy cost, crutch ambulation and lower extremity plaster cast. *Arch Phys Med Rehabil.* 1981; 62:512.

20. Watkins A. Rehabilitation after hemipelvectomy. *J Am Med Assoc.* 1962; 181:793–794.

CHAPTER 7

Upper Limb Prosthetics

Prior to antiseptic surgery and antimicrobial drugs, many amputations of the limbs were caused by fractures. From the thirteenth century forward, knights on horseback provided mobility while archers and spearmen on foot showered the enemies with a hail of arrows and spears. Based on early Chinese fireworks and the writings of Roger Bacon about gunpowder, cannons were developed which lofted large metal balls into castles.

By 1812, Pauly had developed a cartridge containing both powder and ball or bullet that was much more effective at destroying bone and flesh. Many limbs required amputation secondary to these new gunshot wounds. The Crow Indian Two Whistles was shot trying to escape following an unlawful raid, losing his arm at the transradial level.

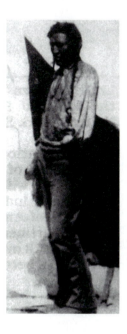

Following completion of reading this chapter, the student will be able to:

1. Compare and contrast the similarities and differences in cause and occurrence between upper and lower limb amputations.
2. Describe the levels of amputation and their relevance to upper limb fitting.
3. Describe the criteria used to determine applicability of body power and externally powered prostheses.
4. Describe the elements and relevance of periprosthetic management of the new upper limb amputee.

Although upper limb prosthetic training is most often provided by the occupational therapist, as noted by Lake, Meier suggests that it is important for all members of the rehabilitation team to develop a basic understanding of this area. The development of multidisciplinary hand teams, which usually include physical therapists who specialize in this area, has also increased interest within the physical therapy community in learning more about the management of higher level losses, as articles by Gaine and others reflect. The fundamentals of training are therefore summarized in this chapter.

AN OVERVIEW OF UPPER LIMB PROSTHETIC PRINCIPLES

Although amputations of the upper limb may be presumed to have occurred from very early times, the first record of an artificial device used for an upper limb amputation is thought to have come from the second Punic War, 218–201 BC. During that conflict, Marcus Sergius, a Roman general, lost his right hand and was fitted with an iron hand that reportedly was used in battle with great dexterity. During the Middle Ages, artificial limbs often appeared as part of a knight's suit of armor, acting to conceal any loss or disfigurement associated with battle.

Incidence

Malone indicates that approximately 6,000 to 10,000 major amputations of the upper limb occur every year in the United States. This does not include the numerous partial finger and thumb amputations that occur during work or recreation. Glattly in 1964 had found approximately a 6 to 1 ratio of lower extremity to upper limb amputations. By 1975, the ratio had increased to approximately 11 to 1. This ratio included both males and females and may be partly explained by a greater increase in the number of lower limb amputees rather than simply a decrease in the number of upper limb amputations.

Etiology

Upper limb amputations occur for the same reasons that all amputations occur. These are trauma, tumor, disease, and congenital deficiencies.

Trauma. Although no comprehensive studies exist on the subject, trauma is undoubtedly the largest producer of upper limb amputations and can include fractures with or without lacerations, electrical and thermal burns, frostbite, and injuries from factory machines or tools and farm implements. Fortunately, as safety practices within industry have improved, the number of traumatic injuries leading to amputation has been decreasing. Improved surgical techniques, including replantation, have also contributed to this decline.

Tumor. The incidence of amputation caused by tumor varied little between 1964 and 1975 according to the two studies cited earlier. Kay and Newman's data demonstrates that approximately 4.5 percent of all the amputations of both lower and upper limb may be attributed to tumors. Nielsen reported an overall rate of 4 percent, but did not break out upper versus lower. Numerous accounts of the locations of primary bone tumors of the upper limb reveal a large number occurring at proximal levels and at young ages (11 to 20 years). This is an unfortunate situation because prosthetic devices for the upper limb are more functional and cosmetic for more distal sites of anatomical loss.

As might be anticipated, significant improvements in cancer detection and treatment in recent decades are believed to have resulted in a gradual decline in the number of individuals for whom upper limb amputation is the only option. According to Torres, it appears that there has been an overall decrease in the incidence of upper limb amputees in the United States and in other countries of the developed world, although this may be due in part to the increased numbers of elderly, dysvascular lower limb amputees.

Disease. Peripheral vascular disease and diabetes do not play a major role in the etiology of amputations in the upper limb. Because the blood flow to the upper limb in dysvascular cases is typically much less impaired than in the lower limb, major limb amputations of the upper limb are only rarely done for vascular reasons. That is not to say, however, that they do not occur. In fact, it is very common to see patients with small vessel disease secondary to diabetes, Lupus (SLE), Raynaud's, or other collagenvascular diseases, who have fingertips missing as a result of dry gangrene. These minor amputations do not require elaborate surgical procedures and rarely require functional restoration via prostheses.

Major limb amputations have been reported for vascular complications secondary to infections produced by drugs injected either into the back of the hand or into the web spaces of the digits. Because of the way the upper extremity is drained on the venous side, infection spreads rapidly. Lymphangitis and cellulitis can quickly overtake the limb, necessitating major surgical intervention and often amputation.

Other examples of upper limb amputations done for reasons of disease are those secondary to major episodes of sepsis, where emboli are released, eventually occluding the major arterial tree of the arm and depriving the more distal components of their blood supply. These can occur following major episodes of sepsis in the very young when complications result from puncture of a major artery as part of treatment.

Congenital Deficiencies. Congenital absences, deficiencies, and in-utero amputations more commonly affect the upper than the lower limbs. Overall, this incidence has remained fairly constant. McDonnell reported in 1989 that these conditions affect one of every 200 newborns and are the most common cause for amputation in children under 5 years of age.

Surgical treatment of congenital malformations of the upper limb is intended to maximize residual function and preserve sensation and movement as much as possible. Special considerations apply when considering amputation in skeletally immature individuals. When possible, preservation of the growth plates is important. Also, disarticulation is preferable to ablation through the diaphysis of the long bones to avoid the risk of painful bony overgrowth. More information on the rehabilitation of pediatric clients may be found in chapter 12.

LEVELS OF UPPER LIMB AMPUTATION

The most distal level of intact anatomy remaining is used to describe upper limb amputations: partial hand [PH], wrist disarticulation [WD], transradial [TR], elbow disarticulation [ED], transhumeral [TH], shoulder disarticulation [SD], and interscauplarthoracic [IST] or forequarter [FQ]. As the amount of anatomic loss increases at the higher levels, the functional loss to the patient increases correspondingly as does the prosthetic challenge. For this reason, the ISO amputation levels are often colloquially characterized as "short, medium, or long" depending on whether the ablation is in the upper, middle, or lower third of the bony segment respectively.

Partial Hand

Partial hand amputations may be considered to be any number of amputations involving any or all of the digits or the radial or ulnar borders of the hand. These are, in fact, the most numerous amputations that occur in either the upper or lower limb, but they often require very little special postoperative treatment and/or prosthetic restoration.

Many articles and books have been written on the topic of partial hand amputations and the surgical considerations relative to these injuries. Partial hand amputations are primarily produced by traumatic episodes that include fractures and soft tissue injuries, or both. It is important to realize that any traumatic injury to the hand may involve the nerves, robbing the hand of its ability to feel as well as move. As the discussion of amputation and prosthetic restoration for upper limb amputations continues, the reader should be aware of the tremendous handicap produced by the absence or diminution of the sensory nerve supply, particularly to the palm of the hand and fingers, in the median nerve distribution.

An important element in the usefulness of any injured hand is the amount of function left in the thumb. Many staged operative procedures for partial hand amputations are directed toward increasing the functional capabilities of the remaining parts, particularly the thumb and small finger because opposition and holding usually require the border digits.

Wrist Disarticulation

The wrist disarticulation level amputation is usually performed when the partial hand residual limb is without thumb or fingers and when the motion afforded by the wrist and palm of the hand has virtually nothing to oppose it. Very often the wrist disarticulation is not performed as a primary amputation, but is done as an elective procedure after a patient discovers that a partial hand prosthesis is cumbersome and not very functional.

According to Tooms, a wrist disarticulation should allow normal distal-radial-ulnar joint motion, thus preserving pronation and supination (Figure 7-1). Although approximately

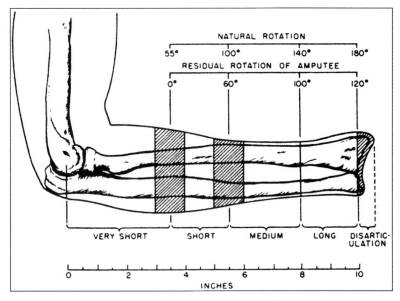

Figure 7-1. Rotation of residual forearm. (*Source:* From Taylor CL. The biomechanics of control in upper extremity prosthetics. *Orthot Prosthet.* 1981; 35:20, with permission.)

50 percent of the pronation-supination is transmitted to the prosthesis, wrist disarticulation remains the amputation of choice in situations where a long lever is advisable or important. Tooms also recommends a long palmar flap, utilizing the skin from the palm of the hand and the fascia under it to pad the distal stump. Burkhalter, Hampton, and Smeltzer indicate it is important that the radial and ulnar styloids be resected slightly to minimize the discomfort the amputee will endure in active pronation-supination within the confines of a hard prosthetic socket. Dr. Burkhalter comments on the scarcity of the true wrist disarticulation amputation. Several years ago, researchers at the University of Iowa Hospitals and Clinics attempted to find and recall all patients since 1930 who had undergone a wrist disarticulation. Upon searching 1.7 million medical records, only 24 patients were identified as having true wrist disarticulation operations. In an unpublished work by Meletiou, he found that wrist disarticulation leads to a high level of function, an excellent employment rate, a high rate of prosthetic use, and a high quality of life.

Transradial Amputation

According to Taylor, a long transradial amputation is defined as one between 8 to 10 inches from the center of the lateral epicondyle to the end of the residual limb. Reportedly, this level allows the amputee to retain between 100 to 120 degrees of pronation-supination (Figure 7-1). By allowing the amputee to utilize the long length of the residual limb as well as pronation-supination, this level provides an excellent opportunity for prosthetic restoration. Assuming a well-healed and equal lateral flap closure, the long transradial amputation provides a functional residual limb for manual labor, farming, industrial work and other similar occupations. It also provides good capability for lifting with the forearm.

As can be seen from Figure 7-1, residual limbs significantly lose pronation-supination as they become shorter. At the medium transradial level, the amputee is well equipped to use standard prostheses to lift moderate weight with the forearm and to utilize the elbow without problems. Residual limbs of medium length allow the prosthetist considerable latitude in configuring the prosthesis. In some situations, the prosthetist might wish to make the prosthetic limb slightly shorter than the contralateral side because this sometimes helps the amputee compensate for a restricted range of motion of the biological elbow or shoulder.

Short and very short transradial amputations result in limbs between 2 and 4 inches in length from the lateral epicondyle. In general, amputations at this length tend to present problems with suspension and range of motion. The bunching of soft tissue in the anticubital fold anteriorly during elbow flexion beyond approximately 100 degrees is also commonly a concern.

Many congenital limb deficiencies occur at the short and very short transradial level and require special consideration due to the short length of the residual limb. In general, residual limbs below the elbow are more functional than an elbow disarticulation assuming that the amputee has intact muscle power on both sides of the elbow joint. Short and very short residual limbs are usually held in a neutral position of pronation-supination for lifting, loading, and other functional activities.

Elbow Disarticulation

Despite the potential functional advantages of self-suspension and enhanced rotational control, Michael has noted that elbow disarticulation remains a controversial and uncommon level due largely to the cosmetic and component limitations inherent in this bulbous residual limb.

In addition to the length consideration, there is also a problem in the medial-lateral dimension, because the condyles of the distal humerus represent a large and bulky end that must somehow be included within a socket. Elbow disarticulation is a level usually reserved for children with growing epiphyses. Studies by Shurr show that bony overgrowth following diaphyseal amputations in children tends to recur, necessitating multiple surgical procedures prior to skeletal maturity. For this reason, amputation through the humerus should be avoided in children with open growth plates.

Transhumeral Amputation

The long or standard transhumeral amputation is defined as one of 50 to 90 percent of the length of a normal humerus and is usually the level of choice for amputation above the elbow. With intact skin, musculature, and nerve supply to the arm, this length transhumeral amputation can provide the muscle power and range of motion necessary to produce very functional results with a conventional prosthesis. Because, as will be discussed shortly, glenohumeral flexion plays an important role in controlling a conventional body powered system, the lever arm of the humerus allows the amputee excellent control over the device. This level may also produce excellent myoelectric signals from the biceps and triceps for operating a myoelectrically controlled system. Additionally, the prosthetist has a great deal of freedom in deciding at what level to place the prosthetic elbow joint and has easy access to the elbow unit for periodic replacement or maintenance.

The medium transhumeral is defined as an amputation of the humerus leaving 30 to 50 percent of its length. Although such residual limbs may still permit adequate functioning of a prosthesis, the lack of length of the humerus places some serious constraints on the placement of the control cables used to operate the prosthetic elbow. When less than 30 percent of the humerus remains, most amputees find there is insufficient leverage to control the socket position, so most short TH amputations are treated functionally as if they were shoulder disarticulations.

Shoulder Disarticulation

The shoulder disarticulation (SD) may be defined as any amputation of the arm from approximately 30 percent of the humerus through the shoulder joint. In cases where the humerus is disarticulated completely, it is obvious that this is a shoulder disarticulation level. However, in those cases where there is a remaining bit of humerus, functionally the patient will be a candidate for a shoulder disarticulation prosthesis even though the anatomical loss is transhumeral. Considering the anatomy, the patient may have up to 30 percent of the length of the upper humerus but will have little motor power available in flexion, extension, or abduction. Therefore, a prosthetic shoulder joint must be considered. As is the case in regard to the hip in the lower limb, shoulder disarticulation amputations are often done for reasons of tumor. It is indeed unfortunate that the tumor invades the limbs near their upper junctions with the body necessitating many prosthetic joints and large and often bulky prosthetic sockets.

Interscapularthoracic or Forequarter Amputation

The most proximal level of amputation surgery in the upper limb is referred to as the forequarter. Like the shoulder disarticulation, it is usually performed because of a tumor. In the forequarter, the clavicle and scapula are usually sacrificed as well as the entire length of the humerus and the rest of the arm. In addition, various lengths of ribs may be sacrificed depending on the nature of the tumor and the reconstruction goals of the surgeon. If the scapula is removed on the amputated side, the range of bilateral scapular abduction is diminished by one-half. As will be seen, this motion is important when body powered systems are used to operate a prosthetic arm. The forequarter amputation would appear to be an ideal level for using an externally powered prosthesis. However, systems utilized at the forequarter level are fraught with difficulties because of the restricted number of motor sites available for myoelectric signal pick up and switch controls are usually necessary. Careful attention to detail on the part of the surgeon is necessary at this level in order that no bony prominences remain under compromised skin. This situation can lend itself to many problems in fitting the very large socket that often encompasses part of the sound side shoulder in an attempt to minimize the tendency for the socket to rotate and fall off.

REHABILITATION OPTIONS

In contrast to the situation with lower limb amputation, a prosthesis is frequently not required for independence when an upper limb absence is present, so long as there is a healthy contralateral limb. Particularly for individuals with congenital high-level, bilateral upper limb deficiencies, Marguardt's decades of experience with European children with severe limb deficiencies due to Thalidomide has shown that independence training using foot skills will be more effective over time than even the most sophisticated prosthetic arms, with few exceptions. Meletiou has verified that a significant percentage of unilateral upper limb amputees choose to function with only the remaining arm, as do some with multiple limb loss. As long as this is the individual's preference, these options should be actively supported with training in alternative ways to accomplish activities of daily living, and should be viewed as successful rehabilitation.

When the patient is interested in a prosthesis, consideration should be given to a passive device. Particularly when there is a high-level loss, use of a lightweight device that restores normal body symmetry may the most practical option. Some prefer the reliability of a prosthesis without many moving parts. A report from Michael, Gailey, Bowker suggests that a passive prosthesis is also popular for selected sports activities, particularly for water, snow, and contact sports.

Active prostheses operate by using torso muscle strength, electrical motors, or a combination of these means. The former is termed a body-powered system while the latter is an externally powered device. Prostheses combining both body and externally powered controls are termed hybrid devices, as noted in Childress and Billock's seminal 1970 work.

Although all three options are equally important aspects of upper limb amputee rehabilitation, this chapter will focus on active prostheses because these are the only devices likely to require use training by the therapist.

BODY-POWERED COMPONENTS AND PROSTHESES

Upper limb components are analogous to those for the more familiar lower limb devices. The typical transradial prosthesis consists of a socket that fits the residual limb, an extension that forms the prosthetic forearm, and an active or passive terminal device. Transradial prostheses have an additional extension forming the humeral segment and some type of elbow device. Shoulder disarticulation and higher levels may also use a prosthetic shoulder joint.

Partial Hand Prostheses
Partial hand prostheses are relatively uncommon and, although books from the time of Bunnell to Bender contain many partial hand, nonstandard prostheses and hooks, these devices are often abandoned as time passes and the amputee grows accustomed to life with something other than a normal hand. Exceptions occur when the amputee is bilaterally involved or when the amputee's occupation or vocation can only be accomplished through the utilization of such a device, which they will use only for that vocation or avocation.

Terminal Devices
A terminal device (TD) is a component used to produce holding or prehension and may be either a hook, hand, or nonstandard device. Terminal devices are usually interchangeable, and applied using a threaded connector. They are typically made of stainless steel or aluminum, sometimes covered with either neoprene or plastizol, and are available in numerous designs. Stainless steel TDs weigh more than aluminum and the level of prosthetic restoration may dictate the type of TD prescribed. The shorter the transhumeral level, the more necessary it is to use a lightweight, aluminum TD. Amputees returning to heavy industrial or farm work usually require stainless steel TDs. In a device described as voluntary opening (VO), biscapular abduction or glenohumeral flexion opens the terminal device and rubber bands close it as the abduction or flexion is reduced. Voluntary-closing (VC) devices work just the opposite but are far less prevalent.

Hooks

Hosmer/Dorrance is the name usually associated with conventional terminal devices. These TDs are identified by numbers, in reverse order of size, with 3 being the largest and heaviest and 12 the smallest and lightest. Hooks may be either canted or lyre shaped. Canted fingers permit better visualization of the object in the TD. The "thumb" of the TD is where the control cable attaches and is the point where the opening force is applied.

Hands

Body-powered hands, like body-powered hooks, are available in either VO or VC configurations. In European countries, many amputees choose to wear a body-powered hand full time even though they offer a relatively inefficient grasp due to frictional losses that are compounded by the rubberized cosmetic glove covering the mechanism. They do offer a more normal appearance to the public than the hook-shaped TDs.

In North America, LeBlanc reports that many upper limb amputees will accept a body-powered hook because of its functional advantages. It is possible to interchange a hook and hand in the same prosthesis, and some amputees find this to be a good compromise. They use the hook in the privacy of their home or during work tasks while wearing a body-powered hand for social occasions. Passive hands are also available and usually offer enhanced cosmesis over those containing an active mechanism.

Transradial and Wrist Disarticulation Prostheses

Transradial and wrist disarticulation sockets often share common design elements. The primary difference is that it is often possible to utilize supra-styloidal suspension in the wrist disarticulation prosthesis, eliminating the need for additional suspension from the control harness. Childress and others have noted that as a general rule, amputees prefer to minimize the control harnessing they must wear.

Conventional TR Socket

Although upper limb sockets are not weight bearing, they must still provide a snug, intimate, total contact fit to permit the amputee to control the prosthesis efficiently and to dissipate the forces inherent in lifting, pushing, and similar activities. A conventional double-wall socket includes the lamination of the socket itself plus a second lamination pulled over the first in order to provide cosmesis, stability, and function. During the casting phase of the fabrication process, the prosthetist pays careful attention to the distribution of pressure around and including the epicondyles, the contact with cut bones, and the olecranon. Adequate relief in the anterior distal socket must be given to the radius so that lifting will not cause high levels of pressure and pain. Attention is also given to the posterior portion of the socket so that lifting will not cause undue pressure on the olecranon. The trimlines of the transradial socket depend a great deal on the length of the residual limb. The shorter the residual limb, the higher or more proximal the trimlines; the longer the residual limb, the lower the trimlines may be. Another consideration for trimlines includes the desire to allow pronation and supination. A high anterior trimline will not allow pronation-supination to occur at the radial ulnar joint of the forearm.

If the terminal device of the prosthesis is ultimately to be positioned near the mouth and if the amputee has restricted range of motion at the elbow, the prosthetist may install the prosthesis in an attitude or angle of preflexion. This preflexion is a combination of the normal hanging angle, or the 10 to 15 degrees in which the elbow normally flexes, coupled with any additional flexion necessary to reach the mouth. Often times the wrist unit may be slightly canted in an anterior-medial direction in order to assist the amputee in getting the terminal device to the midline.

Elbow Hinges

Single pivot stainless steel hinges are used when heavy duty use is anticipated. Because the suspension of the prosthesis is handled primarily by the harness, there is little need to develop an auxiliary suspension on the condyles around the elbow. This allows the amputee full use of the elbow joint in an attempt to gain whatever elbow range of motion possible. Although stainless steel single pivot hinges are very durable, they also eliminate pronation-supination. In contrast, flexible hinges are designed to maintain the available pronation-supination to eliminate the need for prepositioning of the terminal device using the normal hand. The classic application for flexible hinges is at the level of the wrist disarticulation, where the patient theoretically has full pronation-supination available and a good long lever with which to not only flex the elbow, but also pronate and supinate the terminal device. In some cases, however, the amputee cannot tolerate the forces generated distally by the prosthesis on the residual limb. In such circumstances, these forces can be eliminated and absorbed by the use of rigid hinges despite the resulting restriction in pronation-supination.

Self-Suspending Transradial Sockets

The original self-suspending socket was developed in Germany immediately after World War II and is termed the Muenster socket after the city where this concept was first promulgated. According to Fishmann, it was originally intended only for use with unilateral short residual limbs and relied on a trim line proximal to the cubital fold that restricted full flexion.

In subsequent decades, the concept of self-suspension has been further developed and utilization of supracondylar contours and muscle contours has permitted lower trim lines that minimally interfere with elbow flexion only slightly, as advocated by Billock and many others. These modern designs are commonly used for passive or externally powered prostheses where no control harnessing is needed. They may also be used with body-powered terminal devices with a simplified harness.

More recently, Madigan and Fillauer reported the increased utilization of elastomeric silicone suspension sleeves for both upper and lower limb applications. When combined with a special shuttle lock, these sleeves adhere to the residual limb via suction and attach mechanically to the distal aspect of the socket, which has proven very effective as noted by Radocy. It is also sometimes possible to apply a rubber sleeve externally to the prosthesis that crosses the cubital fold and provides self-suspension, as is done with transtibial prostheses.

Split-Socket Prostheses

Sometimes the amputee is physically unable to flex the elbow through a normal range of motion. Particularly in bilateral cases, where the ability to reach the face and head is of functional importance, one of two very specialized split-socket prostheses can be provided. The split socket with step-up hinges (Figure 7-2) consists of a socket within a socket, attached by either step-up or variable-gear elbow hinges. These hinges utilize gear ratios to produce flexion of the prosthesis that is greater than flexion of the elbow joint, often by a factor of two. In a case where the amputee has only 60 degrees of active elbow flexion, by using a geared hinge or

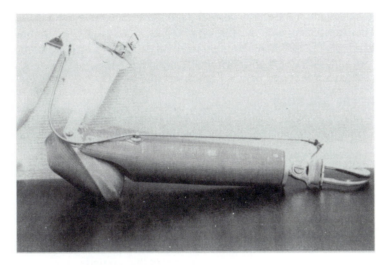

Figure 7-2. The split socket with step-up hinge.

variable step-up hinge, the amputee may develop 120 degrees of elbow flexion in the prosthesis, thus enabling him to bring the terminal device to his mouth. The prosthesis is often a bit uncosmetic and demands a force factor of two times normal in exchange for the added range of motion. Additionally, the control of the forearm section and terminal device of such a prosthesis may be difficult and lifting heavy objects may be contraindicated because objects falling out of the grasp of the terminal device will propel the forearm section toward the midline uncontrolled, potentially hitting and/or injuring the patient.

If an amputee cannot maintain a desired angle of elbow flexion, a stump activated-positive elbow lock is available. This lock allows the patient to develop the appropriate amount of flexion and then lock the hinge at the desired position. Lock activation usually requires motion of the remnant triceps muscle.

In cases where an amputee is unable to produce enough power with the residual limb to flex the elbow, a split housing system or fair lead similar to that used in transhumeral prosthetics may be utilized. This allows a pull on the cable, usually using biscapular abduction, to flex the elbow until around 100 degrees of elbow flexion occurs. The elbow is then locked and further pull on the cable opens or closes the terminal device similar to many transhumeral systems. It is important to understand that split socket prostheses are used very infrequently and only in cases where both patient and prosthetist are willing to accept the inherent trade-offs in force and excursion and realize that full range of motion and terminal device opening may be impossible no matter what prosthetic restoration is provided.

Transhumeral and Elbow Disarticulation Components
As noted previously, transhumeral amputations typically require the addition of some sort of elbow mechanism. The exception is for infants and small children, where a one-piece prosthesis with the forearm fixed at about 90 degrees of flexion is commonly used to reduce the weight and complexity of operation.

The bulk and length of the elbow disarticulation residuum generally precludes the use of anything except external hinges at the elbow joint, with either adjustable friction or a locking mechanism. Compared to the more common internally locking mechanical elbows, such external hinges offer fewer locking positions and reduced durability.

Transhumeral Sockets

The transhumeral socket must be intimately fitted to provide effective control and rotational resistance while the prosthesis is being used functionally. The extent of the trim lines is generally the inverse of the length of the residual limb: shorter residuums require more socket stabilization about the shoulder region. Conversely, longer residuums usually terminate on the proximal humerus allowing a greater range of glenohumeral movement that the longer bony lever arm can control effectively.

The medial wall of the transhumeral socket is flattened so that it lies comfortably against the chest (Figure 7-3). The anterior wall must contour to the residual limb while allowing relief for the cut end of the humerus. Because glenohumeral flexion is used to flex the elbow and open and close the terminal device, it is very important that no undue pressure be allowed on the cut end. Although the lateral and posterior walls primarily cover soft tissue, it is important that they contour exactly the patient's remaining anatomy. The socket must be tight fitting, but at the same time not restrictive. A total contact socket retards swelling of the limb and provides good proprioception relative to the position of the arm and shoulder. Upon inspection of the socket, the medial and lateral dimensions will look relatively flat while the anterior and posterior walls appear slightly rounded in part because of the bulk of the musculature and in an attempt to restore the normal looking anatomy of the biceps and triceps.

Elbow Mechanisms

Internal and external glenohumeral motion is simulated by passive rotation of a turntable mounted just above the mechanical elbow, allowing the amputee to preposition the forearm

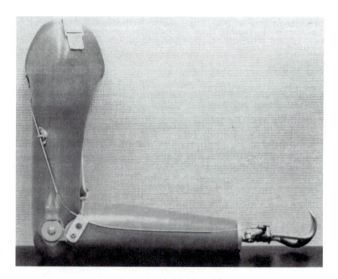

Figure 7-3. Transhumeral socket.

relative to the body. Because most standard transhumeral amputations are between 50 to 90 percent of the length of the humerus, it is possible to utilize the internally locking elbow as the main component of body-powered transhumeral prostheses. In most cases, assuming reasonable muscular control and skin coverage, this provides a very functional level with which to drive the transhumeral prosthesis. The shorter the length of the humerus, the more difficult it is for the amputee to perform activities with the elbow flexed and the terminal device fully open, particularly near the midline or mouth. Although full terminal device opening is not mandatory for most unilateral transhumeral amputees, it remains a goal for many patients even though one normal hand remains. Patients with shorter transhumeral amputations have difficulties performing full terminal device opening near the mouth.

Shoulder Disarticulation Components

As mentioned earlier, the prosthesis for a very short transhumeral amputation is virtually identical to a shoulder disarticulation prosthesis because the length of the humerus is such that it cannot functionally generate useful motion. Available motions for operating the terminal device and/or elbow unit include shoulder elevation and depression as well as biscapular abduction. For all practical purposes, glenohumeral flexion is not available at this level. The socket usually covers the acromion and scapula and must include relief for these bony prominences (Figure 7-4). The socket may be referred to as a shoulder cap in that it covers the shoulder, allowing no motion yet suspending the socket by long trim lines anterior, superior, and posterior. The axillary component is similar to transhumeral sockets in that it must allow easy entry, yet a snug fit with minimal superior displacement.

It is more difficult to generate excursion of control cables as the length of the humerus shortens. Therefore, short transhumeral or shoulder disarticulation amputees have great difficulties activating BP prostheses. Because glenohumeral flexion is no longer available, biscapular abduction must provide the motor power for flexion of the elbow as well as opening of the

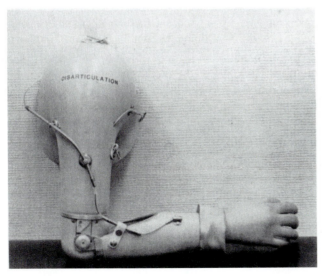

Figure 7-4. Shoulder disarticulation prosthesis.

terminal device. A spring-loaded elbow flexion assist (Figure 7-5), mounted on the medial side of the prosthetic elbow, may be added to aid in elbow flexion. Use of this spring assist permits the prosthetist to position the elbow flexion attachment closer to the elbow center, thereby capturing additional excursion necessary for terminal device opening in full elbow flexion.

From a functional point of view, it must be emphasized that the very short transhumeral and shoulder disarticulation level amputees will utilize their prostheses only for assistance or specific tasks. It is unrealistic to expect body-powered prostheses to significantly contribute to such activities of daily living as feeding and dressing with this level of loss.

Forequarter Components

Different from the shoulder disarticulation, the forequarter amputation requires a more extensive socket usually covering part of the sound side shoulder. The socket on the involved side is also longer and larger than in shoulder disarticulation or transhumeral level. Sauter from Canada developed a fitting frame to replace the solid plastic shoulder cap. This frame allows greater heat loss, excellent cosmesis and suspension, and lightweight fabrication. With all motions of the shoulder gone, available force production and excursion are also gone. Amputees at this level require at least an excursion amplifier (pulley) and often external power. An excursion amplifier is a pulley system geared on a ratio of 2:1. As the amputee pulls with 1 inch of excursion, the amplifier delivers 2 inches of cable movement. The price paid for this excursion is force in that it requires a double amount of force to produce the 2-inch excursion. Harnessing may be customized to each individual patient's needs. Motions available include chest expansion or contralateral shoulder elevation.

In many cases, the forequarter amputee will readily accept a lightweight, passive shoulder cap that restores normal shoulder symmetry and allows the blouse or shirt to hang more naturally. These prostheses are often fitted soon after the amputation (Figure 7-6).

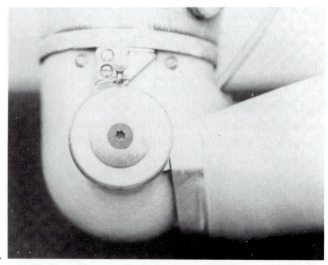

Figure 7-5. Elbow flexion assist.

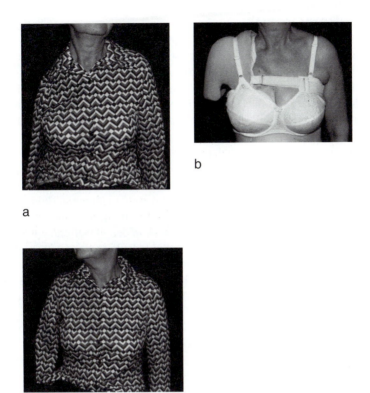

a

b

c

Figure 7-6. The initial prosthesis provided following interscapularthoracic amputation (a) is usually a passive "shoulder cap" prosthesis (b). Such lightweight devices permit the amputee to wear clothing more comfortably and restore torso symmetry (c).

BODY-POWERED CONTROL AND HARNESSING

Body power for prosthetic operation has the inherent advantages of being reliable and intuitive for the user. As Tooms has noted, it is also faster than current externally powered devices, although this gap is closing as improved motor technology is developed each decade.

In addition, Fryer notes that body-powered components are generally lighter and less complicated than externally powered alternatives, making them less expensive and more tolerant of hard use as well. For all these reasons, there is a general preference among rehabilitation professionals to offer body-powered components whenever feasible.

Whenever limitations in strength or excursion make body power impractical, external power is the only active alternative available. This is often the case when high-level amputation has occurred. Additional advantages to external power will be discussed later in this chapter.

Sources for Body Power

Nonelectric prostheses require body power through harnessing of available motions to produce desired prosthetic control or function. Several options are available throughout the upper limb and thorax. In body-powered, cable-driven artificial limbs, two concepts underlie the utilization of functional body power. These two concepts are excursion and force. Force is necessary in order to pull on a cable to produce functioning of the prosthesis. Excursion is important because the distance the cable is pulled will determine the magnitude of the resulting motions at the elbow and hand.

Whether transhumeral or transradial, perhaps the best overall movement in regard to both excursion and force is glenohumeral flexion. Taylor states that between 40 to 60 pounds of force can be generated by the average adult in glenohumeral flexion. This is more than enough to operate and control the prostheses. In addition to excursion, glenohumeral flexion produces good length and may be harnessed easily depending on the length of the humerus.

Another excellent source of body power is shoulder elevation/depression. Shoulder elevation/depression is used primarily for locking and unlocking elbows in short transhumeral, shoulder disarticulation, or forequarter length amputations. Although shoulder elevation produces good excursion and good length, it requires a fixed point, usually at the waist, in order to provide an anchor against which to pull. This anchor often is moveable if connected to either a belt or pants. A more secure means of utilizing shoulder elevation is by means of a peroneal strap or strap that goes through the groin on the opposite side of the amputated shoulder. However, peroneal straps are very uncomfortable for most patients.

Scapular abduction or protraction produces a good excursion with which to operate the terminal device or flex the elbow of a prosthesis. Studies have indicated that 2 inches of cable excursion are needed to open and close a terminal device with the elbow in neutral. Although the strength produced by scapular abduction is generally good, the resulting excursion is limited. However, when both scapulae are available, the required 2 inches usually can be achieved.

Shoulder depression may be used because it produces good force but restricted excursion. Shoulder depression is often harnessed to produce the required 5/8 to 3/4 inch excursion needed to lock or unlock the elbow of a transhumeral prosthesis.

Chest expansion is another motion that may be used because of its good force but only moderate excursion. Chest expansion is most commonly used to lock or unlock the elbow of a shoulder disarticulation or forequarter level amputation.

Combinations of the aforementioned motions may be used in specific situations. For example, in congenital cases, locks of either elbow or shoulder may be accomplished by residual dysplastic hands, particularly ones located in nonanatomical places. Such conditions as phocomelia may also lend themselves to nonstandard applications.

Transradial Harnessing

The most common harness for the transradial amputee is a figure 8 harness and a Northwestern ring. Figure 7-7 demonstrates the figure 8 harness from both the anterior and posterior perspectives. The components of the transradial harness include the axillary loop, which serves as an anchor for the terminal device to pull against; the anterior suspensor strap lying in the delto-pectoral groove on the involved side and maintaining the primary suspension of the prosthesis; and the control attachment strap originating on the ring and lying on the lower third of the scapula, incorporated into the hanger and the cable. The ring lies flat on the back, inferior

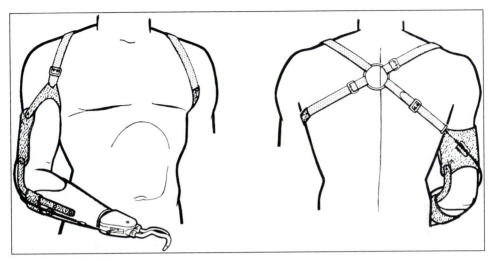

Figure 7-7. Figure 8 harness.

to C-7, and ideally just to the sound side of the center of the spine. It is important that the harness be tight enough to activate the terminal device yet loose enough to be comfortable and allow the amputee freedom of movement of both arms and both shoulders.

As was noted previously, the primary motor source for the transradial figure 8 harness is glenohumerous flexion. An increase in the angle of glenohumeral flexion will open the terminal device; the rubberbands will close it as the amputee extends the shoulder. In the case where the amputee desires to open the terminal device close to the body, biscapular abduction is utilized. Adduction or retraction is then used to allow the split hook to return to its closed position.

Transhumeral Harnessing

The typical harness for the transhumeral prosthesis is a figure 8 harness with a sewn cross point located inferior to C-7 and ideally slightly to the sound side (Figure 7-8). These components are similar to the figure 8 harness used at the transradial level, but with the addition of the anterior suspensory strap and the elbow lock cable strap attached to it. The anterior suspensory strap is composed of two parts, the first of which is a solid webbing strap running posteriorly to anteriorly over the shoulder and through the deltoid- pectoral groove. One inch inferior to the clavicle, this strap connects to a piece of elastic webbing that terminates at the distal portion of the humeral component of the prosthesis, slightly medial to the anterior midline. The elastic acts to return the elbow lock cable after each pull. A solid webbing strap located more superficial to the elastic strap activates the elbow lock. It is important that the axillary loop on the transhumeral harness remain snug and consistent in its location in the sound side axilla as it serves as the anchor from which the other two straps pull.

Standard transhumeral harnessing requires certain motor functions. Those motor sources are biscapular abduction and glenohumeral flexion. Biscapular abduction opens and closes the terminal device whenever the elbow locked, and flexes and extends the elbow when it is unlocked. Studies at New York University indicate that it requires 2 inches of excursion to flex the elbow to full flexion and 2 1/2 inches of excursion to open the terminal device fully at

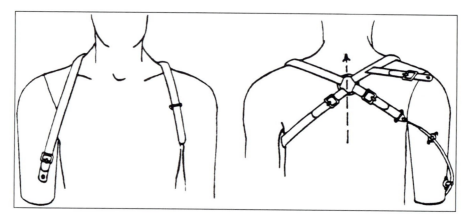

Figure 7-8. Above-elbow harness. (*Source:* From Northwestern University Prosthetic Orthotic Center, 1987, with permission.)

the mouth. Therefore, a total of 4 1/2 inches of excursion is necessary to fully operate a body-powered transhumeral prosthesis. A combination motion of shoulder depression, abduction, and extension produces 5/8 to 3/4 inch of excursion and 2 pounds of force required to activate the elbow locking cable.

The described transhumeral control system is termed dual control, because only two cables are required to operate the elbow and terminal device. A single control cable flexes and extends the elbow and, when the elbow is locked, also opens and closes the terminal device. In order to produce flexion of the elbow, this cable passes slightly anterior to the elbow hinge. The housing through which the cable runs is discontinuous and sometimes referred to as a fair lead. With the elbow unlocked, this fair lead allows the pull on the cable to flex the elbow, pulling the two housings together at the elbow. As was indicated previously, it requires approximately 2-1/2 inches of cable excursion to fully flex the prosthetic elbow.

The distal housing, from the elbow center to the wrist unit, is connected to the forearm by a component called an elbow flexion attachment. This elbow flexion attachment controls the position of the cable relative to the elbow joint and is adjusted by the prosthetist during the fitting process to provide the most optimum terminal device function. The more distal the location of the elbow flexion attachment, the lower the force required to flex the elbow, because the perpendicular distance from elbow center is increased. This also results in a need for greater excursion. On the other hand, moving the elbow flexion attachment more proximal to the elbow center demands more force to flex the elbow, but utilizes less excursion. Because most transhumeral amputees have no problem generating force but some have problems generating excursion, proximal location of the elbow flexion attachment may be advantageous.

EXTERNALLY POWERED CONTROLS, COMPONENTS, AND PROSTHESES

Prior to the 1970s, externally powered prostheses were largely confined to research settings and, according to Childress, had little clinical impact. Michael reports that over the past decades, these components have become increasingly reliable and lighter in weight as battery and motor technology have advanced and they are now part of mainstream prosthetic practice in all developed countries.

Externally Powered Control Options

Electrically operated prostheses are controlled by two primary means. The preferred method, termed myoelectric control, uses special surface electrodes that read the surface EMG signals from antagonistic muscle groups. For example, most transradial (TR) prostheses use signals from the wrist extensor group to open the terminal device while signals from the wrist flexors cause it to close. When two independent muscle sites are not available, a single electrode that responds to the rate or magnitude of the EMG signal can be used to open and close the terminal device, as originally proposed by Corces and Scott.

Simple myoelectric systems open and close the terminal device at a constant speed. In 1995, Parker and Scott reported on more advanced systems that allow the amputee to modulate both the speed of motion and the grip force by varying the magnitude of the EMG signal. Sears and Shaperman have shown that the majority of amputees given the choice preferred the more precise function offered by such proportional myoelectric control.

When more than one electrically powered component is provided, such as when an electric wrist pronator-supinator is provided along with an electric terminal device, the same muscle sites usually control both components. One common strategy is for the amputee to use simultaneous co-contracture and immediate relaxation of both muscle sites to switch the control mode from wrist to terminal device and back.

The second control option is to use some type of electromechanical switch to operate the electrical component. As noted by Kansas and Weaver, most require only a very small movement by the amputee, whether incorporated into a harness or pushed or pulled by a bony prominence of phocomelic digit. Switch control is less intuitive than agonist-antagonist myoelectric control, but is often the only practical alternative for higher level amputees. Switch control is also useful when the amputee's voluntary muscle control is inconsistent, when the skin is fragile or badly scarred and cannot tolerate direct contact with an electrode, and in similar cases where EMG control is not feasible.

Terminal Devices

As is the case with body-powered alternatives, externally powered terminal devices may look like a human hand or more like a mechanical device, each offering characteristic advantages and disadvantages as reviewed by Neal. In fact, a motorized forearm component termed a Prehension Actuator is now available that can open any VO hook while the rubber bands close it when the motor is turned off (Figure 7-9). One of the most commonly used electromechanical devices is the Griefer, which is German for gripper (Figure 7-10).

Electric hands are the most popular externally powered components, as noted by Malone et al and many others, presumably because they offer a powerful grip force with minimal effort by the amputee as well as a pleasing appearance. Unlike body-powered hands, electric hands can be quite functional because the efficiency of the motor can overcome frictional losses without extra amputee effort, resulting in a very secure grip. Advances in control options, including the recent development of microprocessor-controlled TDs based on concepts proposed by Winkler and Bierwirth, have made the use of these devices very simple for the amputee, as noted by Williams.

Figure 7-9. The Prehension Actuator has a small electric motor inside the forearm segment which can be activated by a microswitch or myoelectric signal. The motor opens the body-powered terminal device while the rubber bands close the TD whenever there is no signal to the motor. (*Source:* Photo courtesy of Hosmer-Dorrance Corporation.)

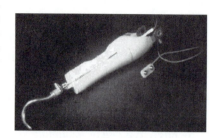

Wrist Disarticulation and Transradial Prostheses

The most common externally powered prostheses are those for these two distal levels of amputation. When used with a self-suspending socket, the result is a prosthesis with no harnessing whatsoever. This translates into increased comfort for the amputee, as well as the ability to use the terminal device functionally in positions that are not possible with harness-actuated devices. For example, the TR or WD amputee can usually open and close the externally powered TD overhead, at arms length to the side, at midline, and even behind the body. Some amputees use both an externally powered hand and gripper, interchanging them according to the task to be performed.

Although originally developed for use by adults, externally powered systems have now been sufficiently miniaturized to be used by teens, children, toddlers, and even infants. Twenty years ago, Sorbye of Sweden began advocating transradial myoelectric fittings when the child is between 2-1/2 and 4 years of age. Subsequent researchers, including Shurr et al, have corroborated that children can successfully use powered arms. Studies by Haag et al have documented that children open and close electric terminal devices as much as 2,000 to 3,000 times per day, suggesting they are being used frequently for functional tasks. Fitting of infants is technically possible, but remains controversial as noted by Meletiou and Stack and McDonnell, and discussed in more detail in chapter 12.

Figure 7-10. The Greifer is the most commonly prescribed electronic hook. It can be easily interchanged with an electronic hand, and offers passive wrist flexion as well as a more powerful grip force than the hand. (*Source:* Photo courtesy of Otto Bock Orthopedic Industry, Inc.)

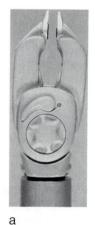 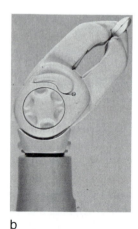

a   b

Elbow Disarticulation and Transhumeral Prostheses

As previously noted, use of body-powered components has a number of advantages including making the prosthesis lighter in weight and faster to operate. For this reason, use of a body-powered elbow joints with an externally powered terminal device is a common strategy to create a hybrid prosthesis, as Billock advocated in 1985. For the person with an elbow disarticulation, this is the only option for an electrical prosthesis because external hinges are the only available articulation. A simplified harness to operate the elbow and provide partial suspension is commonly used in hybrid prostheses for these levels.

The TR amputee has more options. One approach is to first select the terminal device according to the individual's functional goals, and then to decide if a body-powered or electrical elbow is appropriate. For example, if the individual prefers a body-powered hook terminal device due to work conditions but has insufficient excursion to also operate a body-powered elbow, an electric elbow is clearly a logical choice. Conversely, if the same individual prefers an electric hand, the available excursion may be sufficient to operate a body-powered elbow successfully. Very high-level amputees may lack sufficient excursion to operate any body-powered components and then a fully electric system is the only active prosthesis possible. For others, a fully electric arm is an attractive option because it requires far less effort and gross motion to operate than prosthesis with any body-powered components (Figure 7-11).

Shoulder Disarticulation and Higher Level Prostheses

As discussed in the section on body power, it is very difficult for most shoulder disarticulation or higher-level amputees to operate a fully body-powered prosthesis. For that reason, use of at least one electric component is often advocated when these individuals desire an active prosthesis, as discussed by Pinzur. Myoelectric control of the terminal device is generally preferred, when feasible; switch control of terminal device and/or electric elbow is also possible.

Functional Use of Externally Powered Components

Prosthetic components are prescribed based on the clinical experience of the team members; as noted by Sears, no absolute criteria for successful use have been identified to date. In an effort to ascertain factors that influence long term functional use of upper limb prostheses, a number of studies have been conducted over the years, as reviewed by Wright et al.

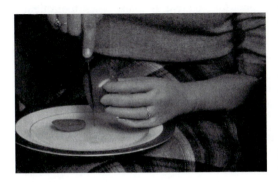

Figure 7-11. Many amputees, particularly those with higher level loss, prefer an externally powered prosthesis due to the ease of operation, powerful grip, and pleasing appearance offered by this technology. The transhumeral prosthesis depicted here provides proportional control of the electronic elbow, wrist, and hand from two antagonist EMG site. (*Source:* Photo courtesy of Motion Control, Inc.)

Northmore-Ball et al studied 43 traumatic transradial amputee workman who were provided with both body and externally powered prostheses in the 1970s. Although these amputees wore the myoelectric arm 91 percent of the time in social situations, they only wore them 15 percent of the time at work for fear of damaging the cosmetic glove covering the electric hand.

Stein and Waller compared a cohort of 20 myoelectric wearers and 16 body-powered wearers performing various functional tasks using both electric- and body-actuated prostheses. The body-powered hook was twice as fast as the myoelectric hand available in the early 1980s, although both were slower in functional tasks than the intact biological hand. Sixty percent of the TR amputees in this study preferred the myoelectric prosthesis over the body-powered one.

In more recent studies, Trost reported in 1993 on a group of 25 amputees who had been fitted with a myoelectric arm 18 years previously. Eleven still wore the electric arms, five exclusively and six alternately with a body-powered system. Five wore a body-powered arm exclusively and seven no longer wore any prosthetic device. In a shorter retrospective review of 20 adults and children fitted with myoelectric devices, Dalsey et al found that 10 of 12 children and 6 of 8 adults continued to wear their prostheses long term. They also noted that these myoelectric prostheses were relatively durable in clinical use.

Atkins et al have studied a group of 21 children and 66 adults who were fitted with electric prostheses. They documented good success when children were fitted with TR prostheses at an early age, but noted that individuals with bilateral upper limb loss often returned to using body-powered devices over time.

This latter finding corroborates a report by Millstein et al who found that the highest failure rate following myoelectric fitting was among those with bilateral upper limb loss. It appears that bilateral powered fitting should be approached with caution, presumably because body-powered TDs are inherently lighter and more reliable due to their simplicity. Some experts advocate fitting bilaterals with a body-powered system on one side and an electric or hybrid arm on the opposite side.

PERIOPERATIVE MANAGEMENT OF THE NEW AMPUTEE

Preoperative Care
Although a smaller number of upper limb amputations are done on an elective basis compared to the lower limb, it is good practice for the clinic team members to visit with the elective upper limb amputee prior to the surgical procedure. Many of the questions and concerns discussed in chapter 1 are also of concern to the upper limb patient. In many cases, the patient's questions deal with the timing of certain procedures and the availability of prosthetic restoration with or without "bionics."

Postoperative Care
As with the lower limb amputee, post-operative programs for upper limb amputation include exercise, compression wrapping, and provision of preparatory prostheses.

Exercise. Depending on the level of amputation, the muscles about the joint proximal to the amputation must be mobilized and exercised as early as medically possible. These exercises will prevent the negative effects of disuse and will assure good functioning of muscles and joints in preparation for prosthetic restoration. Specifically, transradial patients need to emphasize elbow range of motion, particularly in extension. They also must strengthen the muscles about the shoulder, particularly the abductors and external rotators, for these two groups are commonly ignored by the patient resulting in adhesive capsulitis or other disuse problems. In the case of the transhumeral amputee, all muscles about the shoulder need emphasis, particularly the abductors and extensors.

It is important in the transhumeral and higher-level amputee to educate and acquaint the patient with the movement known as biscapular abduction as early as possible. This motion is not commonly used by normal adults to perform any activity of daily living and therefore most amputees find this difficult to learn at first. In addition, shoulder elevation and depression may also be introduced.

Compression Wrapping. Although the upper limb amputation site is not a weight-bearing residuum, there is a need to apply consistent compressive dressings in order to reduce volume and remove edema from the residual limb. This may be done using a compression bandage or stump shrinker. If a compression bandage is used, it is best applied in a figure 8 fashion similar to that done for TT amputees. The keys to any compression wrap are to apply pressure more distally than proximally, to make oblique turns rather than circular turns, and to complete coverage of the limb as quickly as possible. In the shorter transhumeral amputations, it may be necessary to incorporate some compression bandage around the other axilla to secure and suspend the wrap. It is important in the long transradial and the long transhumeral residual limbs not to choke the remaining extremity by circumferential pressure creating a tourniquet. In the shoulder disarticulation or forequarter level, wrapping may serve primarily to hold surgical dressings in place rather than to promote any great amount of volume reduction.

Preparatory Prostheses. Preparatory prostheses in the upper limb are perhaps more important than in the lower limbs and certainly the timing of such prostheses is critical. In elective surgical cases, preparatory prostheses need to be discussed with amputees prior to amputation so that they understand the goals as well as the specific details of the hardware to be used. Studies by Malone, Burkhalter, and others indicate there may be a critical period of time following unilateral upper limb amputation in which preparatory prostheses must be fitted. If upper limb amputees are allowed to develop one-handed skills and are not fitted early with temporary or preparatory prostheses, the likelihood of those amputees wearing and using an upper limb prosthesis is significantly reduced. Malone et al reported on elective amputations done for brachial plexus injuries where myoelectrically controlled prostheses were delivered promptly, in a preparatory system, allowing the client to quickly learn the control and use of the prosthesis. In nonelective upper limb amputations, it is often difficult to fit early prostheses to patients with multiple skin flaps or staged procedures. However, it is still important that patients be fitted as soon as medically indicated with preparatory prostheses.

Preparatory prostheses may be made of plaster, plastic, or any of the newer resin-impregnated casting materials. The length of these devices is not absolutely critical. It is critical for these devices to be functionally a part of the amputee's early rehabilitation program. In addition to beginning the process of residual limb maturation and exercise, temporary or preparatory prostheses may assist the amputee in activities of daily living such as feeding, dressing, or helping in the room while still in the hospital or at home following discharge.

To maximize the chances for a successful functional fitting of an upper limb prosthesis, a check socket is frequently utilized. Check sockets may be made of several materials. Included in this group are plaster or clear plastics such as Surlyn. It is important that the prosthetist evaluate the height and position of the trim lines so that any compromise between range of motion, suspension, and function can be made and, more importantly, be understood by the amputee prior to the final delivery of the prosthesis. Once the check socket has been fitted and evaluated by both prosthetist and patient, a positive model is made from the check socket and the definitive prosthesis is made from that positive model.

REFERENCES

1. Atkins DK, Donovan WH, Muilenberg A. Retrospective analysis of 87 children and adults fitted with electric prosthetic componentry (abstract). *J Assoc Child Prosthet Orthot Clin.* 1993; 28:2.
2. Bender LF. *Prostheses and Rehabilitation After Arm Amputation.* Springfield, IL: Charles C. Thomas; 1974.
3. Billock JN. The Northwestern University supracondylar suspension technique for below-elbow amputations. *Orthot Prosthet.* 1972; 26(4):16–23.
4. Billock JN. Upper limb prosthetic management hybrid design approaches. *Clin Prosthet Orthot.* 1985; 9(1):23–25.
5. Bunnell S. *Surgery of the Hand,* 3rd. ed. Philadelphia: Lippincott; 1956.
6. Burkhalter WE, Hampton FL, Smeitzer JA. Wrist disarticulation and below-elbow amputation. In: *Atlas of Limb Prosthetics, AAOS.* Saint Louis: Mosby; 1981; 183–191.
7. Childress D. Historical aspects of powered limb prostheses. *Clin Prosthet Orthot.* 1985; 9(1):2–13.
8. Childress DS, Billock JN. An experiment with the control of a hybrid prosthetic system: Electric elbow, body-powered hook. *Bull Prosthet Res.* 1970; 10(14):62–77.
9. Childress DS, Billock JN. Self-containment and self-suspension of externally powered prostheses for the forearm. *Bull Prosthet Res.* 1970; 10(14):4–21.
10. Dalsey R, Gomez W, Seitz WH et al. Myoelectric prosthetic replacement in the upper-extremity amputee. *Orthop Rev.* 1989; 18:697–702.
11. Dorcas DS, Scott RN. A three-state myo-electric control. *Med Biol Eng.* 1966; 4:367–370.
12. Fishman S, Kay HW. Munster-type below-elbow socket, an evaluation. *Artificial Limbs.* 1964; 8(2):4–14.
13. Fryer CM, Michael JW. Body-powered Components. In: Bowker JH, Michael JW, eds. *Atlas of Limb Prosthetics,* 3rd ed. St Louis: Mosby-Yearbook; 1992.
14. Gaine WJ, Smart C, Bransby-Zachary M. Upper limb traumatic amputees: Review of prosthetic use. *J Hand Surg.* 1997; 22B:73–76.
15. Glattly HW. A statistical study of 12,000 new amputees. *South Med J.* 1964; 57(1):1373–1378.
16. Haag GM, Klasson B. Miniaturized electronic event counter. *Scand J Rehab Med.* 1978; 60(suppl 6):28–32.
17. Kanas J, Weaver S. Toddler use of a switch controlled electric hand shoulder disarticulation prostheses. A case study (abstract). *J Assoc Child Prosthet Orthot Clin.* 1990; 25:29.
18. Kay HW, Newman JD. Relative incidence of new amputations. *Orthot Prosthet.* 1975; 29(2):3–16.
19. Lake C. Effects of prosthetic training on upper-extremity prosthesis use. *J Prosthet Orthot.* 1997; 9:3–9.
20. LeBlanc M. Use of prosthetic prehensors. *Prosthet Orthot Int.* 1988, 12:152–154.
21. Madigan RR, Fillauer KD. 3–S prosthesis: A preliminary report. *J Pediatr Orthop.* 1991; 11:112–117.

22. Malone JH, Childers SJ, Underwood J, Leal JH. Immediate postsurgical management of upper-extremity amputations: Conventional, electric, and myoelectric prosthesis. *Orthot Prosthet.* 1981; 35(2):1–9.

23. Marquardt E, Fisk JR. Thalidomide children: Thirty years later. *J Assoc Child Prosthet Orthot Clin.* 1992; 27:3–10.

24. McDonnell PM, Scott RN, McKay LA. Incidence of congenital upper-limb deficiencies. *JRBK J Assoc Child Prosthet Orthot Clin.* 1988; 23:8–14.

25. Meier RH. Upper limb amputee rehabilitation. *Phys Med Rehabil: State Art Rev.* 1994; 8:165–185.

26. Melendez D, LeBlanc M. Survey of arm amputees not wearing prostheses: Implications for research and service. *J Assoc Child Prosthet Orthot Clin.* 1988; 23:62–69.

27. Meletiou S. The functional outcome of the wrist disarticulation: A long-term follow-up. Unpublished.

28. Meredith JM. Comparison of three myoelectrically controlled prehensors and the voluntary-opening split hook. *Am J Occup Ther.* 1994; 48:932–937.

29. Michael JW, Gailey RS, Bowker JH. New developments in recreational prostheses and adaptive devices for the amputee. *Clin Orthop.* 1990; 256:64–75.

30. Michael JW. Amputations. In: *Orthopaedics: A Study Guide.* Spivak J et al, 1999.

31. Michael JW. Upper limb powered components and controls: Current concepts. *Clin Prosthet Orthot.* 1986; 10:66–77

32. Millstein S, Heger H, Hunter G. A review of the failures in use of the below elbow myoelectric prosthesis. *Orthot Prosthet.* 1982; 36(2):29–34.

33. Nader M. The artificial substitution of missing hands with myoelectrical prostheses. *Clin Orthop.* 1990; 258:9–17.

34. Neal M. Coming to grips with artificial hand design. *Design Eng.* 1993; March: 26–27, 29, 32, 34.

35. Neilsen PE et al. Arterial blood pressure in the skin measured by a photoelectric probe and external counterpressure. *Vasa.* 1973; 2:35.

36. Northmore-Ball et al. The below elbow myoelectric prosthesis: A comparison of the Otto Bock myoelectric prosthesis with the hook and functional hand. *J Bone Joint Surg (Br).* 1980; 62:363–367.

37. Parker PA, Scott RN. Myoelectric control of prostheses. *Crit Rev Biomed Eng.* 1995; 13:283–310.

38. Pinzur MS, Anbelats J, Light TR et al. Functional outcome following traumatic upper limb amputation and prosthetic limb fitting. *J Hand Surg.* 1994; 19A:836–839.

39. Radocy R, Beiswenger WD. A high-performance variable-suspension, transradial (below-elbow) prosthesis. *J Prosthet Orthot.* 1995; 7:65–67.

40. Sears HH, Shaperman J. Proportional myoelectric hand control: An evaluation. *Am J Phys Med Rehabil.* 1991; 70:20–28.

41. Sears HH. Approaches to prescription of body-powered and myoelectric prostheses. *Phys Med Rehabil Clin North Am.* 1991; 2:361–371.

42. Shurr DG, Cooper RR, Buckwalter JA, Blair WF. Juvenile amputees classification and revision rates. *Orthot Prosthet.* 1982; 36:23.

43. Shurr DG, Cooper RR, Buckwalter JA, Blair WF. The terminal transverse congenital deficiency of the forearm. *Orthotics & Prosthetics.* 1981; 3:22–25.

44. Sorbye R: Myoelectric prosthetic fitting in young children. *Clin Orthop.* 1980; 148:34–40.

45. Stack DM, McDonnell PM. Conditioning 1–6 month old infants by means of myoelectrically controlled reinforcement. *Int J Rehabil Res.* 1995; 18:151–156.

46. Stein RB, Waller M. Functional comparison of upper limb amputees using myoelectric and conventional prostheses. *Arch Phys Med Rehabil.* 1983; 64:243–248.

47. Taylor C. The biomechanics of the normal and of the amputated upper extremity. In: *Human Limbs and Their Substitutes.* Klopsteig PE, Wilson PD, eds. New York: McGraw-Hill; 1954; 169–221.

48. Tooms RE. Amputation surgery in the upper limb. *Orthop Clin North Amer.* 1972; 3(2):383–395.

49. Torres MM. Incidence and causes of limb amputations. *Phys Med Rehabil: State Art Rev.* 1994; 8:1–8.

50. Trost FJ. A long term follow-up on amputees with myoelectric prostheses (abstract). *J Assoc Child Prosthet Orthot Clin.* 1993; 28:30

51. Williams TW. One-muscle infant's myoelectric control. *J Assoc Child Prosthet Orthot Clin.* 1989; 24(2/3):53–56.

52. Winkler W, Bierwirth W. Eine klinische studie uber die automatisierte griffsteuerung mit dem suva-sensor (A clinical study on an automatic grip control devices using the suva-sensor). *Orthop Tech.* 1996; 47:955–957.

53. Wright TW, Hagen AD, Wood MB. Prosthetic usage in upper extremity amputations. *J Hand Surg.* 1995; 20A:619–622.

CHAPTER 8

Lower Limb Orthoses

Steel, and then aluminum, became the materials of choice for leg orthoses from the 1920s until 1968. Such braces, worn by Franklin D. Roosevelt, were hand-made by the highly skilled orthotists of that era who fashioned each individual part from raw metal stock. The knee joints locked while the ankles allowed free motion in dorsiflexion but prevented plantarflexion beyond 90 degrees. All cuffs were lined with leather, and straps and buckles provided the closures.

Roosevelt's leg braces

Stricken with polio at the prime of his life, Franklin Roosevelt did not let his disability deter him from realizing remarkable achievements. Exercise, particularly swimming, became a vital part of Roosevelt's treatment and general conditioning. As early as the summer of 1923, he wrote to a friend:

"During the past six weeks I have been swimming three times a week—first in the Astor pool and lately in the pond on our place. The legs work wonderfully in the water and I need nothing artificial to keep myself afloat. As a matter of fact I see continuous improvement in my knees and feet. When I left Boston I understood [Dr.] Lovett to say that I need use the braces only for convenience, and I have therefore worn them very little; especially as my arms are so strong that I hoist myself about from chair to chair. However, Eleanor is just back from Newport where she saw Lovett, and he seemed horrified that I had not worn them more. Hence, I shall begin the strenuous life and the braces again. Honestly, I think the rest from them has been a good thing for these six weeks, and has done me not a particle of harm."

On loan from the National Archives and Records Administration, Franklin D. Roosevelt Library, Hyde Park, New York

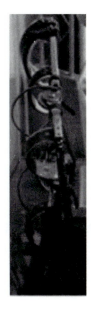

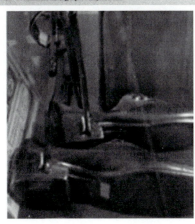

Following completion of reading this chapter, the student will be able to:

1. Differentiate among the terms custom fitted, custom fabricated, and pre-fabricated when describing lower limb orthoses.
2. Discuss the concept of total contact orthoses.
3. Discuss three types of hip orthoses used for pathologies of the hip.
4. Discuss the importance of the ground reaction forces when using a knee-ankle-foot orthosis (KAFO) with an unlocked knee joint.

As was explained in chapter 1, by international agreement, orthoses are named by the body segments encompassed. Shuch and Pritham have concisely summarized this terminology in their 1995 article. To insure that the prescribed orthosis is clinically useful to the patient, it is equally important for rehabilitation professionals to have both clear functional goals as well as realistic biomechanical control expectations. Although decisions about the fabrication details are usually best left to the orthotist's discretion, all clinic team members need a basic understanding of the issues involved. This chapter will highlight the basic considerations leading to the selection of a specific orthosis for a particular client, and offer examples of commonly encountered designs to illustrate application of these principles.

FUNCTIONAL GOALS

Lower limb orthoses can offer one or more of the following functions:

1. Maintenance or correction of body segment alignment
2. Assistance or resistance to joint motion
3. Axial loading of the orthosis and therefore relief of distal weight bearing forces
4. Protection against physical insult

It is imperative that every orthosis prescribed can be described using at least one of the goals previously listed. If not, then it is highly likely that the orthosis will fail to satisfy the clinic team's expectations. Prescription of an orthosis without a clear functional goal in mind is the most common cause for failure of the orthosis to achieve the desired outcome. Consultation with the ABC certified orthotist is recommended prior to finalizing the prescription whenever the goals or biomechanical function expected are not completely clear.

BIOMECHANICAL CONTROL OPTIONS

Once the general functional goals have been determined, then the biomechanical control options necessary to reach these goals can be specified. Because most orthoses influence one or more skeletal articulations, it is generally useful to specify the type of joint control desired, as shown in Table 8-1.

TABLE 8-1. BIOMECHANICAL CONTROL OPTIONS

Permit free motion (in one plane)
Enhance desired motion
Resist undesired motion
Limit motion (to a fixed or variable range)
Stop motion (removable stop = lock)

Source: Michael, JW. Orthotic treatment of neurologic deficits. In: *Handbook of Neurorehabilitation.* Couch J, Good D, eds. New York: Marcel Dekker, Inc; 1994.

As Perry has noted, the orthosis should ideally only control pathological movements, carefully avoiding interference with normal or compensatory motion. For that reason, the available joint controls are listed in descending order of preference—from the least restrictive to the most restrictive. Biotechnical matching of the design of the orthosis to the individual's needs is a difficult challenge as there are often no strict guidelines. Collaborative discussion between experienced rehabilitation team members has proven to be the most effective method to make such clinical judgments.

MAJOR IMPAIRMENTS TREATED WITH ORTHOSES

Table 8-2 lists common impairments that are frequently managed effectively with orthoses. It should be noted, however, that there are no diagnosis specific orthotic devices; the notion of cerebral palsy braces is now recognized as obsolete. Modern orthoses are prescribed based on their biomechanical capabilities to reduce or eliminate the pertinent functional deficits in each individual case.

The Moss Rehabilitation Hospital in Philadelphia notes that this is only possible based on an accurate and complete evaluation of the patient's current capabilities, taking into account the prognosis for a given condition to improve, remain stable, or worsen over time. Use of a standardized form can aid in recording all necessary information in a concise format. It is crucial to thoroughly understand the relationship between the patient's clinical performance and the physical findings. In particular, the rehabilitation team must clearly distinguish between

TABLE 8-2. MAJOR IMPAIRMENTS REQUIRING LOWER LIMB ORTHOSES

Problems at Birth	Diseases	Trauma
Cerebral palsy	Cerebral vascular accident	Spinal cord injury
Spina bifida	Muscular dystrophy	Fracture
Long bone malformations	Arthritis	Head injuries
Hemophilia	Multiple sclerosis	Muscle, cartilage, and tendon
Osteogenesis imperfecta	Scoliosis	rupture
Club foot	Legg-Calvè-Perthes	
	Poliomyelitis	

Source: Adapted from *Lower Limb Orthotics, A Manual.* Philadelphia, Pa: Rehabilitation Engineering Center, 1978.

primary functional losses and volitional or compensatory deviations, because the latter does not require orthotic management.

Even when the orthosis successfully mitigates the primary loss, it is often helpful for the therapist to teach the patient explicitly that the compensation is no longer needed. For example, some individuals may persist in flexing the hip joint excessively (to increase ground clearance of the limb in the swing phase) based on years of habituation to untreated flaccid ankle equinus even though a plastic leaf-spring orthosis now brings the foot to neutral reliably with every step. Such compensations typically decrease gradually over time, but the extinction of such energy-consuming habits is hastened by good therapy training.

FABRICATION CONSIDERATIONS

Once a clear, functional, biomechanically feasible purpose has been determined for the orthosis, it must then be designed and fabricated or selected from available alternatives, and then fitted properly to the patient. Such technical factors are generally the domain of the experienced orthotist, but it is useful for all rehabilitation personnel to have a basic understanding of the choices involved.

Prefabrication Versus Custom Fabrication

The first decision is whether a prefabricated device might be adequate or if a custom-made orthosis is required. In general, simple problems and temporary impairments may be amenable to treatment using prefabricated orthoses, provided the overall shape of the limb is essentially normal and protective sensation is present. Absence of sensation or the existence of significant physical deformity are general contraindications to the use of premade orthoses due to the risk of iatrogenic injury to the patient from a poorly fitting device.

Prefabricated devices are further subdivided into those provided without alteration in standard sizes (often available off the shelf (OTS) from pharmacy or medical equipment stores) and those requiring significant alterations to custom fit them to the patient. Soft supports available in several sizes, right or left, are a common example of OTS prefab devices. For short-term applications where minimal support is required, such devices may be sufficient, and they are comparatively inexpensive.

Most custom-fitted prefabricated orthoses are made from a high-temperature thermoplastic material (such as polypropylene) which can be trimmed, sanded, polished, and remolded with local heating to optimize the fit for an individual patient's anatomy. Probably the most common application of this level of technology would be the provision of a prefabricated plastic AFO in the presence of recent peroneal palsy that is expected to resolve. The misuse of such devices by delivering them unaltered, particularly when done by personnel who lack the training and laboratory equipment to modify them appropriately, is a deplorable waste of health care resources that should be avoided.

For definitive treatment, custom-made orthoses are generally preferred because they fit more precisely and therefore provide superior biomechanical control to prefabricated solutions. Particularly when significant fixed deformity is present, it may be less costly to create a custom orthosis rather than to extensively modify a prefabricated one.

Custom Made-to-Measurement Versus Custom Made-to-Patient Model

Custom orthoses may be further categorized as to whether they are made based on measurements of the involved limb segment or based on a three-dimensional impression of the body part. Although plaster-of-Paris bandages have been traditionally used to create an intimate impression of the limbs and trunk, use of various electronic digitizing techniques is gradually becoming viable as an alternative. Regardless of the input source, careful fabrication of the orthosis followed by meticulous custom fitting to the individual's needs are the hallmarks of the provision of quality orthotic care.

In the lower limb, measurements are frequently used to create a blueprint for a minimal contact orthosis consisting of small bands that contact the body, connected to rigid bars of metal alloy that stabilize the orthosis. Originally made from very heavy steel, such orthoses are now made from lighter alloys of aluminum or titanium whenever feasible. The minimal contact style of orthosis has the general advantages of being cooler in hot weather and accommodating fluctuating limb volumes fairly well, due to the small surface area in contact with the leg. Metal alloys are also quite rigid.

A three-dimensional positive model (usually of plaster) is the foundation for the fabrication of total contact-style orthoses. Although use of thermoplastic materials is common, such devices may also be laminated from thermosetting resins with appropriate internal reinforcement fibers. Thermoplastic orthoses are commonly preferred by the patients because the large surface area in contact with the body makes them thin, light, and requires less pressure for a given amount of biomechanical control provided. Thermoplastics offer toughness and flexibility in many orthotic applications as well.

Of course, an orthosis can be created with whatever degree of contact is necessary, so these distinctions are not absolute. Hybridization, combining the versatility of custom-molded plastic shells with the rigidity of metal joints, is increasingly common. Finally, the growing utilization of laminated carbon fiber-reinforced orthoses worldwide promises to blur these traditional distinctions even further.

EXAMPLES OF ORTHOSES

This section of the chapter will highlight selected orthoses to illustrate the range of options available. It is not intended to be a comprehensive review of all possible orthoses.

Foot Orthoses

The foot is the foundation for the lower limb, and proper positioning of the ankle-foot complex is the sine qua non of lower limb orthotic management. As a general rule, alignment of the foot with the calcaneus centered beneath the talus is recommended whenever appropriate, because, as Root states, this has traditionally been considered to be a neutral posture. Carlson and Berglund report that when the foot cannot be passively placed in the desired position, then the foot orthosis (FO) serves as a "shim" to bridge the distance from the fixed position of the sole of the foot to the floor.

The shoe is an important adjunct in the orthotic management of lower limb pathologies. Poorly fitted or badly designed shoes must be avoided because they can diminish or negate the effectiveness of even a well-fitted orthosis. On the other hand, as noted by Helland, a properly designed shoe can enhance orthotic function and provide significant support to the involved limb. Custom-made shoes, which have an interior that is molded to a model of the affected foot, may be considered a subset of FOs because they provide equivalent functional support. Placing a custom-made FO within a commercially made shoe is less costly, when feasible.

In addition to the treatment of structural deformities from disease or injury, custom foot orthoses are commonly utilized to reduce the risk of ulceration when insensitivity is present due to diabetic or other neuropathies. Glancy has observed that they may also be of value in the treatment of athletes when the repetitive stresses of competition or training result in various pain syndromes. Chapter 11 will review this specialty area within orthotic practice in more detail.

Ankle-Foot Orthoses
The AFO is probably the most commonly utilized lower limb orthosis in clinical practice. Although the traditional metal and leather braces are still used selectively in North America, they have been largely superseded by custom-molded plastic devices in recent years.

Single and Double Bar AFOs
Metal and leather AFOs typically consist of one or more bands covering half the circumference of the lower leg, connected to the shoe, usually with some type of hinge or joint at the ankle. Single bar designs are common in pediatrics while the double bar style predominates in adults due to its greater inherent strength (Figure 8-1).

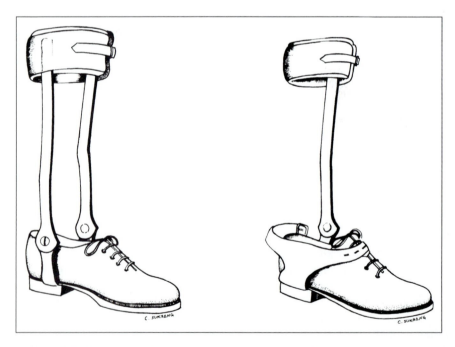

Figure 8-1. Traditional dual bar and single bar metal minimal contact design ankle-foot orthoses attached to shoes. The single bar AFO has a leather T-strap to provide a medially-directed corrective force at the ankle.

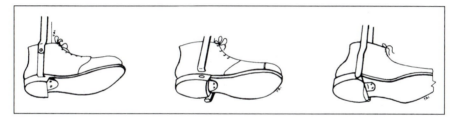

Figure 8-2. Shoe attachment options for traditional AFOs.

The metal superstructure may be attached permanently to the shoe via the "stirrup," which is a U-shaped piece of metal secured permanently between the heel and sole of the shoe. Particularly when combined with an extended steel shank reinforcing the sole of the shoe, this is the strongest construction and therefore preferred for many heavy-duty applications. The superstructure may be removable if a caliper plate or split stirrup is provided, which makes donning and doffing and interchanging shoes much easier. For many patients, having the orthosis attached to the shoe itself is inconvenient and undesirable (Figure 8-2). As noted by Bensman and Lossing, a hybrid orthosis with a molded plastic FO attached to the metal superstructure is one design that provides orthotic control independently of the footwear chosen, and the more intimately fitted contours of the total contact style foot section can provide enhanced varus or valgus control of the subtalar joint (Figure 8-3).

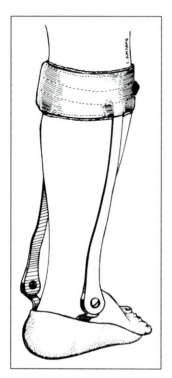

Figure 8-3. An example of a hybrid design with a molded thermoplastic foot segment attached to a double bar metal superstructure.

These orthoses are typically fabricated with a double-adjustable ankle joint, as shown in Figure 8-4. The anterior and posterior channels in the ankle joint affect dorsiflexion and plantarflexion motion respectively. If the channels are open, then free sagittal plane motion is permitted. Placing a spring in the channel, which pushes against the stirrup, adds an assist/resist to the motion. Introducing a rigid pin in the channel limits motion to the desired range or eliminates it altogether. The spring resistance and the position of the limiting pins can be incrementally varied using the adjustment screws that close the top of each channel. As Shurr has observed, these myriad ankle control options make orthoses utilizing this joint among the most easily adjustable options available.

Prefabricated "training braces" using ankle joints of these types are sometimes used for evaluation purposes with different patients. Unfortunately, the inadequate fit and excessive flexibility of such one-size-fits-all devices degrades the biomechanical control provided and permits only a very gross approximation of the function that can be expected from a well-fitted and properly fabricated custom orthosis. For this reason, most experienced rehabilitation teams rely on the judgment and experience of the clinic team and find such temporary devices of very limited value.

Total Contact AFOs

Ankle-foot orthoses made from high temperature thermoplastic, molded intimately to a rectified positive model of the affected limb, are commonly provided and offer excellent clinical results for a broad spectrum of biomechanical deficits. Patient acceptance is high due to the light weight (150–200 grams average) comfort, control, and relatively cosmetic appearance offered by such devices. By careful selection of the plastic material and its thickness, as well as the fabrication technique and trimlines, the orthotist is able to provide a wide range of biomechanical control to meet individual needs. Figure 8-5 illustrates three functionally different AFOs all made from polypropylene material.

The "trimline" refers to the edges of the orthosis (Figure 8-6). As a general rule, the farther the orthosis encompasses the limb segment circumference, the more rigidly it resists motion. Showers and David were among the first to observe that selective reinforcement of critical areas is also possible using specialized contours or by adding various reinforcement materials prior to fabrication.

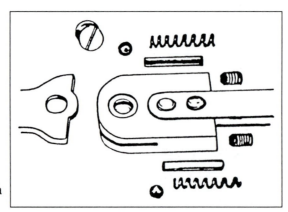

Figure 8-4. Elements of a double-adjustable ankle joint.

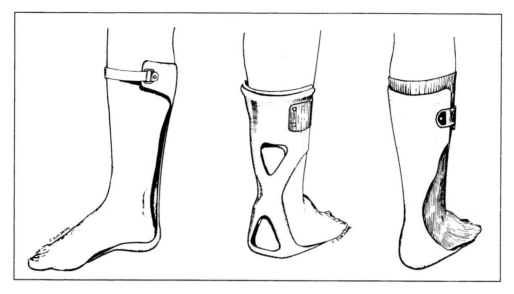

Figure 8-5. Variations in the thickness and contours of the plastic material significantly alter the biomechanical function the AFO provides. The polypropylene orthoses depicted here provide dorsiflexion assistance but vary in the amount of coronal plane stability offered.

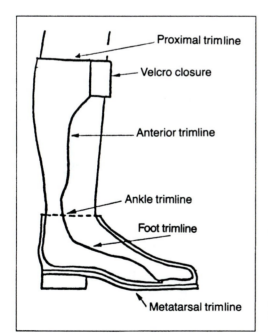

Proximal trimline

Velcro closure

Anterior trimline

Ankle trimline

Foot trimline

Metatarsal trimline

Figure 8-6. Trimlines in these key areas affect the stiffness and range of mobility permitted within the orthosis. (*Source:* Adapted from *Lower Limb Orthotics.* Rehabilitation Engineering Center, Moss Rehabilitation Hospital, Philadelphia, 1978.)

The primary limitations to total contact plastic AFOs are that they cannot accommodate large volume fluctuations and that they are inherently warmer to wear than minimal contact designs. Although early reports from McCollough and others advised that the original primitive designs were too flexible to manage pronounced spasticity, more recent authors including Rogers and Vanderbilt report that contemporary innovations have demonstrated conclusively that the ability to increase the circumferential containment makes total contact designs the preferred approach in such cases.

Articulated Plastic AFOs

In recent decades, much work has been done to expand the applicability of plastic total contact AFOs. The use of plastic AFOs incorporating various ankle joints is increasing in popularity, particularly for pediatric applications, largely due to the excellent clinical acceptance by the patients who use them. Figure 8-7 illustrates the inherent versatility of this design when applied to dynamically changing conditions such as gait recovery following cerebral vascular accidents.

In this illustrative example, the foot segment is initially rigidly anchored to the tibial shell posteriorly. By temporarily loosening the machine screw and inserting the wedge deeper, prior to tightening the fastener, the clinician can vary the dorsiflexion angle incrementally. Such an adjustable solid ankle AFO is often useful in preventing extensor or flexor synergy patterning that is common early in stroke recovery.

Presuming the patient's volitional control gradually returns, it is often possible to loosen the machine screw slightly thereby allowing a limited range of motion. The patient can then practice controlling the ankle voluntarily, secure in the knowledge that the limited motion AFO will prevent them from entering into that range of ankle motion that will trigger their spasticity.

In some cases, voluntary control gradually improves but the knee sometimes snaps back into hyperextension in late stance phase. Discarding the machine screw and wedge converts

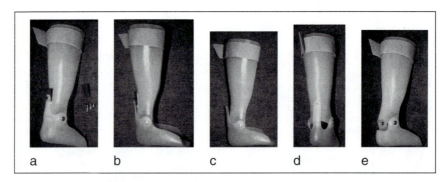

Figure 8-7. An example of an articulated plastic AFO that can be altered to provide progressively less control as the patient's condition improves. a = solid ankle design with adjustable dorsiflexion angle. b = AFO allowing a limited range of ankle motion in the sagittal plane. c = AFO with plantarflexion stop. d = AFO with plantarflexion resist. e = AFO with free sagittal plane motion to control the swing phase inversion/eversion.

the articulated AFO into a design that provides a plantarflexion stop and allows dorsiflexion motion. This can be useful to provide a kinesthetic reminder to the patient when the knee starts to hyperextend, from the pressure against the calf of the posterior shell, while the free dorsiflexion movement helps keep the gastroc-soleus complex from contracting. If the posterior tab that stops plantarflexion motion is trimmed into a thin strip, it then acts as a spring resist and the device becomes a plantarflexion resist/free dorsiflexion AFO.

Ideally, the patient eventually recovers full volitional control over their limb during the stance phase, but some swing phase inversion often persists, and results in initial contact on the lateral border of the foot. Trimming the posterior overlap off the footplate now allows unrestricted sagittal plane motion while holding the foot in a neutral position throughout the gait cycle in the coronal plane. In this configuration, the device is an AFO offering free sagittal plane motion while controlling inversion/eversion.

Although Ford, Grotz, and Shamp originally described a progressive neurophysiological design for CVA management, any of these AFO configurations are appropriate for a variety of pathological conditions presenting similar biomechanical deficits. This case example illustrates the functional versatility of these total contact, articulated orthoses.

Floor Reaction AFO

Orthotist Jimmy Saltiel of Israel designed an orthosis for himself that permitted safe ambulation despite complete paralysis of his knee, ankle, and foot secondary to poliomyelitis. His insight was to use ground reaction forces generated by a solid ankle AFO to prevent his knee from collapsing into flexion. A schematic is depicted in Figure 8-8. The trimlines anterior to the malleoli result in a very rigid device. Contact of the anterior foot plate during stance generates a ground reaction force that acts to hold the broad anterior panel firmly against the proximal shin. Much like having the palm of one's hand pushing against the tibia with every step, this force resists forward tibial motion and thereby discourages knee collapse.

As Yang et al have observed, this illustrates a very important but often subtle principle in the biomechanics of orthoses: The device often influences the next higher biological joint, and this can be used for therapeutic purposes in selected cases. Saltiel's brilliant application of this principle has now helped tens of thousands of people worldwide who might otherwise have received the logical, but biomechanically unnecessary, knee-ankle-foot orthosis (KAFO) with a locked knee to manage their leg paralysis. Colloquially termed the "floor reaction AFO," Harrington et al have proposed that it be configured to allow free plantarflexion in cases where the pretibial muscles remain functional, and that variant is termed an "articulated floor reaction" AFO (Figure 8-9).

Yang et al also noted that prerequisites for successful application of such ground reaction orthoses include a biologically stable knee, the absence of any significant knee contractures, a cooperative patient, and good voluntary hip extensors on the involved side. If any of these essentials are absent, use of a knee-ankle-foot orthosis is indicated. Whenever a solid ankle orthosis is provided, Glancy and Lindseth suggest that careful consideration should be given to modifying the sole of the shoe using a soft heel and rocker sole, to optimize the patient's gait.

Unweighting AFO Designs

Other examples of specialized AFOs would be those designed to partially unweight the ankle or foot by transferring some of the vertical loading onto the orthosis. According to McIlmurray

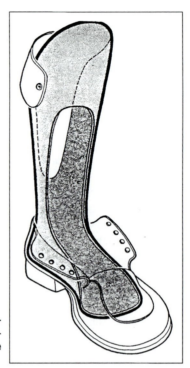

Figure 8-8. One configuration of a solid ankle AFO designed to stabilize the knee using ground reaction forces.

and Greenbaum these were originally termed Patellar Tendon Bearing or PTB orthoses, based on the assumption that prosthetic weight-bearing principles could be applied to non-amputated limbs (Figure 8-10), but studies by Lehmann et al now make it clear that circumferential containment and restriction of ankle motion are the primary features that unload the ankle rather than the contours about the knee per se.

Carlson et al recently reported a resurgence in interest in a lace-closure orthosis that uses the inverted cone contour of the distal calf musculature to unweight the ankle-foot complex, as shown in Figure 8-11. Figure 8-12 illustrates a specialized design utilizing a bivalve shin closure in combination with a forefoot support platform to fully unload the calcaneus bilaterally. The small platform extensions that contact the floor are called "patten bottoms." They transmit the ground reaction forces from the floor to the shell structure of the orthoses.

Figure 8-9. Articulated AFO that allows free plantarflexion, but limits dorsiflexion. This articulated floor reaction design is only feasible if the patient can actively dorsiflex the foot voluntarily.

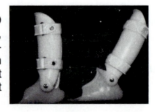

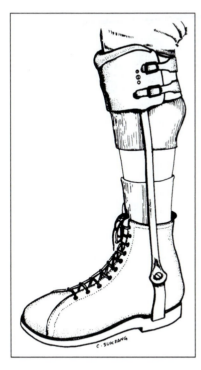

Figure 8-10. Traditional PTB AFO attached to a high-top shoe reduces stress and loading on the foot and ankle. Biomechanically similar designs of total contact thermoplastic materials are more common today.

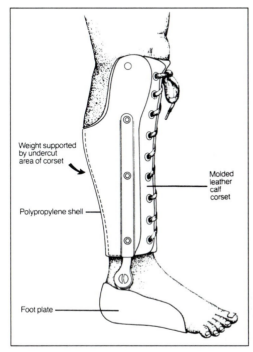

Weight supported by undercut area of corset

Molded leather calf corset

Polypropylene shell

Foot plate

Figure 8-11. Calf corset style AFO partially unweights the ankle and foot by transferring weight bearing forces onto the gastroc-soleus musculature.

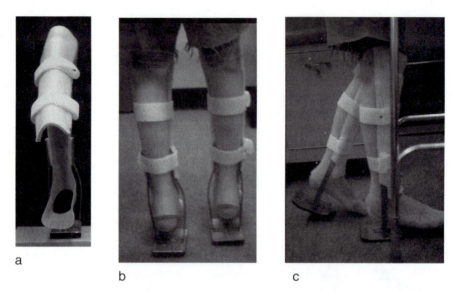

a

b   c

Figure 8-12. An alligator-mouth design solid ankle AFO, so named because of the way the hinged anterior panel opens for donning and doffing. The heel cutout insures that the calcaneous is non-weight bearing, as the forces are transmitted from the patten bottom on the ground through the side bars and onto the shin musculature. The forefoot plate also allows some weight bearing through the talus.

KNEE ORTHOSES

Knee orthoses (KOs) were originally intended only to support damaged joints and were custom molded to a model of the affected leg. The lever arms were as long as was physically possible to decrease the force per unit area as much as possible and the intimately fitted contours inherently provided three dimensional control.

In general, KOs should be used whenever the pathology is limited to the knee joint itself and the rest of the leg is essentially normal. Liu et al have documented that the longer the lever arms and the more rigid the hinges provided, the greater the biomechanical control the orthosis can offer. Virtually any musculoskeletal deficiency about the knee may be amenable to treatment with a knee orthosis, including genu varum, valgum, and recurvatum, as Hoffer et al have reported. Although dual sidebar designs predominate, studies by Lindenfeld et al have found that single upright designs can also be effective, particularly in providing enhanced mediolateral control.

KOs for Athletes

Along with the rise of sports medicine as a subspecialty, interest in using KOs for part-time protection during vigorous activities has increased in recent decades. As reported by Nicholas, this lead to a multitude of standardized configurations, originally popularized by the Lenox Hill proponents, and later to the development of literally hundreds of similar prefabricated designs. When KOs are used for such sports-related applications, they are often classified into somewhat arbitrary "rehabilitation" and "functional" genres, as noted by the *American Academy of Orthopaedic Surgeons,* in their classic text, *Atlas of Orthotics.*

A rehab KO is typically used immediately following reconstructive surgery to protect the repaired ligaments from overloads during the active healing phase. It is often worn only intermittently thereafter, primarily during sports competitions when the risk of reinjury is increased. Studies by Bos et al and others intended to document the effectiveness of custom-made KOs versus prefabricated designs have resulted in inconsistent findings to date. Functional KOs are often intended to be worn long term in lieu of surgical reconstruction of the damaged knee structures. The severity of the deficit and the magnitude of the activities attempted determine whether such KOs are worn full-time or only during selected activities. It is common to use knee joints that limit the range of motion at the knee in both of these applications.

The most controversial application of KOs in sports is the use of prophylactic braces intended to prevent injuries before they occur. Johnson and Paulos have observed that a spate of scientific studies offering conflicting conclusions about the effectiveness of using such devices for this purpose have been published recently. According to Levine et al, there is a clear consensus emerging that prefabricated orthoses with short lever arms or flexible joint bars are biomechanically incapable of providing significant protection in impact situations. In fact, although it can be demonstrated that a well-designed and well-fitted KO can significantly reduce the stresses on the knee under laboratory conditions, Lina et al advised it is not at all certain that this is sufficient to provide useful biomechanical protection in real-life situations. Some researchers, including McNair et al, have speculated that the sports KO may function, at least in part, by proprioceptively cueing the wearer, allowing them to use their muscle strength more effectively to stabilize the knee.

Non-Articulated KOs

As a general rule, non-articulated knee orthoses are intended for short-term use because the inability to bend the knee makes sitting and rising from a chair difficult. Probably the most common KO in this group is termed a knee immobilizer, because it circumferentially encompasses the leg and restricts knee motion in all directions. Prefabricated designs that use plastic or metal stiffeners inside a textile shell provide the least support, but may be sufficient for temporary support of mild sprains and strains. When more positive biomechanical control is required, or when better self-suspension is necessary, Pritham and Stills have reported that a custom-molded knee cylinder made from high temperature thermoplastic can be beneficial. The long leverage offered by intimate fitting from the ischium to the malleoli, and the self-suspension from contouring in the supracondylar fossa, account for the superior stabilization offered by this custom orthosis.

Another common prefabricated KO is sometimes called the Swedish knee cage, and is shown in Figure 8-13. Due to the very short lever arms, this device provides only minimal support. In addition, the *Atlas of Orthotics* notes that it has been criticized for its bulky appearance at the knee and protrusion of the bars above the thigh when sitting. Although sometimes used temporarily to provide limited resistance to genu recurvatum, this orthosis is rarely appropriate for long-term use. A variation with pivoting bands is available that offers improved cosmesis, but it suffers from the same leverage limitations.

Figure 8-14 illustrates a simple design consisting of two straight metal bars with swivel bands at each end that contact the leg posteriorly. This orthosis is sometimes premade but may

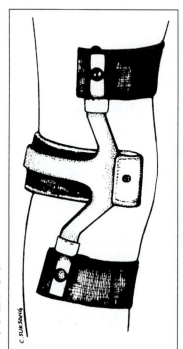

Figure 8-13. Despite the limited control offered by the short lever arms, the Swedish knee cage is sometimes used to provide mild resistance to genu recurvatum, particularly for short-term problems.

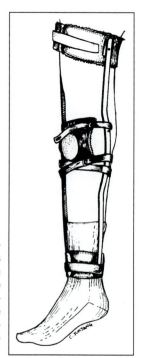

Figure 8-14. A simple knee orthosis consisting of swivel cuffs connected to solid bars can be used to temporarily stabilize the knee or to reduce knee flexion contractures. Tightening the anterior straps above and below the knee creates a powerful knee extension force.

be custom fabricated for best results. Adjustable anterior infrapatellar and suprapatellar straps (or the functionally equivalent "knee cap" pictured) stabilize the leg inside the orthosis. This design is sometimes used for temporary stabilization of the knee during preliminary ambulation training. In the presence of knee flexion contractures, the anterior straps can be gradually tightened over time, ideally immediately following manual ranging by the therapist, to gradually work out the contracture.

Off-The-Shelf KOs

Despite the manufacturer's sometimes flamboyant claims, OTS soft supports provide very limited biomechanical control of the knee. Elastic splints, in particular, function primarily as gentle reminders to favor the knee and as a covering to retain warmth from the body. One design using the counterforce of elastic straps to resist lateral patellar subluxation has been demonstrated to be effective in some cases.

Hinged prefab KOs are commonly used for short-term postoperative support, particularly during the initial healing phase. Even when metal hinges with stops are added, the knee is free to move several additional degrees under load due to deformation of the textile sleeve, so only gross motion is restricted.

KNEE-ANKLE-FOOT ORTHOSES

Conceptually, a KAFO consists of the combination of a KO and an AFO. Because the least orthosis necessary is the best orthosis, the use of KAFO and higher orthoses is only justified when a lesser device would be inadequate biomechanically.

Single and Double Bar KAFOs

As was the case with AFO designs, single bar styles are common in pediatric practice while the stronger double bar configuration is typical for adult applications. Such minimal contact orthoses share the advantages of the similar AFO designs: cooler in warm climates, able to accommodate some limb volume fluctuations, and rigidity from the strength of the side bars chosen.

Figure 8-15 depicts the biomechanical control options available in knee joints. The single axis or polycentric hinges allow a free range of normal knee motion in the sagittal plane; most incorporate hyperextension stops in the event the knee is suddenly overloaded in extension. The offset single axis joint is a special application that stabilizes the orthotic hinge in extension during stance phase by using ground reaction forces. When the leg is unweighted, the knee is free to flex normally during the swing phase. Figure 8-16 illustrates the most common application of this knee joint: as part of a KAFO designed to reduce (but not eliminate) genu recurvatum in the paralytic leg. Stabilizing the patient's knee in slight extension eliminates pain from distension of the posterior capsule while simultaneously insuring that the ground reaction force [GRF] is sufficiently anterior to stabilize the knee despite weak or absent quadriceps musculature.

When necessary, the knee can be locked during ambulation and unlocked for sitting. The ring or drop lock is probably the most commonly used design in the United States. As the knee reaches full extension in standing, gravity pulls the metal ring down around the hinge and prevents motion. It is manually unlocked when the wearer uses the hand to raise the lock. In some cases, a remote release via a cable or lever is provided.

Orthotic Knee Joint Options

	Examples	Biomechanical Control	Typical Application
Single Axis	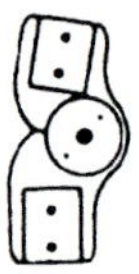	Coronal plane HOLD fixes genu varum-valgum; Saggital plane = Free flexion-extension; integral hyperextension stop	Mild to moderate genu varum or valgum
Offset	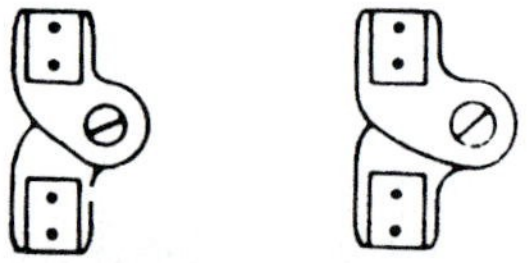	Coronal plane HOLD fixes genu varum-valgum; Saggital plane = Free flexion-extension; integral hyperextension stop	Moderate genu recurvatum
Polycentric	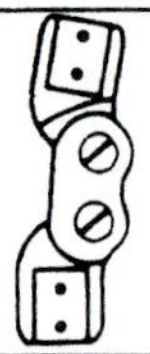	Coronal plane HOLD fixes genu varum-valgum; Saggital plane = Free flexion-extension; integral hyperextension stop	Usually, self-suspending orthoses - to track the knee axis more closely
Lock	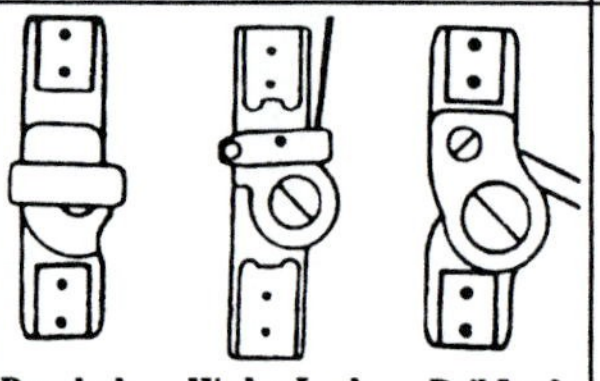 Droplock Wedge Lock Bail Lock	Coronal plane HOLD fixes genu varum-valgum; Saggital plane = removable LOCK in full extension	Paralysis, severe paresis, severe genu varum/valgum or recurvatum
Lock + Variable Flexion	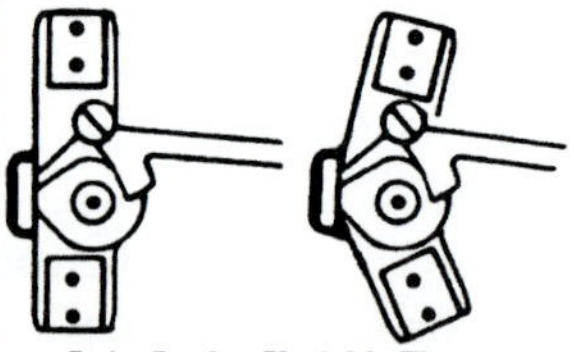 Swiss Lock + Variable Flexion	Coronal plane HOLD fixes genu varum-valgum; Saggital plane = removable LOCK, in variable degrees of flexion	Usually, spastic paralysis with reducible knee flexion contractures

Figure 8-15. Orthotic knee joints offer several basic biomechanical control options.

Another option is to link the locking joints with a flexible or rigid U-shaped bar that resembles the handle on a bucket. This characteristic appearance gave rise to the colloquial term bail lock. It is also sometimes referred to as a Swiss or Schweitzer style of locking joint.

Hahn described one special KAFO design developed at the Craig Rehabilitation Institute to allow adults and children with paraplegia to stand hands-free, by locking the knees in extension and the ankles in slight dorsiflexion. This Scott-Craig KAFO is depicted in Figure 8-17. One advantage to this minimal contact design is that it is easier for the person with paraplegia to apply than alternatives with posterior calf bands or plates. The chief disadvantage is that,

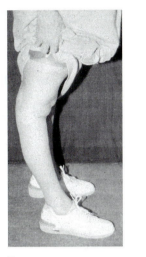
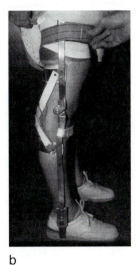
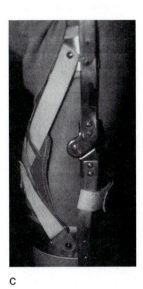

a

b

c

Figure 8-16. Offset knee joints depicted here allow the paralyzed knee to move into slight extension so the ground reaction force while walking will stabilize the knee; the joint stops and the posterior "sling" prevent further hyperextension. When the orthosis is unweighted during the swing phase, the knee can flex freely.

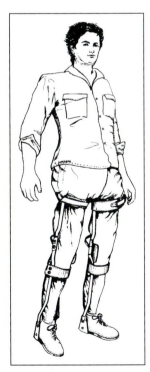

Figure 8-17. These Scott-Craig design KAFOs stabilize the lower limbs with the knees locked in extension and the ankles in a fixed, slightly dorsiflexed position. The shoes are specially reinforced to provide a stable base of support. This configuration allows the paraplegic individual hands-free standing, as depicted here, and also permits a swing-through gait with the use of forearm crutches.

for sufficient structural strength, the shoes and stirrups must be specially reinforced, which adds significant weight to these KAFOs.

Total Contact KAFOs

The use of total contact plastic shells in KAFO design is increasingly common worldwide. Analogous advantages to those inherent in the plastic AFO include lower pressures for a given magnitude of biomechanical control, and the thin, tough, flexible nature of the plastic material. It is common to make a hybrid orthosis that incorporates rigid metal alloy bars or their equivalent in carbon fiber reinforced plastic and metal knee and/or ankle joints. Figure 8-18 shows one example of a laminated carbon fiber KAFO illustrating one of a myriad of trimlines that are possible with modern engineered plastic construction.

Unweighting KAFOs

For many decades, experts such as Tacchdjian and Jouett and Curtis et al believed that partially unweighting the leg and holding it in abduction would reduce the risk of malformation of the femoral head in the presence of Legg-Calvè-Perthes disease. Shaw has described one example, the Toronto orthosis shown in Figure 8-19 developed at the Hugh MacMillan Centre. The awkward and energy-consuming gait that resulted, combined with the lack of any convincing outcome data, resulted in the gradual demise of these devices.

Occasionally, the use of an ischial containment or quadrilateral style brim is advocated to partially unweight the knee, shin, ankle, or foot. Due to the compressibility of the soft tissues in the thigh, this is often difficult to achieve, particularly in obese individuals. More frequently, adding such an intimately fitting proximal segment into the KAFO design will enhance rotational stability by encapsulating more of the pelvic bony structure in the device. This is often helpful when treating paraplegic limbs with severe atrophy following childhood disease processes such as poliomyelitis

Shaw and others originally believed that use of such prosthetic contours in orthoses designed to treat long bone fractures was essential. Later researchers such as Zucker have shown

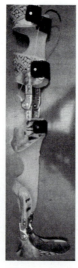

Figure 8-18. The high strength of modern reinforced plastics permits the orthotist to vary the trimlines according to the patient's functional needs, as illustrated by the laminated carbon fiber-reinforced KAFO shown here. (*Source:* Otto Bock Orthopedic Industry, Inc.)

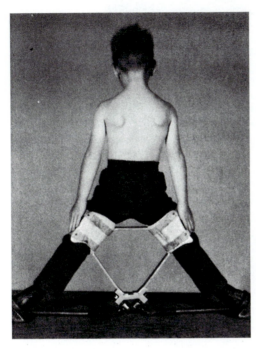

Figure 8-19. The Toronto orthosis is intended to hold the femurs in abduction and external rotation, to reduce the risk of femoral head deformation during the consolidation phase of Legg-Calvè-Perthes disease. It is uncommon today to use such extensive bracing.

that no external orthosis can prevent telescoping of unstable fragments, that secure circumferential containment provides the biomechanical control to biologically splint mid-shaft fractures, and that intermittent vertical loading on the bone actually enhances the healing process.

HIP ORTHOSES

Hip orthoses (HpO) are used most frequently to resist spastic adduction, to provide postoperative motion control following surgical hip replacement, or to treat hip dysplasias. Due to the volume of soft tissue about the torso and upper thigh, it is virtually impossible to prevent small degrees of hip motion in any direction or to provide significant rotational control of the lower limb.

Hip Dysplasia Orthoses

According to Fujioka et al, the Pavlik harness is the most popular orthosis for nonoperative treatment of infantile developmental dysplasia of the hip (DDH) worldwide. This prefabricated device is designed to restrict hip adduction and extension movements that would allow the femoral head to rotate outside the acetabulum while permitting other movements. Alternative designs that accomplish similar biomechanical goals to treat DDH include abduction pillows and abduction splints such as the original Lorenz and subsequent Ilfield devices, as well as numerous subsequent variations (Figure 8-20).

Although Wang et al reports the containment theory in the treatment of juvenile Legg-Calvè-Perthes disease is now being challenged, this childhood disease is still sometimes managed with a hip orthosis which holds the legs in abduction. Figure 8-21 illustrates one example.

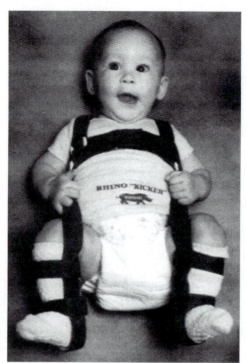

Figure 8-20. Cloth harness designed by Pavlik is a common treatment for developmental dysplastic hip disorders. The more rigid splints advocated by Lorenz and others hold the hips in a similar position.

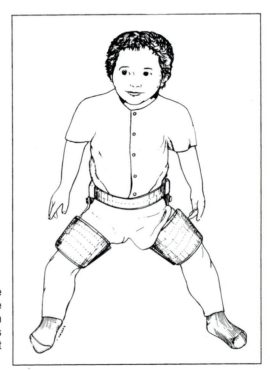

Figure 8-21. Scottish-Rite design hip orthosis holds the femurs in abduction. Although controversial, this orthosis is sometimes still used to treat Legg-Calvè-Perthes disease.

Hip orthoses to control abduction or adduction are rarely used full-time or long term. They are sometimes used nocturnally to resist spastic "scissoring" and thereby reduce the frequency of hip subluxation, dislocation, or urinary disturbances, as noted by Nakamura and Ohamu. Lima et al have reported that for adults, prefabricated or custom-made HOs are often applied for a few weeks following total hip replacement surgery to limit gross motion in the acute healing phase. It is virtually impossible for a hip orthosis to prevent redislocation or re-subluxation, but some clinicians including Naef believe it may reduce the risk, particularly following total joint revision surgery. Figure 8-22 shows one example of a post-operative HO design.

HIP-KNEE-ANKLE-FOOT ORTHOSES (HKAFO) AND HIGHER-LEVEL DEVICES

For the first three-quarters of this century, patients with paraplegia were often provided with bilateral KAFOs connected to a metal pelvic band by locking hip joints. Figure 8-23 depicts a unilateral version of such an HKAFO. When the entire lower body is locked rigidly, the resulting swing-to or swing-through gait is laborious and energy consuming. Follow-up studies of both children (by Hoffer et al) and adults (Hawran and Biering-Sorenson) fitted with HKAFOs documented that only a small percentage use such devices long term. As a result, such restrictive orthoses are rarely prescribed today.

Reciprocating Gait Orthoses

One high level lower limb orthosis that has been successful in treating people with paraplegia links left and right KAFOs such that flexion of one hip causes extension of the opposite hip. Colloquially termed reciprocating gait orthoses by Douglas et al, these devices use flexible cables or pivoting bars to allow paraplegics the option of ambulating foot over foot while using external aids such as a walker or forearm crutches for balance. Figure 8-24 shows one example of this technology. The extension to support the paralyzed trunk makes this device a Lumbar-Sacral-Hip-Knee-Ankle-Foot Orthosis or LSHKAFO in the ISO terminology.

The outcome of using this system by children with myelodysplasia has been studied in some detail. According to McCall and Schmidt, it appears that these patients have a strong preference for reciprocal gait even though the RGO also permits swing-to or swing-through gait, because holding one hip joint steady in effect stabilizes the opposite hip. Yngve et al noted that while reciprocal gait is more energy efficient, swing gaits are usually faster. Many children will swing through to cover short distances within the classroom but use the reciprocating gait to cover longer distances, such as trips to the library, with less exertion.

There are also several similar HKAFO devices intended for use by adults with acquired lower limb paralysis. Figure 8-25 illustrates one design by Wallace Motlock, C.O. (who designed the original reciprocating orthosis several decades ago while practicing in Toronto). As reported by Winchester et al, this design uses a pivoting isocentric linkage connected by lateral bars to floor reaction-style AFOs that fit over the patient's shoes. One advantage of this orthosis, which can also be designed to fit inside the shoes, is that the patient can don the system easily while seated in a wheelchair.

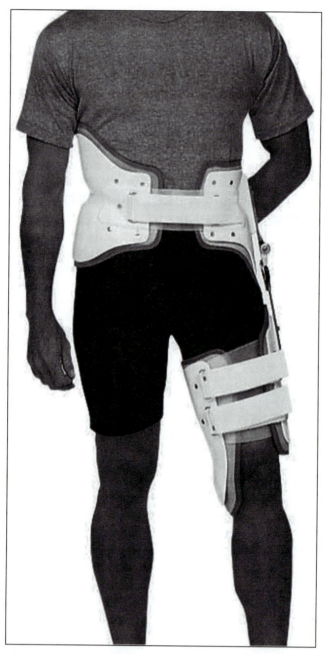

a

Figure 8-22. Examples of an HKO and HKAFO used immediately following total hip replacement to reduce the risk of subluxation in the postoperative phase. The HKAFO provides rotational control due to the purchase on the foot, which the HKO cannot.

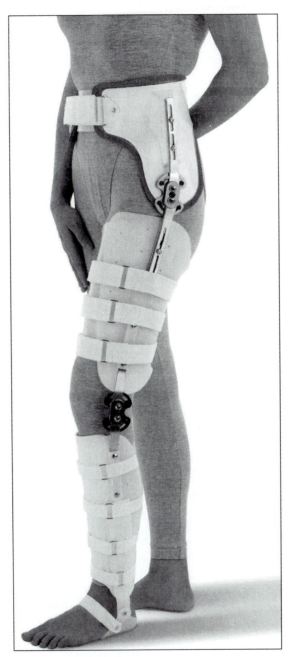

b

Figure 8-22. continued

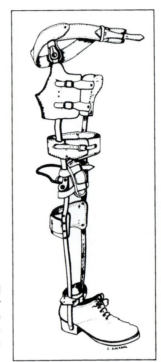

Figure 8-23. The traditional HKAFO that locks all the lower limb joints has been shown to have a very high long-term rejection rate and is therefore rarely prescribed today.

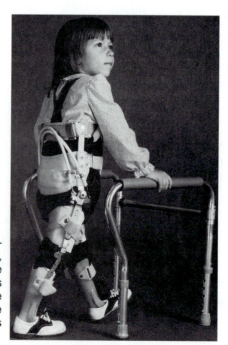

Figure 8-24. Children tolerate extensive bracing well, and often ambulate despite higher-level paralysis, as this photo depicts. Because of the extensions to stabilize the paralyzed trunk, this device is termed an LSHKAFO.

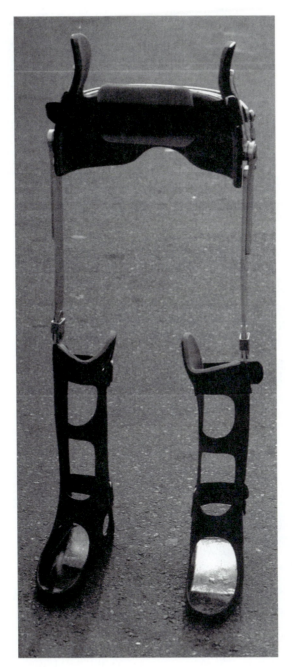

a

Figure 8-25. This isocentric-style orthosis is particularly easy to don from a seated position in a wheelchair.

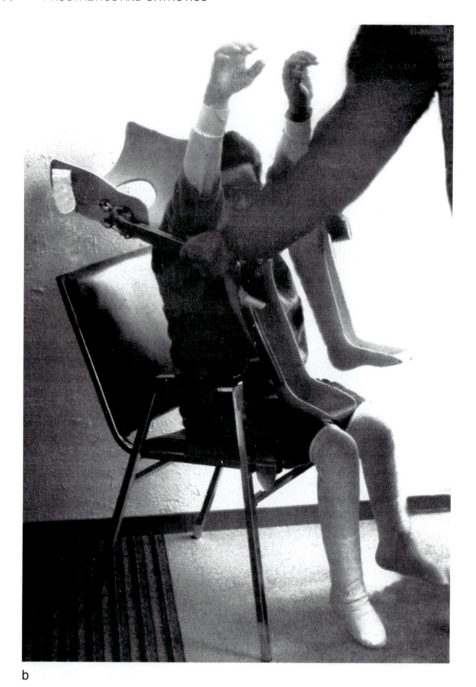

b

Figure 8-25. continued

Another variation on this theme, shown in Figure 8-26, uses the force of gravity to cause the leg to swing forward slowly. According to Stallard et al, the more rigid construction of this hip guidance orthosis (HGO) has shown to result in a more energy efficient gait for adults than the RGO designs attached to relatively flexible thermoplastic KAFOs. It appears that the increased efficiency results because the HGO construction resists adduction so completely that the patient needs less lateral shift to advance first one leg and then the other. Major et al have

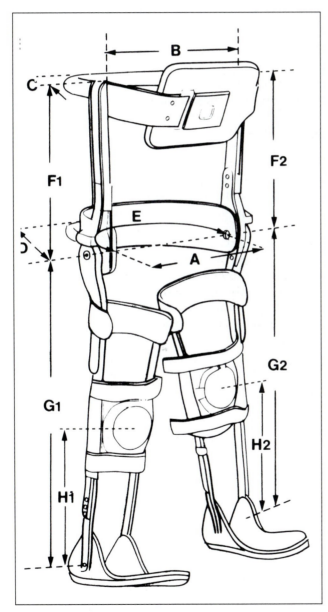

Figure 8-26. The rigid construction of this hip guidance orthosis has been shown to make paraplegic locomotion less energy consuming than walking with other reciprocating orthoses. Despite the bulk and weight of this orthosis, which is worn over clothing and normal shoes, British follow-up studies have shown a good long-term acceptance rate by selected paraplegic adults.

reported long-term follow up of British patients using this device suggesting that a significant majority choose to wear this complex orthosis regularly for specific tasks when ambulation is important to the user.

Finally, some centers are experimenting with the addition of functional electrical stimulation of paralyzed surface muscles to provide motion along with RGO or other orthoses to stabilize the paralyzed limbs. Grant et al reports it appears that this may allow paraplegics to walk more quickly or as Solomonow notes for greater distances than with orthoses alone, but Sykes et al have observed that the postulated energy advantages have not been shown to date.

OTHER LOWER LIMB ORTHOSES

Clearly, it is impossible to describe more than a fraction of the possible permutations in lower limb orthoses in one chapter, or even in one text. The devices highlighted here are representative of the scope and range of orthoses encountered in clinical practice or discussions, but they do not necessarily represent the "best" solution for any individual.

Clinician preferences, based on training and experience, frequently influence local practice patterns. For example, in the hot and humid climate of the southern states, minimal contact orthoses are often favored because many patients report these configurations are cooler and therefore more comfortable than total contact plastic equivalents. In the cooler northern climes, thermoplastic orthoses are more likely to predominate because excessive perspiration is seldom an issue.

All members of the rehabilitation team are encouraged to ask for the rationale underlying the provision of a particular orthosis for a specific individual's needs. In all cases, there should be a clear and realistic biomechanical justification for the function of each prescribed device. Fabrication details and specific variations should be based on a complete physical evaluation and discussion with the patient of the plusses and minuses of the equivalent alternatives that are pertinent to their deficits. To illustrate this concept, Figure 8-27 shows several differing ways to manage flaccid equinus with an orthosis.

REFERENCES

1. *American Academy of Orthopaedic Surgeons, Orthotics Atlas.* St. Louis, MO: Mosby; 1975.
2. Baker BE. Knee bracing. *Curr Opin Orthop.* 1992; 3:805–808.
3. Bensman A, Lossing W. A new ankle-foot orthosis combining the advantages of metal and plastics. *Orthot Prosthet.* 1979; 33(1):3–10.
4. Beynnon BD, Pope MH, Wertheimer CM et al. The effect of functional knee-braces on strain on the anterior cruciate ligament in vivo. *J Bone Joint Surg.* 1992; 74A:1298–1312.
5. Bobecchko W, McLaurin C, Motlocch W. Toronto treatment in Legg-Perthes disease. *Art Limbs.* 1968; 12(2):36–41.
6. Bos RPMJ, Grady JH, Vierhout PAM et al. A comparison of two custom-made and two off-the-shelf rigid knee orthoses in the treatment of ACL-deficient knees. *J Prosthet Orthot.* 1997; 9:25–32.
7. Bowen JR, Guille JT, Puniak MA et al. Prospective evaluation of various methods of treatment for Legg-Calve-Perthes disease (abstract). *Orthop Trans.* 1993/94; 17:1096.
8. Bronkhorst AJ, Lamb GA. An orthosis to aid in reduction of lower limb spasticity. *Orthot Prosthet.* 1987; 41(2):23–28.

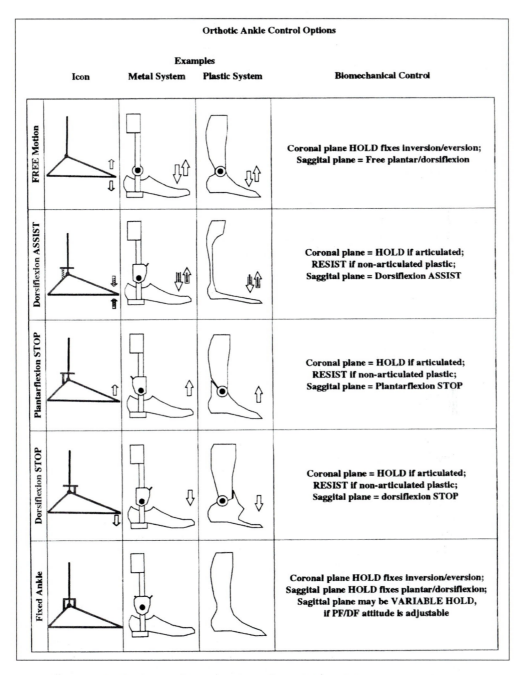

Orthotic Ankle Control Options

Examples

Icon	Metal System	Plastic System	Biomechanical Control
FREE Motion			Coronal plane HOLD fixes inversion/eversion; Saggital plane = Free plantar/dorsiflexion
Dorsiflexion ASSIST			Coronal plane = HOLD if articulated; RESIST if non-articulated plastic; Saggital plane = Dorsiflexion ASSIST
Plantarflexion STOP			Coronal plane = HOLD if articulated; RESIST if non-articulated plastic; Saggital plane = Plantarflexion STOP
Dorsiflexion STOP			Coronal plane = HOLD if articulated; RESIST if non-articulated plastic; Saggital plane = dorsiflexion STOP
Fixed Ankle			Coronal plane HOLD fixes inversion/eversion; Saggital plane HOLD fixes plantar/dorsiflexion; Sagittal plane may be VARIABLE HOLD, if PF/DF attitude is adjustable

Figure 8-27. There are often several possible orthotic solutions to managing a particular biomechanical deficit, as illustrated here in the case of flaccid equinas. The certified orthotist, with input from the other clinic team members, usually discusses the advantages and limitations of each approach with the patient to determine the optimal orthosis for each individual.

9. Carlson JM, Berglund G. An effective orthotic design for controlling the unstable subtalar joint. *Orthot Prosthet.* 1979; 33(1):39–49.

10. Carlson JM, Hollerbach F, Day B. A calf corset weightbearing ankle-foot orthosis design. *J Prosthet Orthot.* 1991; 4(1):41–44.

11. Curtis B, Gunther S, Gossling, Paul S. Treatment for Legg-Perthes disease with the Newington ambulation-abduction brace. *J Bone Joint Surg.* 1974; 56A(6):1135–1146.

12. Douglas R, Larson P, D'Ambrosia R, McCall R. The LSU reciprocation-gait orthosis. *Orthopedics.* 1983; 6(7):834–839.

13. Ford G, Grotz RC, Shamp JK. The neurophysiological ankle-foot orthosis. *Clin Prosthet Orthot.* 1986; 10:15–23.

14. Fujioka F, Terayama K, Sugimoto N et al. Long-term results of congenital dislocation of the hip treated with Pavlik harness. *J Pediatr Orthop.* 1995; 15:747–752.

15. Glancy J. Orthotic control of ground reaction forces during running (a preliminary report). *Orthot Prosthet.* 1984; 38(3):12–40.

16. Glancy J, Lindseth RE. Solid ankle orthosis. *Orthot Prosthet.* 1972; 26:14.

17. Grace TG, Skipper BJ, Newberry JC et al. Prophylactic knee braces and injury to the lower extremity. *J Bone Joint Surg.* 1988; 70A:422–427.

18. Grant MH, Andrews BJ, Delargyma MA et al. Use of FES in crutch-aided locomotion (abstract). *J Biomech.* 1992; 25:731.

19. Hahn HR. Lower extremity bracing in paraplegics with usage follow up. *Paraplegia.* 1970; 8(3):147–153.

20. Harrington ED, Lin RS. Gage JR Use of the anterior floor reaction orthosis in patients with cerebral palsy. *Orthot Prosthet.* 1983–84; 37(4):34–42.

21. Hawran S, Biering-Sorensen.The use of long leg calipers for paraplegic patients: A follow-up study of patients discharged 1973–82. *Spinal Cord.* 1996; 34:666–668.

22. Helfand AE. Basic considerations for shoes, shoe modifications, and orthoses in foot care. *Clin Podiatry.* 1984; 2:431–440.

23. Hicks JE, Leonard JA, Nelson VS et al. Prosthetics, orthotics and assistive devices: 4. Orthotic management of selected disorders. *Arch Phys Med Rehabil.* 1989; 70:S210–S217.

24. Hoffer M, Feiwell E, Perry R, Perry J, Bonnett C. Functional ambulation in patients with myelomeningocele. *J Bone Joint Surg (Am).* 1973; 55:137–148.

25. Hong C, San Luis EB, Chung S. Follow-up study on the use of leg braces issued to spinal cord injury patients. *Paraplegia.* 1990; 28:172–177.

26. Ilfeld FW. The management of congenital dislocation and dysplasia by the means of a special splint. *J Bone Joint Surg.* 1957; 39A:99–110.

27. Johnston JM, Paulos LE. Prophylactic lateral knee braces. *Med Sci Sports Exerc.* 1991; 23:783–787.

28. Klasson BL. Carbon fibre and fibre lamination in prosthetics and orthotics some basic theory and practical advice for the practitioner. *Prosthet Orthot Int.* 1995; 19:74–91.

29. Lehmann JF, De Lateur BJ, Price R. Weight-bearing and other orthoses for skeletal and joint insufficiency. *Phys Med Rehabil Clin North Am.* 1992; 3:185–192.

30. Levine RS, Begeman P, King AI. An analysis of the projection of lateral knee bracing using a cadaver simulation of lateral knee impact (abstract). *Orthop Trans.* 1988; 12:744.

31. Lima D. Overview of the causes, treatment, and orthotic management of lower limb spasticity. *J Prosthet Orthot.* 1989; 2:33–39.

32. Lima D, Magnus R, Paprosky WG. Team management of hip revision patients using a post-op hip orthosis. *J Prosthet Orthot.* 1994; 6:20–24.

33. Lindenfeld TN, Hewett TE, Andriacchi TP. Decrease in knee joint loading with unloader brace wear in patients with medical compartment gonarthrosis (abstract). *Orthop Trans.* 1996/97; 20:107.

34. Liu SH, Lunsford T, Gude S et al. Comparison of functional knee braces for control of anterior tibial displacement. *Clin Orthop.* 1994; 303:203–210.
35. Liu SH, Mirzayan R, Bowen R et al. Comparison of off the shelf and custom functional knee braces in controlling anterior tibial displacement (abstract). *Orthop Trans.* 1995; 19:565.
36. Lorenz, A. Die Sogenannte Angeborene Huftvenenkung. *Ihre Pathologie und Therapie.* Stuttgart: Ferdinand Euke; 1920.
37. Major RE, Stallard J, Farmer SE. A review of 42 patients of 16 years and over using the ORLAU Parawalker. *Prosthet Orthot Int.* 1997; 21:147–152.
38. Marans HJ, Jackson RW, Piccinin J et al. Functional testing of braces for anterior cruciate ligament-deficient knees. *Can J Surg.* 1991; 34:167–173.
39. McCall R, Schmidt W. Clinical experience with the reciprocal gait orthosis in myelodysplasia. *J Pediatr Orthop.* 1986; 6:1157–1161.
40. McCollough NC. Current status of lower limb orthotics. *Orthop Dig.* 1975; 3:17–29.
41. McIlmurray WJ, Greenbaum W. A below-knee weight-bearing brace. *Orthop Prosthet Appl J.* 1958; 12(2):81–82.
42. McNair PJ, Stanley SN, Strauss GR. Knee bracing: Effects on proprioception. *Arch Phys Med Rehabil.* 1996; 77:287–289.
43. Michael, JW. Orthotic treatment of neurologic deficits. In: *Handbook of Neurorehabilitation.* Couch J, Good D, eds. New York: Marcel Dekker, Inc; 1994.
44. Millet CW, Drez DJ. Principles of bracing for the anterior cruciate ligament-deficient knee. *Clin Sports Med.* 1988; 7:827–833.
45. Naef M, Burckhardt A, Hageli W. TL Die konservative behandlung der rezidivierenden huftprothesesnluxation mit der huftgelenksorthese nach Hohmann (the conservative treatment of retrogressive hip prosthesis dislocation with the hip joint brace according to Hohmann). *Med Orthop Tech.* 1990; 110:230–234.
46. Nakamura T, Ohamu M. Hip abduction splint for use at night for scissor leg of cerebral palsy patients. *Orthot Prosthet.* 1980; 34(4):13–18.
47. Nicholas JA. Bracing the anterior cruciate ligament deficient knee using the Lenox Hill derotation brace. *Clin Orthop.* 1983; 172:137–142.
48. Perry J. Pathological gait. In: *Orthotics Atlas.* St. Louis, MO: Mosby; 1975.
49. Pritham C, Stills M. Knee cylinder. *Orthot Prosthet.* 1980; 33(4):11–17.
50. Purvis JM, Dimon II JH, Meehan PL, Lovell WW. Preliminary experience with the Scottish Rite Hospital abduction orthosis for Legg-Calvè -Perthes disease. *Clin Orthop Rel Res.* 1980; 150:49–53.
51. Randall F, Miller H, Shurr D. The use of prophylactic knee orthoses at Iowa State University. *Orthot Prosthet.* 1983–84; 37(4):54–57.
52. Rehabilitation Engineering Center. *Lower limb orthotics: A manual.* Philadelphia, PA: Moss Rehabilitation Hospital, 1978.
53. Requa RK, Garrick JG. Clinical significance and evaluation of prophylactic knee brace studies in football. *Clin Sports Med.* 1990; 9:853–869.
54. Rogers JP, Vanderbilt SH. Coordinated treatment in cerebral palsy - where are we today? *J Prosthet Orthot.* 1989; 2(1):68–81.
55. Root ML. Development of the functional orthosis. *Clin Podiatr Med Surg.* 1994; 11:183–210.
56. Rosman N, Spira E. Paraplegic use of walking braces: A survey. *Arch Phys Med Rehabil.* 1974; 55:310–314.
57. Rubin G, Dixon M, Danisi M. VAPC prescription procedures for knee orthoses and knee-ankle-foot orthoses. *Orthot Prosthet.* 1977; 31(3):9–25.
58. Saltiel J. A one-piece laminated knee locking short leg brace. *Orthot Prosthet.* 1969; 23(2):68–75.
59. Sarmiento A, Sinclair WF. Application of prosthetics-orthotics principles to treatment of fractures. *Artificial Limbs.* 1967; 11(2):28–32.

60. Schuch CM, Pritham CH. International Standards Organization terminology: application to prosthetics and orthotics. *J Prosthet Orthot.* 1994; 6:29–33.

61. Shamp JK. Neurophysiologic orthotic designs in the treatment of central nervous system disorders. *J Prosthet Orthot.* 1989; 2:14–32.

62. Shaw JL. Application of prosthetic-orthotic principles to the treatment of tibial fractures. *Artificial Limbs.* 1972; 16(1):51–54.

63. Showers D, David L. A reinforcing technique in orthotics and prosthetics. *Orthot Prosthet.* 1982; 32(2):108–112.

64. Shurr D. Metal vs. plastic AFO—A therapist's view. *Clin Prosthet Orthot.* 1983; 7(1):4.

65. Sitler M, Ryan J, Hopkinson W et al. The efficacy of a prophylactic knee brace to reduce knee injuries in football: A prospective, randomized study at West Point. *Am J Sports Med.* 1990; 18:310–315.

66. Solomonow M. Performance of walking orthosis for paraplegics (abstract). *Gait Posture.* 1995; 3:86.

67. Stallard J, Major RE, Butler PB. The orthotic ambulation performance of paraplegic myelomeningocele children using the ORLAU ParaWalker treatment system. *Clin Rehabil.* 1991; 5:111–114.

68. Stallard J, Major RE, Patrick JH. The use of the Orthotic Research and Locomotor Assessment Unit (ORLAU) ParaWalker by adult myelomeningocele patients: A seven retrospective study - preliminary results. *Eur J Pediatr Surg.* 1995; 5(Suppl 1):24–26.

69. Sykes L, Campbell IG, Powell ES et al. Energy expenditure of walking for adult patients with spinal cord lesions using the reciprocating gait orthosis and functional electrical stimulation. *Spinal Cord.* 1996; 34:659–665.

70. Tacchdjian MA, Jouett LD. Trilateral socket hip abduction orthosis for the treatment of Legg-Calvé-Perthes' disease. *Orthot Prosthet.* 1968; 2(2):49–62.

71. Wang L, Bowen JR, Puniak MA et al. An evaluation of various methods of treatment for Legg-Calve-Pethes disease. *Clin Orthop.* 1995; 314:225–233.

72. Warren CG, Lehmann JF, Delateur BJ. Pelvic band use in orthotics for adult paraplegic patients. *Arch Phys Med Rehabil.* 1975; 56:221–223.

73. Winchester PK, Carollo JJ, Parekh RN et al. A comparison of paraplegic gait performance using two types of reciprocating gait orthoses. *Prosthet Orthot Int.* 1993; 17:101–106.

74. Yang G, Chu D, Ahn J, Lehneis H, Conceicao R. Floor reaction orthosis: Clinical experience. *Orthot Prosthet.* 1986; 40(1):33–37.

75. Yngve D, Douglas R, Robert J. The reciprocating gait orthosis in myelomeningocele. *J Pediatr Orthop.* 1984; 4:304–310.

76. Zamosky I. Shoe modifications in lower-extremity orthotics. *Bull Prosthet Res.* 1964; 10(2):54–95.

77. Zucker RS. Rehabilitation of fractures of the lower extremity. *Phys Med Rehabil: State Art Rev.* 1995; 9:161–174.

CHAPTER *9*

Spinal Orthoses

The colloquial names of many orthotic and prosthetic items are derived from the identity of those physicians, surgeons, orthotists, and prosthetists who first developed or promulgated the design, or from people who first needed or wore some similar device. Such is the case with the Minerva jacket. Minerva was the Roman goddess of medicine, but also the goddess of war. According to Bulfinch's mythology, Minerva leaped from Jupiter's brain in complete armor. Included in this costume was her helmeted head and aegis or breast-plate. Since the early cervical spine casts nearly covered the entire head, they became known as the Minerva cast or Minerva jacket. Modern thermoplastic versions of this orthosis are still used for immobilization of the cervical and upper thoracic spine.

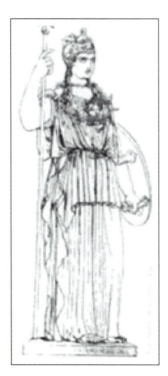

Following completion of reading this chapter, the student will be able to:

1. Describe the common functional elements of a spinal orthosis and their respective anatomical relevance to trim lines.
2. Describe the concept of the burst fracture, distinguish it from a compression fracture, and identify the implications for spinal orthotic treatment.
3. Discuss common orthotic treatment options for upper, middle, and lower cervical spine injury, and identify an appropriate orthosis for each level of injury based on the published literature.
4. Discuss the role of spinal orthoses in the treatment of idiopathic scoliotic.

This chapter will present a brief historical perspective on spinal orthoses, a consideration of the intended functions of spinal orthoses, and an overview of the components of spinal orthoses. Commonly prescribed spinal orthoses and clinical studies supporting their effects and effectiveness in the overall treatment of spinal disorders will also be highlighted.

HISTORICAL PERSPECTIVE

The history of spinal orthoses may be traced to the ancient Greeks and Egyptians. Early records indicate that these cultures used bark that was cut circumferentially from a tree and then placed around the body of the patient with a spinal deformity or problem (Figure 9-1). The configuration of the bark very much resembles the design and purpose of modern spinal orthoses that utilize metal, fabric, and plastic contoured to produce the desired function. Today, plastics of many kinds have replaced metal in many spinal orthoses. Lightweight and washable plastics are easily molded, usually remoldable, and offer the patient a cosmetic and comfortable orthosis.

FUNCTIONS OF SPINAL ORTHOSES

In 1961, Lucas and Bresler described the spine as a modified elastic rod. When the base was fixed with only the intrinsic or ligamentous components in place, the largest load it could withstand without buckling was 2 kg. Clearly the extrinsic musculature plays a very important part in the overall stability of the human spine. In cases where the intrinsic structures are inadequate, a spinal orthosis may be required to provide extrinsic stability.

Clinical reasons for the use of spinal orthotics include immobilization, support, and correction/prevention of deformity. Immobilization orthoses are classically used for a large group of conditions, including trauma with or without surgical fixation or reconstruction. During this time, there is a need to limit motion of portions of the spinal column. Because spinal

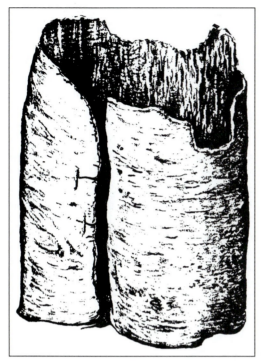

Figure 9-1. Ancient tree-bark spinal orthosis.

orthoses may be worn for a period of weeks or months, the material chosen and the fit are particularly important to both patient compliance and comfort.

Supportive orthoses may be thought of as those that provide temporary care in cases of pain in the cervical or thoracolumbar region of the spine. Principles employed in supportive orthoses are an increase in intra-abdominal pressure, a kinesthetic reminder or restraint of painful range of motion, and the application of pressure over the largest possible surface area. Cervical orthoses are almost always supportive or immobilizing, because most pathologies create instability rather than deformity of the cervical spine. Such supportive orthoses may be custom fabricated, or prefabricated and custom fitted to each patient. Their successful use depends on choice of the appropriate orthosis following a complete diagnostic workup and professional custom fitting. Corrective orthoses include a large group of devices used primarily in growing children for spinal diseases such as scoliosis and kyphosis.

COMPONENTS OF SPINAL ORTHOSES

Despite differing overall designs and functions, almost all spinal orthoses are composed of various combinations of simple functional parts or components. This chapter will review those components, first for traditional metal and leather designs, and later for more contemporary thermoplastic devices.

Thoracic Band

The most proximal component of any lumbosacral orthosis (LSO) or thoracic lumbosacral orthosis (TLSO) is the thoracic band (Figure 9-2). For maximum leverage, the superior border of this component should be located 1 inch inferior to the more inferior angle of the scapula. The lateral borders of the thoracic band are the midaxillary trochanteric lines (MATLs). The thoracic band allows attachment of other components, including the lateral uprights, the paraspinal uprights, or shoulder straps.

Pelvic Band

The pelvic band usually represents the most distal component of a spinal orthosis (Figure 9-3). It lies inferiorly at the level of the sacrocoxygeal junction. Laterally the pelvic band extends to the MATL at the level between the greater trochanter and the iliac crest. In order for the pelvic band to be fitted properly, the contours over the buttocks should flow into the concavity of the gluteus maximus, allowing proper end support. This also gives rise to other components, such as the paraspinal uprights, the lateral uprights, and the apron or corset.

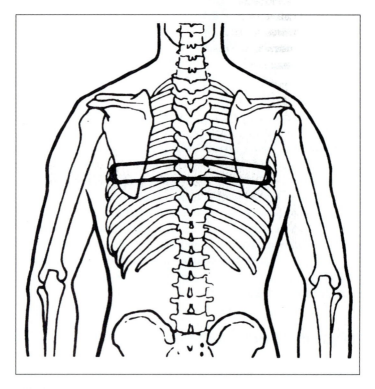

Figure 9-2. Thoracic band.(*Source:* Reproduced by permission from Berger N, Lusskin R. Orthotic components and systems. In: *American Academy of Orthopaedic Surgeons: Atlas of Orthotics.* St. Louis, MO: Mosby; 1975.)

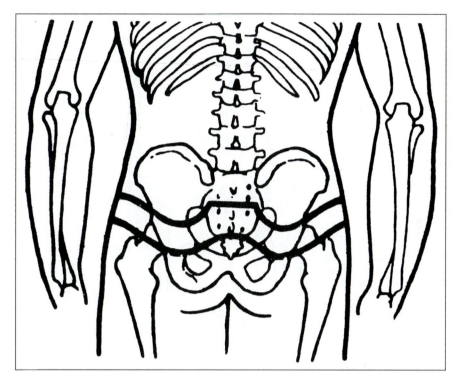

Figure 9-3. Pelvic band. (*Source:* Reproduced by permission from Berger N, Lusskin R. Orthotic components and systems. In: *American Academy of Orthopaedic Surgeons: Atlas of Orthotics.* St. Louis, MO: Mosby; 1975.)

Paraspinal Uprights

Paraspinal uprights, or bars, are positioned parallel to the spine, being careful not to touch the transverse processes of the vertebrae (Figure 9-4). They are bounded on the superior end by the thoracic band and on the inferior end by the pelvic band. These paraspinal bars may either be contoured to the lumbar lordosis or bridged to encourage lumbar spine flexion.

Lateral Uprights

Lateral uprights, or bars, follow the MATL and connect the pelvic band and the thoracic band (Figure 9-5). The lateral uprights connect the posterior half and the anterior half, providing attachment points for the apron or abdominal support.

Abdominal Support or Apron

The abdominal apron, or corset, makes up the anterior portion of many orthoses (Figure 9-6). It lies superiorly 12 mm inferior to the xyphoid process of the sternum and inferiorly 12 mm superior to the symphysis pubis. The corset may be constructed of either nylon or cotton duck material and usually is made with straps and buckles to allow the patient to adjust the abdominal compression. The corset extends to the lateral borders of the orthosis at the MATL.

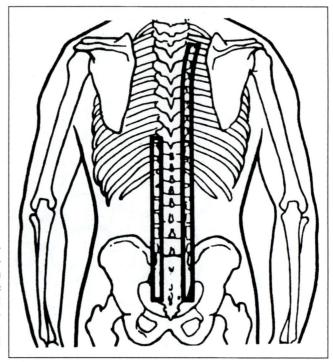

Figure 9-4. Paraspinal uprights or bars. (*Source:* Reproduced by permission from Berger N, Lusskin R. Orthotic components and systems. In: *American Academy of Orthopaedic Surgeons: Atlas of Orthotics*. St. Louis, MO: Mosby; 1975.)

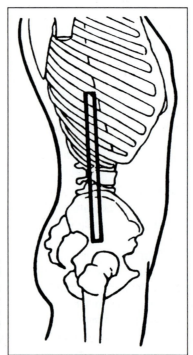

Figure 9-5. Lateral uprights, or bars. (*Source:* Reproduced by permission from Berger N, Lusskin R. Orthotic components and systems. In: *American Academy of Orthopaedic Surgeons: Atlas of Orthotics*. St. Louis, MO: Mosby; 1975.)

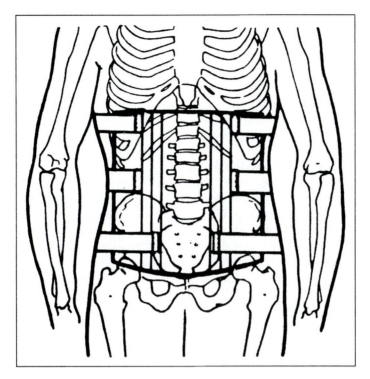

Figure 9-6. Abdominal support or apron. (*Source:* Reproduced by permission from Berger N, Lusskin R. Orthotic components and systems. In: *American Academy of Orthopaedic Surgeons: Atlas of Orthotics.* St. Louis, MO: Mosby; 1975.)

The corset may also be a stand-alone orthosis and is widely prescribed for low back pain. According to Ewing, corsets have been recorded as early as 1530 for Catherine of Medici. Perry, in her classic article on use of spinal orthoses found that the most often prescribed orthosis was the abdominal corset.

Component Similarities Using Total Contact-Plastic Spinal Orthoses

It is important to understand and appreciate the structure, location, and function of the aforementioned orthotic components, even though today the more commonly used orthoses are plastic. The trim lines of plastic spinal orthoses incorporate the basic components as part of their integrated design, offering similar biomechanical functions.

Because these plastic orthoses, whether custom made from a patient model or custom fitted, are total contact in nature, the pressure or force per unit area is less than would be the case with their metal counterparts. This may account for the increased comfort reported with thermoplastic orthoses, although the trade-off is often more perspiration secondary to increased retention of body heat.

Most of the commonly prescribed metal spinal orthoses have total contact-plastic counterparts. The reader is advised to consider the biomechanical function desired and patient needs when evaluating trim lines and fit of either type of orthosis.

COMMONLY PRESCRIBED SPINAL ORTHOSES

Spinal orthoses are described functionally by their ISO nomenclature denoting the body segments covered, often modified by noting the primary biomechanical control features. In the clinic setting, they are often referred to by their historic name.

Spinal orthoses can be designed to resist anterior, posterior, lateral, and rotary trunk movement, or a combination of these motions. These controls are often abbreviated using the capital letters A, P, L, and R.

Chair-Back: LSO, AP Control

The components of the chair-back orthosis are a pelvic band, a thoracic band, two paraspinal bars, and an abdominal corset or apron (Figure 9-7). Biomechanically the orthosis is a combination of two three-point pressure systems. One system consists of two anteriorly directed forces from the thoracic and pelvic bands and a posteriorly directed force from the corset. The reverse is also true. There are two posteriorly directed forces from the corset and an anteriorly directed force from the paraspinal bars. Using these force systems, motions of lumbar flexion and extension are resisted, and the intra-abdominal pressure is raised.

Raney Flexion Jacket: LSO, APLR Control

Raney, in 1969, reported on his experience with the Royalite flexion jacket. The orthosis that now bears his name (Figure 9-8) was a by-product of the original Hauser flexion jacket, the first jacket used to flex the lumbar spine. The orthosis was developed by a patient who was an engineer with back pain that was not improved by fitting with a chair-back orthosis. The engineer added a new front panel that included a concave aluminum dish pressing into the abdomen to his existing chair-back orthosis and experienced immediate pain relief. These

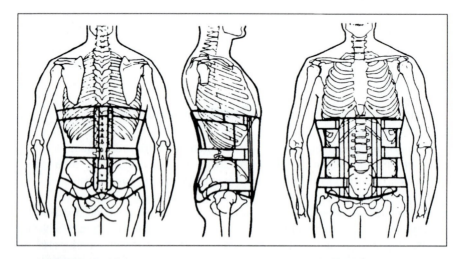

Figure 9-7. Chair-back LSO. (*Source:* Reproduced by permission from Berger N, Lusskin R. Orthotic components and systems. In: *American Academy of Orthopaedic Surgeons: Atlas of Orthotics.* St. Louis, MO: Mosby; 1975.)

orthoses were made of aluminum until lighter weight Royalite plastic was developed. Raney hypothesized that by flexing the lumbar spine, pressure was transferred to the anterior portion of the intervertebral disc, noting that it was the posterior portion of the disc was irritated in many cases. Results from over 1,500 cases indicated that use of the Raney flexion jacket yielded relief of symptoms. The modern Raney flexion jacket is a custom-fitted spinal orthosis with a hard, anterior shell to maintain the lumbar spine in a flexed position.

Williams: LSO, AL Control
The Williams LSO is an example of a metal analogue of the Raney plastic LSO. The Williams LSO consists of a pelvic and thoracic band, a corset, and lateral/oblique bars (Figure 9-9). These lateral/oblique bars allow the hinged orthosis to pivot on the thoracic band, thus allowing flexion of the lumbar spine and distal motion of the orthosis. Pulling on the anterior straps attached to both sides of the oblique bars causes the pelvis to be flexed and pulled anteriorly. The abdominal corset causes increased intra-abdominal pressure, which has been shown to unload the lumbar spine.

Knight: LSO, APL Control
The Knight LSO is very much like the chair-back except that in addition to the chair-back components, the Knight also has two lateral bars. Therefore, in addition to the three-point pressure systems of anteroposterior forces, there is limitation of lateral flexion via the lateral bars.

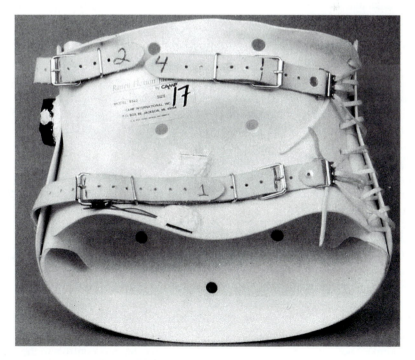

Figure 9-8. Raney flexion LSO.

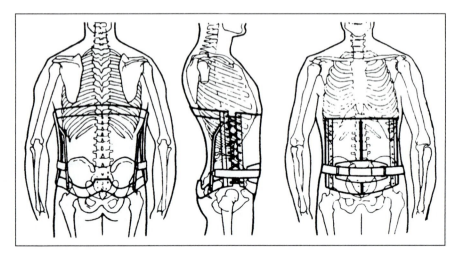

Figure 9-9. Williams LSO. (*Source:* Reproduced by permission from Berger N, Lusskin R. Orthotic components and systems. In: *American Academy of Ortho-paedic Surgeons: Atlas of Orthotics*. St. Louis, MO: Mosby; 1975.)

In 1970, Perry published the results of a study regarding the prescription of orthoses for spinal disorders. In this study, chair-back and Knight LSOs were mentioned by 54 percent of the respondents and Williams mentioned by 19 percent. No other orthosis was mentioned in more than 4.6 percent of the responses.

Jewett: TLSO with Anterior Control

The Jewett hyperextension orthosis is composed of components that have not previously been discussed (Figure 9-10). These components include a sternal pad and pubic pad anteriorly and a posteriorly located lumbar pad. The two anterior pads direct forces in the posterior direction, while the lumbar posterior pad directs one force anteriorly. This orthosis is used for patients who need to limit flexion or anterior motion following injury to the body of a vertebra, such as often occurs following a compression fracture. Because the Jewett has no lateral bars, lateral bending is not significantly restricted.

The C-35 from Camp, the CASH orthosis from Storrs, and many other manufacturers' devices offer similar biomechanical control to that of the Jewett, and are referred to generically as a TLSO, anterior control.

Body Jackets: TLSO, APLR control

The TLSO body jacket, which was formerly made from leather, then iron and steel, is now made of lightweight plastics (Figure 9-11). These devices are either custom fabricated from a model impression of each patient or custom fitted from either prefabricated shells, or from measurements generated from a CAD CAM system. Thermoset plastics have the advantage of being better contoured to the model but are more labor intensive and therefore, more expensive than thermoplastic equivilents.

Total contact body jacket orthoses offer similar biomechanical controls to the older style metal and leather designs but distribute forces over the largest possible area by using the

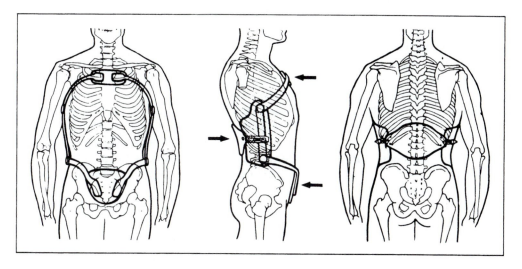

Figure 9-10. Jewett TLSO, anterior control. (*Source:* Reproduced by permission from Berger N, Lusskin R. Orthotic components and systems. In: *American Academy of Orthopaedic Surgeons: Atlas of Orthotics.* St. Louis, MO: Mosby; 1975.)

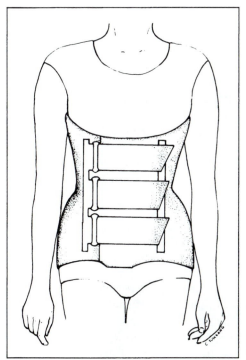

Figure 9-11. TLSO body jacket.

principle of total contact. Depending on the amount of material removed from the model, the amount of intra-abdominal pressure and pelvic position may also be controlled.

For many reasons, TLSO body jackets are the orthosis of choice for many patients. They may be easily washed, readily modified, and are quite cosmetic, being easily hidden under most loose-fitting clothes. TLSO body jackets may have a variety of opening styles depending on the patient's needs. Anterior or posterior openings with Velcro closures are typical, while bivalved styles, with straps on either side for easy entry and exit, are also available. Cotton T-shirts are often used to provide a comfortable interface between the padded foam lining and the skin. Cervical attachments may be added to TLSOs in cases of concomitant cervical spine injuries, converting them into CTLSO orthoses (Figure 9-12). TLSO body jackets may also be made using CAD-CAM techniqes, from a series of measurements or from a digital replica of the patient's torso.

Cervical Orthosis Components

Cervical orthoses do not have components in the same sense that thoracolumbar spinal orthoses do. Nachemson makes a distinction between two groups of cervical orthoses: the cervical orthosis (CO) dealing with the region of C1-2, and the cervical thoracic orthosis (CTO) dealing with levels C-3 to T-1. Spinal kinematic studies suggest that flexion and extension occur mainly at the level of C5-6, while 80 percent of the rotation occurs at C1-2. This is borne out by a quick examination of the anatomy and the configuration of the cervical vertebrae.

A large percentage of cervical orthoses in use today are prefabricated. Nachemson classifies cervical orthoses as soft, reinforced, or rigid. A soft cervical collar is usually made of

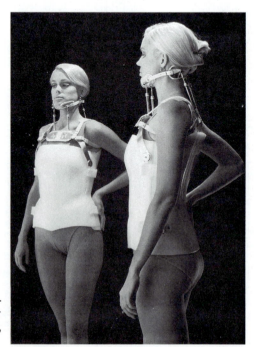

Figure 9-12. TLSO with cervical attachment. (*Source:* Becker Orthopaedic, Troy, MI, with permission.)

polyurethane foam or foam rubber and is encased in a knitted material like stockinette. Rear closure is usually accomplished using Velcro.

The Philadelphia collar is an example of a reinforced CO made of polyethylene foam reinforced with plastic struts anteriorly and posteriorly (Figure 9-13). These orthoses are available in a range of adult and pediatric sizes, based on the distance from chin to chest and neck circumference. There are two styles available, with or without a cutout for an intubation tube.

Another example of a reinforced cervical orthosis is the Sternal-Occipitomandibular Immobilizer (SOMI) (Figure 9-14). The SOMI consists of three pieces: a sternal yoke, the anterior mandibular support, and the occipital support. These CTOs are easily fitted, particularly when the patient is recumbent, and are available in adult and pediatric sizes.

The most rigid cervical orthosis is the Halo (Figure 9-15). Originally developed for polio patients, it has become widely used for the unstable cervical spine, usually at the C1-2 level, although it may be used for instability at more inferior levels, including the upper thoracic spine.

EFFECTS AND EFFECTIVENESS OF SPINAL ORTHOSES

In addition to the intended clinical functions of immobilization/motion control, support, and prevention/correction of skeletal deformity, several other consequences of the application of spinal orthoses have been described and/or studied. Not all effects of spinal orthotics are positive. Potential negative effects include skin breakdown due to the intimate fit, psychologic dependency, and weakened muscles or aggravated symptoms, thought to be a by-product of

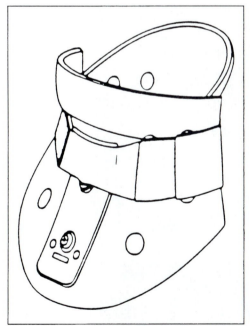

Figure 9-13. Philadelphia collar.

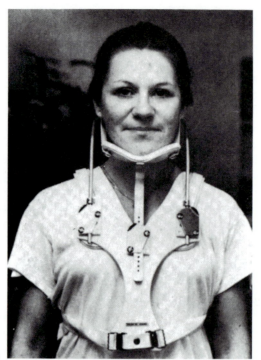

Figure 9-14. SOMI.

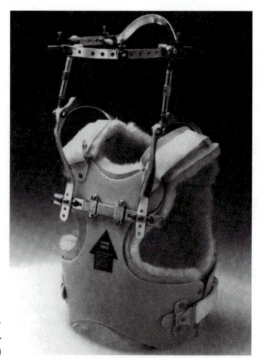

Figure 9-15. Halo. (*Source:* Fillauer Orthopaedic, Chattanooga, TN, with permission.)

inactivity or lack of motion. Reports of the effects and effectiveness of spinal orthoses are summarized in the following sections.

Immobilization/Motion Control/Support

The normal anatomy of the human spine dictates to some extent what motions occur. For example, although there is motion of the thoracic spine, it is more limited than either the cervical or lumbar regions. Due to the thoracic spine construction, motion into flexion is greater than extension. Lateral bending of the spine increases as the spinal level moves inferiorly, but axial rotation decreases from superior to inferior. The lumbar spine allows flexion and extension, but little pure rotation due to the construction and position of the facets.

White and Panjabi refer to the "low stiff viscoelastic transmitter" when describing the medium between the orthosis and the skeletal structures of the spine. Because of the skin and soft-tissue interface, it is impossible for even the most rigid orthosis to completely immobilize the spine. To this end, even the Halo has been shown by Johnson et al to allow some cervical-sine motion. Because slight bone movement at fracture sites is known to stimulate bone healing, some motion may be desirable in orthotic applications. It remains the responsibility of the health care professional to understand the goal of each orthotic application to provide the best system consistent with the case.

In an effort to mobilize young children with paraplegia, HKAFOs like the RGO and ARGO may be used (chapter 7), often combined with a TLSO body jacket to externally support the paralytic spine. It should be noted, however, that no spinal orthosis has proven effective in preventing the progression of *paralytic* scoliotic curves. Campbell, in 1999, reported on the long term progression of paralytic scoliosis in a paraplegic individual who wore RGOs while a growing youngster. Previous reports by Raycroft and Curtis describe the 52 percent incidence of paralytic scoliosis in 103 children with spina bifida but no other congenital vertebral anomalies. A higher incidence is related to the more cephalad location of the lesion, and therefore more extensive trunk paralysis.

Banta and Hamada, in 1976, reported on 268 patients with a 4-year follow up indicating that those patients with defects in the thoracic and lumbar spine developed scoliosis 100 percent of the time by the ages of 10 to 14 years.

In 1999, Campbell questioned the efficacy of RGOs and HGOs to alter the course of scoliosis or to retard the eventual onset of hip and knee flexion contractures in a young, ambulatory population. He presents a case for a more complete biomechanical analysis of each individual patient to treat the spinal deformity as well as the paraplegia.

Management of Thoracolumbar Fractures.
Holdsworth in 1963 was the first to use the term burst fracture to describe a spinal fracture from extreme axial loading that caused the body of the vertebra to explode, thus threatening stability of the spine. The burst fracture may involve one or both of the bony end plates of the vertebral body and may or may not produce a loose bone fragment that can retropulse or move posteriorly to cause compression on the spinal cord and neurologic deficits.

In 1983, Denis developed a three-part classification of spinal fractures. Instability of the first degree involves the risk of increasing kyphosis, as often seen in compression fractures. Such fractures may be safely treated with an anterior control TLSO spinal orthosis.

Instability of the second degree involves a burst fracture with the risk that further collapse of the fracture may lead to increased neurologic deficit. Denis believed that early ambulation or sitting upright, even in a motion-limiting TLSO, could cause further neurologic problems due to instability under axial loading. He reported on 20 percent, or 6 of 29, cases of non-operatively treated burst fractures without initial neurologic deficit that later developed deficits. Prior to Denis's report, most fractures of thoracic and lumbar vertebrae were treated with either a TLSO or LSO with anterior control, using orthoses like the Jewett. In light of these findings, many surgeons altered their postfracture treatment program to include a TLSO body jacket to control the fracture in all planes. The jacket is often lined with 1/4-inch foam padding to allow for minor changes in body size or configuration, because many of these patients wear their orthoses for 3 to 6 months and some longer. In cases where high thoracic and/or concomitant cervical fractures occur, cervical extensions may be added to these orthoses without difficulty. Most patients are able to don and doff the TLSO independently.

A study from the University of Iowa found that neurologically intact burst fractures may be successfully treated nonoperatively using bed rest for 6 weeks followed by the use of a TLSO body jacket for up to 6 months. According to this study, there were no complications, and the occurrence of postinjury back pain or deformity was very small.

McEvoy and Bradford reported a retrospective review of 399 fractures of the spine. Of these, 53 were followed for at least 1 year, 22 of whom were treated nonsurgically and 31 operatively. All had burst fractures. Thirty-eight had neurologic deficits. The patients without deficit were treated with body jackets or casts and showed good results. At follow up averaging 3 years, 68 percent were neurologically improved, although back pain was more common in the surgical group. These findings suggest that patients with burst fractures may be treated nonsurgically with TLSO body jackets with good results.

Presently the issue whether to brace a "fixed" fracture is an open question. The record of most instrumentation for spinal fixation is good. The presence of severe fractures or systemic diseases might cause the surgeon to want the peace of mind of some extra spinal protection. Patients with Potts' disease, diabetes, rheumatoid arthritis, or severe spinal osteoporosis are likely to heal fractures slowly. Osteomyelitis of the spine is always a concern. Spinal metastases almost always require spinal orthoses following surgery, whether spinal instrumentation was implanted or not.

Control of Thoracolumbar Spine Motion.

Orthotic intervention may be considered adjunctive treatment; sometimes it is used only after other treatments fail to provide the desired relief. Fidler and Plasmans in 1983 compared lumbosacral motion while using four spinal orthoses. These four orthoses were the canvas corset, the Raney LSO, the Baycast TLSO, and the Baycast TLSO with leg spica. Results indicated that the corset reduced the lumbar spine motion by one-third; the Raney and Baycast TLSO reduced motion by two-thirds; while the Baycast with spica was most effective. The Baycast with spica restricted angular movement below the third lumbar level including the lumbosacral junction. There was no restriction of lumbosacral junction motion with the LSOs or the Baycast jacket alone, since both lacked the leg extension. Therefore, if the orthotic goal is to reduce motion at the level of the lumbosacral junction, a TLSO with leg spica must be used.

To evaluate the role of primary orthotic treatment, J. Weinstein and K. Spratt reported on patients presenting with either spondylolisthesis or retrolisthesis who were randomly assigned to either a flexion or extension orthosis protocol. The method involved a very complete diagnostic evaluation to measure spondy or retro displacement. This evaluation provided the baseline from which follow-up evaluations could be compared. A Raney flexion orthosis or TLSO with anterior control orthosis was randomly assigned and fitted by an experienced orthotist. Evaluation of treatment outcomes was assessed using a visual-analogue pain scale (VAS), a disability questionnaire (DQ), and the organic pain-behavior composite (OPBC). Results indicated that compliance of orthosis wearing was relatively good, with 60 of 65 (92 percent) returning for at least one of two follow-up visits. Even though only 55 percent of patients returned for both follow-up visits, 31 of 65 (48 percent) were found to be compliant, wearing the orthosis at least 100 hours in one month or 400 hours in 4 months. Females were found to be less compliant than males, although most of the females (8 of 10) were treated in flexion orthoses. None of the noncompliant subjects had been assigned an inappropriate orthosis, as judged by radiographic follow up. A general tendency was for improvement over time, regardless of assignment protocol or amount of vertebral-body translation. Patients in extension orthoses demonstrated greater improvement as compared to all other patients for each of the three outcome criteria.

Cervical Spine Immobilization/Control. Soft collars provide kinesthetic reminders to immobilize the cervical spine. Hartman et al reported that soft collars restrict only 5 percent to 10 percent of flexion and extension and provide no restriction to axial rotation. Johnson et al studied 44 normal subjects wearing three of six possible cervical orthoses. These six were the soft collar, the Philadelphia collar, the four-poster orthosis, the SOMI, the Yale, and the Halo. Like Hartman et al, Johnson et al found the soft collar to be a useful reminder but little else. The Philadelphia collar was biomechanically better than the soft collar, but was not effective in controlling rotation. The four-poster orthosis was found to be equal to other CTOs in controlling flexion, especially of the middle cervical vertebrae. Similar to other CTOs, it was not effective in controlling rotation, lateral bending, and flexion and extension of the upper cervical spine. The other CTOs provided better fixation of the orthosis on the thorax and, thus, better cervical control. The Yale orthosis was the product of this study, since it was the best overall motion-restriction device tested, even though it lacked support at the C1-2 joint. Interestingly the SOMI was very successful at controlling motion at the C1-2 and C2-3 joints. Because the SOMI works well in controlling upper-level flexion, and because it is easily fitted in the supine position, it is often the orthosis of choice where upper cervical level flexion is a potential problem.

Johnson found the Halo, originally used at Rancho Los Amigos, to be the best overall orthosis in controlling rotation of the cervical spine, even though it did not completely eliminate all spinal motion. Because acutely injured patients often cannot tolerate the amount of distraction necessary to completely immobilize the spine, a very small amount of motion occurs even with the Halo in place.

The two most common clinical problems associated with the Halo are pin loosening and infection. Lind et al studied the effects of the Halo orthosis on vital capacity. In neurologically intact patients, the Halo reduced the vital capacity by 10 percent, although the reduction was regained after removal of the Halo.

In 1984, Lunsford reported on 10 normal women, fitted with four cervical orthoses: the Philadelphia, the Malibu, the Miami J, and the Newport Extended Wear. An elastic tensiometer controlled the consistency of resistive force. Motion was measured and restriction of motion reported as a percentage of normal. Allowed range of motion in degrees was reported. The

Malibu restricted saggital flexion by 50 percent. Saggital extension was limited by 57 percent. The Malibu was best at transverse plane motion restriction, limiting motion by 61 percent.

Deformity Prevention and Correction

The TLSO or CTLSO orthoses are used for problems or diseases of the thoracic or thoracolumbar spine, depending on the nature of the pathology and its anatomic location. Perhaps the best known diseases treated with these orthoses are idiopathic scoliosis and juvenile kyphosis. In these cases, the orthosis acts as a corrective device, applying forces in given directions to produce changes in the musculoskeleton as the child grows.

The forces needed to correct a coronal plane deformity of the thoracic spine have been measured to be 3 to 5 kg. Andriacchi et al demonstrated that ribs provide stability, and this principle is used routinely with CTLSOs of the Milwaukee type (Figure 9-16) by applying lateral superomedially directed forces with thoracic pads. This biomechanical model has been developed by Patwardhan et al in a classic work that should be required reading for anyone involved in the management of these patients.

Use of orthoses for idiopathic scoliosis and kyphosis is often based on the concept of active movement away from the pads, thus producing active correction. However, in neurologically based scolioses and kyphoses, patients may be unable to actively pull away from the pads, thus requiring a more passive treatment principle. CTLSOs and TLSOs are used in this patient group to allow supported sitting and to reduce the rate of further skeletal collapse. Radiographs of this patient group reveal "drooping ribs" that angle acutely and often nearly parallel to the

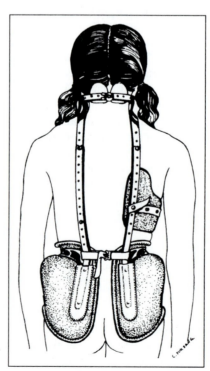

Figure 9-16. CTLSO, Milwaukee type.

bodies of the vertebrae. In these cases, the lateral pads or lateral walls of the TLSO or body jacket provide little corrective force. Generally, the higher the apex of the cervical or thoracic curve the more difficult it is to control, the less effective the treatment, and the greater the chance of curve progression over time.

The literature in this area is ever evolving. There are critics who oppose the use of orthoses because there are cases where curve progression continues despite proper bracing and surgical stabilization is eventually necessary. There are some who argue that most small curves (30 degrees or less) deserve careful observation and a trial using orthotic treatment. The natural history of scoliosis has yet to be completely elucidated. Retrospective studies show that about 30 percent of all idiopathic scoliotic curves will eventually arrest without surgical stabilization. The clinical problem is how to prospectively determine who will arrest and who will progress and which treatment to provide.

Weinstein and Ponseti have written an excellent review on idiopathic scoliosis, indicating that double curves are at a greater risk for progression than single curves. The older the patient is at the time of presentation, the less likely it is that the curve will progress. Curves detected before menarche tend to progress more than those detected postmenarche, 66 percent to 33 percent. The lower the Risser sign and the larger the initial curve at detection, the higher the risk of progression.

It was once thought that after skeletal maturity was reached, there was no further curve progression, but recent studies have demonstrated that this is not always the case. Weinstein and Ponseti found that 68 percent of the curves in their study progressed after skeletal maturity unless they were less than 30 degrees. In thoracic curves, the Cobb angle, apical vertebral rotation, and the Mehta angle were important prognostic factors. In lumbar curves, the degree of apical vertebral rotation, the Cobb angle, the direction of the curve, and the relationship of the fifth lumbar vertebra to the intercrest line were of prognostic value. Curves that measured between 50 and 75 degrees at skeletal maturity, particularly thoracic curves, progressed the most, an average of 1 degree per year for 40 years. However, by further follow up, it was shown that these curves caused no more back pain than in the normal population and required no life-saving surgery or other procedures, contrary to what has been stated by some authors.

Weinstein and Ponseti state that few long-term studies demonstrate brace effectiveness, because most do not document long term curve progression after bracing has been discontinued. The most common response to bracing is a moderate amount of correction while the orthosis is worn, with slow, steady progression of the curvature back to the original magnitude of the curve. According to Weinstein and Ponseti, this occurs, in 80 percent of braced patients regardless of the curve pattern.

In 1984, Miller et al reported on 255 patients aged 8 to 17 years with idiopathic scoliosis curves of 15 to 30 degrees. Divided into two groups, they were treated with either a CTLSO or no orthosis. Results showed a nonsignificant trend, suggesting that CTLSOs reduced the progression of the curve. However, because 75 percent of the curves were nonprogressive, it is possible that no bracing would have been equally successful. The orthosis did prevent progression of 5 percent of the patients at a mean rate of 8 percent per year. Unfortunately these patients were not easily identified prospectively; thus, withholding treatment was not justified.

Gardner et al discussed the search for prognostic indicators in the progression of scoliosis curves. The series of 70 unselected patients revealed that braced patients from 10 to 55 degrees did better than nonbraced. Best mean correction measured at 13 months following brace cessation was 41 percent. In the braced group, 33 percent of the curves progressed and 24 percent reduced at least 5 degrees. Untreated patients progressed in 43 percent of cases, while 14 percent had curves that improved at least 5 degrees.

Winter et al reported on 95 patients with thoracic curves of 30 to 39 degrees treated by CTLSOs from the same orthotic laboratory and treated with the same protocol. Follow up averaged 2 1/2 years or until surgery. Of the 95, 15 (16 percent) eventually underwent surgery. For the 80 who did not, curve progression began at 33 degrees and at follow up was 31 degrees. This reflects a pattern of similar studies, but does not speak to the issue of difficult curves or curves that tend to progress in a high percentage of patients. A case report of a 57-degree T5-11 curve treated by brace is reported. The follow-up curve measured at 40 degrees. The authors suggest that no other explanations exist except that the CTLSO was effective.

Bassett and Bunnell evaluated the influence of the axillary level Wilmington brace (Figure 9-17) on spinal decompensation in adolescent idiopathic scoliosis. The concept of decompensation involves the relationship of a plumb line between the seventh cervical vertebra and the gluteal crease. The greater the distance between the two structures, the greater the decompensation. Ideally, the compensated curves will align over one another. Seventy-one patients with greater than 1 cm of decompensation were included in this study. Average follow up was 2 years. There was no correlation between the Cobb angle pretreatment and the decompensation post-treatment. Results indicated that improvement averaged 1.4 cm for thoracic curves; 1.4 cm for thoracolumbar; 1.5 cm for double-structural curves, with decompensation in 27 patients (38 percent) less than 1 cm. Six cases increased an average of 1.2 cm. The authors concluded that the Wilmington brace was successful in treating scoliosis.

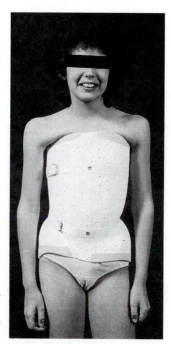

Figure 9-17. TLSO, Wilmington type. (*Source:* Basset G, written communication, with permission.)

The Rosenberger scoliosis orthosis (Figure 9-18) is a low-profile, custom-molded orthosis used in the treatment of idiopathic scoliosis. It uses a snugly fitted end-support section and high counterforce trimlines on the concavity of the curve to aid the righting reflex. A corrective strap is located inside the jacket to reduce the curve by adding a transverse load in the posterolateral quadrant. Worn 23 hours a day, it is used with apices below T6. Gavin et al reported on 12 patients with curves averaging 25 to 35 degrees, mean 28.1 degrees. Initial reduction ranged from 23 percent to 100 percent, with a mean of 42.1 percent. Longer-term postbrace results were not presented.

Emans et al reported on 295 patients treated with the Boston, low-profile TLSO system with at least 1 year postbracing follow up. Prebrace curves ranged from 20 to 59 degrees using the Cobb method. Mean treatment time was 2.9 years. Mean best in-brace correction was 50 percent, with mean postbrace correction of 11 percent. Follow-up comparison with prebrace angles demonstrated 49 percent unchanged (5 degrees), 39 percent correction of 5 to 15 degrees, 4 percent corrected 15 degrees or more, 4 percent lost 5 to 15 degrees, and 3 percent lost more than 15 degrees. Twelve percent eventually required surgery. Their data indicated that partial brace compliance appeared as effective as full-time wearing. Emans et al concluded that Boston orthoses without a cervical superstructure appeared as successful as those with superstructure, for curves with apices below T7.

Scheuermann's kyphosis, or epiphysitis, is a disease for which the literature indicates consistent successful orthotic treatment. Montgomery and Erwin reviewed 203 cases of Scheuermann's kyphosis. Sixty-two were fitted with Milwaukee-type CTLSOs. Thirty-nine were followed in the orthosis for an average of 18 months. The mean curve was reduced from 62 degrees to 41 degrees. Further follow up revealed a loss of correction of 15 degrees, indicating that 18 months of brace wearing was not enough.

Dr. Robert Winter writes that during the 1990s, many studies, such as those by Fernandez-Filiberti et al and Longstein and Winter, have confirmed that the natural history of idiopathic scoliosis can be positively effected by spinal orthotic fitting. He continues that orthotic care should begin with the curve between 20 and 29 degrees, as measured using the method of Cobb. Studies by Longstein and Winter that compare curves treated at 20 to 29 degrees 30 to 39 degrees, show better results with earlier treatment.

In the earlier treatment, the goal was to maintain the curve at the magnitude it began. Orthoses were not expected to correct curves beyond the original magnitude. Current treatment at

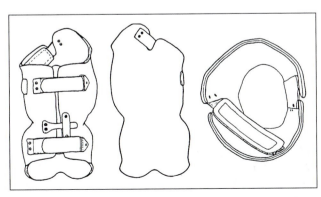

Figure 9-18. TLSO, Rosenberger. (left) Anterior view of the orthosis, including trimline, opposition gradients, and high axillary wall. (middle) Posterior trimline, with unique superior aspect. (right) Transverse view, showing placement of corrective strap. (*Source:* Gavin T, Bunch WH, Dvonch VM. The rosenberger scoliosis orthosis. *J Assoc Child Prosthet/Orthot Clin.* 1986; 21:37, with permission.)

the University of Iowa using the Rosenberger orthosis demonstrate that it is possible to reduce an immature curve under 30 degrees to near zero. Care must be taken to not decompensate the curve, or push or pull the upper spine out of line with the top of the sacrum. The goal must be to correct and hold each curve as much as possible, without malaligning it over the sacrum.

Secondary Effects of Spinal Orthoses

Nachemson and Morris studied in vivo effects of abdominal compression on intradiscal pressure. By using a very tight abdominal corset worn to the point of tolerance, intradiscal pressure was reduced by 30 percent.

Norton and Brown inserted K wires into the spinous processes of lumbar vertebrae and posterosuperior iliac spines. Sitting was found to produce lumbar flexion of L5 and S1. Application of a long dorsal-lumbar orthosis focused forces near the T-L junction, too proximal to affect the lumbar spine. Flexion at the L5-S1 joint was greater in the orthosis, causing increased motion at the ends of the supported levels. These orthoses only reduced interspace flexion but did not eliminate it. While using an inflatable corset, the intradiscal pressure was lowered by 25 percent. This finding suggests that the clinical results using corsets and orthoses may be due partially to compression of the abdomen, thus decreasing the load on the vertebral column.

Waters and Morris studied electrical activity of the trunk muscles with and without spinal orthoses. In standing, both a chair-back orthosis and corset caused decreased activity or had no effect, while during walking, neither orthosis had any effect. During fast walking, there was increased muscle activity while wearing the orthoses.

THE FUTURE OF SPINAL ORTHOTICS

Undoubtedly, future studies will continue to elucidate important factors involved in the evaluation and treatment of spinal disorders. With the use of improved imaging techniques, evaluation and follow-up will be more precise and specific. The role of nonsurgical interventions will be more thoroughly evaluated and understood, and as new materials and designs are developed, the place of spinal orthotics in the treatment regimen will become clearer.

Idiopathic scoliosis orthoses will continue to evolve as further studies indicate necessary changes. Electronic compliance monitoring will answer the questions concerning how many hours the orthoses need to be worn daily in order to alter the natural history of this disorder. Such monitors are now available and need to be implemented clinically. Much credit for continual improvements in orthotic treatment goes to Thomas Gavin and Associates at Loyola University in Chicago for the exemplary research they have published to help all of us understand this very complicated disease and its orthotic treatment.

REFERENCES

1. Andriacchi T, Schultz A, Belytschco T, Galante J. A model for studies of mechanical interaction between the human spine and rib cage. *J Biomech.* 1974; 7:497.
2. Banta JV, Hamada JS. The natural history of spine deformity in myelomeningocele: A study of 130 patients. *J Bone Joint Surg.* 1976; 58A:279.

3. Bassett GS, Bunnell WP. Influence of the Wilmington brace on spinal decompensation in adolescent idiopathic scoliosis. *Clin Orthop Rel Res.* 1987; 223:164–169.

4. Campbell JH. Outcome study: The progression of spinal deformity in paraplegic children fitted with reciprocating gait orthoses. *JPO.* 1999; 11(4):79–84.

5. Denis F. The three column spine and its significance in the classification of acute thoracolumbar spinal injuries. *Spine.* 1983; 8:817.

6. Emans JB et al. The Boston bracing system for idiopathic scoliosis. *Spine.* 1986; 11(8):792–801.

7. Ewing E. *Fashion in Underwear.* London: Batsford; 1971.

8. Fernandez-Filiberti R, Flynn J, Ramirez N, Trautman M, Alegria M. Effectiveness of TLSO bracing in the conservative treatment of idiopathic scoliosis. *J Ped Orthop.* 1995; 15:176–181.

9. Fidler MW, Plasmans MT. The effect of four types of support on the segmental mobility of the lumbosacral spine. *J Bone Joint Surg.* 1983; 65A(7):943–947.

10. Gardner ADH et al. Some beneficial effects of bracing and a search for prognostic indicators in idiopathic scoliosis. *Spine.* 1986; 11:779.

11. Gavin T, Bunch WH, Dvonch VM. The Rosenberger scoliosis orthosis. *Int Clin Info Bull.* 1986; 21(3–4):35–38.

12. Hartman JT, Palumbo F, Hill BJ. Cineradiography of the braced normal cervical spine: A comparative study of five commonly used cervical orthoses. *Clin Orthop.* 1975; 109:97–102.

13. Holdsworth FW. Fracture, dislocations, and fracture dislocations of the spine. *J Bone Joint Surg.* 1963; 45 B:6.

14. Johnson RM, Hart DL, Simmons EF, Ramsby GR, Southwich WO. Cervical orthoses—A study comparing their effectiveness in restricting cervical motion in normal subjects. *J Bone Joint Surg.* 1977; 59A:332.

15. Johnson RM, Owen JR, Hart DC, Callahan RA. Cervical orthoses: A guide to their selection and use. *Clin Orthop.* 1981; 154:34, 35.

16. Lind BJ, Nordwall A, Sihlbom H. Manuscript in preparation.

17. Longstein JE, Winter RB. The Milwaukee brace for the treatment of adolescent idiopathic scoliosis: A review of 1020 patients. *J Bone Joint Surg.* 1994; 76A:1207–1221.

18. Lucas DB, Bresler B. Stability of the ligamentous spine. Technical Report No. 40, Biomechanics Laboratory, University of California, San Francisco and Berkeley: January 1961; 41.

19. Lunsford TR, Davidson M, Lunsford BR. The effectiveness of four contemporary cervical orthoses in restricting cervical motion. *JPO.* 1994; 6(4):93–99.

20. McEvoy RD, Bradford DS. The management of burst fractures of the thoracic and lumbar spine. *Spine.* 1985; 10(7):631–637.

21. Miller JAA, Nachemson AL, Schultz AB. Effectiveness of braces in mild idiopathic scoliosis. *Spine.* 1984; 9(6):632.

22. Montgomery SP, Erwin WE. Scheuermann's kyphosis—long-term results of Milwaukee brace treatment. *Spine.* 1981; 6(1):5–8.

23. Nachemson A, Morris JM. In vivo measurements of intradiscal pressure, a method for the determination of pressure in the lower lumbar disc. *J Bone Joint Surg.* 1964; 46A:1077.

24. Nachemson AL. Orthotic treatment for injuries and diseases of the spinal column. *Phys Med Rehabil.* 1987; 1(2):11–24.

25. Norton PL, Brown T. The immobilizing efficiency of back braces. *J Bone Joint Surg.* 1957; 39A:111–139.

26. Patwardhan A, Vanderbs R, Knight GW, Gogan WJ, Levine PD. Biomechanics of the spine. In: *Atlas of Orthotics.* Bund W, ed. St. Louis, MO: Mosby; 1985; 139–150.

27. Perry J. The use of external support in the treatment of low back pain. *J Bone Joint Surg.* 1970; 52A:1440.

28. Raney FL. The royalite flexion jacket. *Spinal Orthotics.* Committee on Prosthetics Research and Development National Academy of Sciences. Monograph. 1969; 85.

29. Raycroft JE, Curtis BH. Spinal curvature of myelomeningocele. AAOS Symposium on Myelomeningocele. Saint Louis, MO, 1972.
30. Waters RL, Morris JM. Effects of spinal supports on the electrical activity of muscles of the trunk. *J Bone Joint Surg.* 1970; 52A:51.
31. Weinstein J, Sprett KQ. Personal communication; 1988.
32. Weinstein SL, Ponseti IV. Curve progression in idiopathic scoliosis. *J Bone Joint Surg.* 1983; 65A(4):447–455.
33. White A, Panjabi M. *Clinical Biomechanics of the Spine.* Philadelphia, PA: Lippincott; 1978.
34. Winter RB, Lonstein JE, Drogt J, Noren CA. The effectiveness of bracing in the nonoperative treatment of idiopathic scoliosis. *Spine.* 1986; 11:790, 791.

CHAPTER 10

Upper Limb Orthoses

The hand surgeon is a relatively new subspecialty allowing a surgeon of orthopaedics, plastics, or microvascular surgery to concentrate on the needs of the patients with hand injuries. Although Sterling Bunnell is usually credited as being the "Father of Hand Surgery," many others have been responsible for equally important advances in this field. Dr. Adrian E. Flatt was a British Royal Air Force surgeon whose many contributions include the development of finger joint prosthetic arthroplasty and innovative changes in the treatment of the congenital hand. His interest in upper limb orthoses and their role in the postoperative care of patients with such problems is particularly noteworthy.

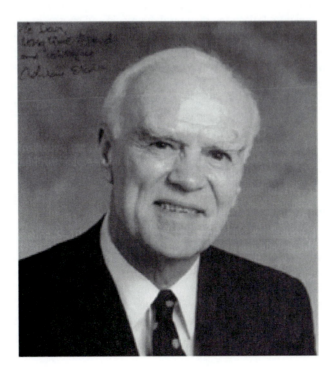

Following completion of reading this chapter, the student will be able to:

1. Discuss the rationale for making the decision as to whether to use low-temperature versus high-temperature materials for upper limb orthotics.
2. Describe the purposes for hand splinting and their relevance to design and materials.
3. Describe four common designs of hand orthoses, their indications, and the treatment expectation.

This chapter will present a limited discussion of the etiology of problems requiring upper extremity orthotics, a brief review of hand functions, and a discussion of orthotic components. It is acknowledged that entire books and atlases have been written on this subject. No attempt will be made here to cover other than the very basics of care.

UPPER EXTREMITY ORTHOSES

The hand is one part of the human anatomy that, more than any other, is treated by many health care professionals. Reasons for treatment by such a diverse group vary, perhaps even for well-intended philosophies. The hand may be cared for initially by a general practitioner, an orthopaedic surgeon, a hand surgeon, a plastic surgeon, a general surgeon, or a traumatologist or emergency room physician. Following the initial diagnosis and treatment plan, the patient may be cared for by a physical therapist, an occupational therapist, a hand therapist, a nurse, and/or an orthotist/prosthetist. Depending on the availability and organization, hand patients are cared for by a diverse group with equally diverse goals and philosophies. Whoever agrees to care for hand patients needs only two basic prerequisites: basic knowledge of hand anatomy, kinesiology, and current care; and a desire to work closely with the managing physician or surgeon and the patient.

ETIOLOGY

Problems leading to the use of hand orthoses can be categorized into three general groups: trauma, congenital problems, and reconstruction following disease.

Trauma

By far the most common patient etiology is the hand-trauma group. These injuries occur in all parts of life including accidents, work-related mishaps, burns, and injuries associated with other injuries, such as the Volkmann's ischemic contracture associated with the fracture of the humerus and subsequent severance of the brachial artery. Many hand-trauma cases also occur while working around the house. A large group of hand injuries come from farm accidents. Recent reports from the Institute of Medicine reveal that farming is the most dangerous occupation in the United States.

Congenital Problems

Congenital hand defects come in a varied array of groups, including the syndactyly or webbed fingers; central defects, where central or middle digits are absent; and polydactyly, or too many fingers. Larger hand-and-arm conditions include radial and ulnar club hand and brachydactyly, or short fingers, with concomitant dysplasia of the entire extremity.

Disease

The reconstructive patient may carry a variety of diagnoses, usually the destructive, collagen-vascular diseases like rheumatoid arthritis, or lupus erythematosis. The patients often undergo numerous surgical procedures to reconstruct the deformed hand, bone, joints, soft tissue, tendons, or skin. Many postoperative situations call for the expertise of a therapist knowledgeable in the care of hands.

TYPES OF HAND SPLINTS

Splints connote many very different things to caregivers, patients, and surgeons. The role of provision of such a splint may be shared, just as the postinjury or postoperative care may be shared. Generally splints occur in two forms, either temporary or definitive.

Temporary Versus Definitive Splints

Temporary splinting is often thought to be done for a primary purpose. It may be altered upon change in condition; should be lightweight, strong, easily donned and doffed; cost little; and provide all biomechanical forces necessary to treat the pathology or need. Needless to say, few, if any, splints rate high in all categories.

From an orthotist's point of view, the time such a splint is needed must be established early, by the surgeon in cooperation with the therapist so that construction and materials may be consistent with such goals. This will prevent situations in which a definitive splint is made for a problem only requiring temporary materials. Generally temporary splints may be constructed of plaster, fiberglass cast, low-temperature thermoplastics, or moldable sheet thermoplastics. Aluminum, steel, or thermosetting resins are usually not considered temporary.

Static Versus Dynamic Splints

In addition to being temporary or definitive, hand splints are also designed to be static or dynamic. Generally speaking, static splints are thought to be resting, or positional splints, used to position or hold a hand or wrist. Dynamic splints are splints that provide a dynamic force, generally utilizing energy-storing materials like rubber bands, spring steel, wound, coiled wire, or plastic with memory. By the design of the splint, a portion of the hand is held or secured while the dynamic force is gently applied. Often this is done to reduce or "direct" the results of scar tissue.

Dynamic splints may direct forces at the small joints of the fingers, the wrist, or the entire hand and wrist. Due to the anatomy of the hand, advantage may be gained by prepositioning the wrist, to attain the desired stretch of the finger. An example of this is the tenodesis effect. When the wrist extends, the fingers flex (metacarpophalangeal, MCP). This natural occurrence may be harnessed to provide useful motion and function.

The purposes of hand splinting may be considered in three groups. These groups are not exclusive as often hand splinting, and indeed, hand care involves goals that may descend from all subgroups. These subgroups are:

1. Immobilization, protection, and/or support. Examples of immobilization, protection, or support would include a fresh burn with skin graft, an acute rheumatoid wrist, or a wrist fracture with finger laceration.

2. Positioning. Positioning often includes sequelae of diseases that cause paralysis where the goal is to maintain positioning, and to maintain motion via passive exercise, while awaiting motor return as with a CVA.

3. Prevention of deformities. Prevention of deformities includes disease or injury that produces imbalance injuries where absent lumbricals may produce an intrinsic minus hand and splinting may assist.

4. Assistance in functional motions. Assistance in functional motion usually involves help with activities of daily living. These tasks may include the use of wrist extension splints to allow mid-sagittal activities where the radial nerve is absent. Another example includes the use of tenodesis splints, as with the C5 quadriplegic, where wrist extension harnessed produces finger flexion and, therefore, useful prehension.

HAND FUNCTIONS

There are four phases of hand function: reach, prehension, carry, and release. Reach requires good range of motion (ROM) in all joints, proximal stabilization, and muscle power in the extensor groups. Following reach, to get the hand to the mouth, 10 to 15 degrees of glenohumeral flexion is required. In the absence of flexion, more wrist flexion must be used.

Prehension may also be referred to as grip. Prehension patterns are primary functions of the hand. There are three main categories: pinch, grasp, and hook. Pinch may be tip, palmar, or lateral. Tip places the object between index finger tip and thumb, with the key to the definition including interphalangeal (IP) and distal interphalangeal (DIP) joint flexion. Tip pinch is usually used for smaller articles, and often employs decreased strength. Palmar prehension, or three-jawed chuck, is the most commonly used form, accounting for 60 percent of all hand activities. This form uses the thumb, index, and long fingers, with the thumb pad placed directly under the fingers. It uses the median nerve, and motor and sensory distribution. Lateral prehension, or key grip, positions the thumb over the flexed proximal interphalangeal (PIP) joint of the index finger. It is called key grip because often keys are placed in locks in this fashion. Severe rheumatoid arthritics who have lost collateral structures of the MCP joints of index through small finger often rely on this grip. Normally, and in patients with rheumatoid arthritis (RA), key or lateral prehension generates more force than tip or palmar.

Tip, palmar, and lateral are prehensions used to manipulate objects to function during activities of daily living. Cylinder, spherical, and hook are gross grasps used to hold rather than to manipulate. Cylinder grasp fashions the hand around a cylinder with the MCP slightly flexed, the PIPs flexed to 75 degrees of flexion, and the thumb opposed under the index and long fingers. Spherical grip may be described as in holding a tennis ball, with the thumb slightly abducted and extended, rather than opposed as in cylinder grasp. Hook grip is often thought of as the "link grip," linking ape prehension with human, and using all fingers, particularly the PIP joints, without using the thumb.

Often students new to the anatomy and kinesiology of the hand confuse thumb extension and abduction. Abduction of the thumb carpometacarpal (CMC) joints involves motion away from the plane of the palm, usually including partial opposition, at least under the index and long pads, as in palmar prehension. Thumb extension of the CMC joint involves motion in the plane of the palm. Note that extension of the thumb joint may occur with the thumb CMC joint either abducted/opposed or extended.

Conditions Affecting the Use of Hand Splints

Any therapist or orthotist working in the area of hand care should be acquainted with the basic science involved in stiffness, and scarring associated with edema. Many sources are available. One resource of note is *Hand Rehabilitation,* in the *Clinics in Physical Therapy* series, edited by Christine A. Moran, RPT. Others may include Hunter and Mackin, Tubiana, and the *AAOS Symposium on Tendon Surgery in the Hand,* edited by Dr. James Urbaniak. Complete reading of these references will allow the new hand therapist a thorough basis for the treatment provided.

Prior to working with fresh tendon injuries, the reader is referred to the excellent work of Evans and Thompson in the 1993 *Journal of Hand Therapy.* Specifics of techniques for 165 tendon injuries reveal excellent results following active motion as redefined.

Of note in distal radial fracture treatment is the work of Laseter and Carter published in 1996. This is must reading prior to caring for patients in need of orthotics for fracture care.

The physiology of scar formation is important in hand care. Following injury, surgery, or infection in the hand, protein-rich exudate invades the narrow passages between layers of tissue in the hand. Because the body uses fibroblasts to seal off infection, normal blood does not carry away the fibroblasts. If the tissue planes do not move, either due to pain, surgical implants, edema, or hand splints, fibrosis occurs very early on. Thus, although hand splints may assist hand care by preventing unwanted motion, this goal must be carefully considered along with the concomitant outcome of stiffness via protein-rich exudate and immobilization.

A. E. Flatt believes that scar formation and remodeling occurs from Day 1 through 18 months post injury. He states that scar formation is always present following the 18-month time period, with the amount and severity of loss of motion and function determined by the genetics of patient, the type and severity of injury, number of surgical procedures in a relatively short period of time, postoperative care, therapist/patient cooperation, and appropriate orthotic management.

Hardy quotes Weber and Davis in her chapter on scar formation: "Hand therapy is behavioral modification of the fibroblast during the healing response." Gribben, in her chapter on splinting, raises nine questions to be answered prior to splinting any patient:

1. Identification of primary, secondary, and association problems?
2. What do I expect to accomplish through the use of a splint?
3. What splint components are integral to correction of the problems?
4. What splint design will best encompass these components?

5. Should the splint be static or dynamic?

6. Should the base be volar or dorsal?

7. What joints should be included in the splint?

8. What is the patient's level of cognition? Is it adequate for correct wearing, and usage of the splint?

9. What is the patient's emotional status?

Once a decision to splint has been agreed upon by all team members (including the patient), a design must emerge. So-called off-the-shelf splints are denounced by many and used by most. However, OTS or noncustom devices of all kinds suffer from the old adage of "fitting everyone, and therefore no one." Fortunately, there is some middle ground, because many patients may be successfully custom-fitted using readily available and premade orthoses.

There are many who believe custom-made orthoses are necessary for each and every patient. In such cases impressions made from plaster or alginate may be used, as well as patterns formed, and orthoses constructed. Obviously, the very large and very small and one-of-a-kind cases require custom design as well as construction. The ultimate answer to custom versus custom-fitted hand orthoses rests with the skill and clientele of the therapist, the numbers of support staff available, and/or the availability of an interested and knowledgeable orthotist.

UPPER EXTREMITY ORTHOTIC COMPONENTS

There are numerous prefabricated splints and splinting systems available to the practicing therapist. These include systems like those from LMB (Lois Barber), Smith and Nephew Roylan, and North Coast. A complete system of hand orthoses available in America today is the Mannerfelt system, developed by Lutz Biedermann, CPO, of West Germany. It is available in three sizes of rights and lefts. Consistent with lower limb orthotics and prosthetics, the Mannerfelt system is modular, allowing all components to be added as needed or removed if unnecessary.

Examples of Splinting Systems

Figure 10-1 demonstrates one version of a long opponens. The long opponens contains at least a short-opponens hand piece and a wrist/forearm component, either attached solidly, or with a spring tension to produce wrist dorsiflexion. Another version of the wrist joint produces spring-assisted ulnar deviation, used for rheumatoid arthritics. This may also be referred to as a forearm-based splint dynamic extension.

Figure 10-2 demonstrates the short-opponens splint, which acts to support the arches of the metacarpals, both transversely and longitudinally. In addition, it may position the thumb CMC and MP or IP joints and prevents contracture of or stretches the thumb-index web space. This is also referred to as a thumb-adduction stop. Lastly, the short opponens provides a point from which more distal components may attach.

Figure 10-3 demonstrates the dynamic finger-extension assist. This component is used when finger joint MPs are stiff or radial nerve injury renders extension difficult or impossible. Because finger flexors still function, patients are able to hold light objects without active extensors. When stiff PIP finger joints affect finger MCP joint motion (hyperextension), a

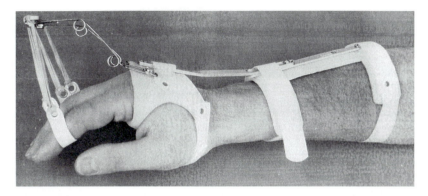

Figure 10-1. A long opponens wrist-hand orthosis. (*Source:* Becker Orthopaedic, with permission.)

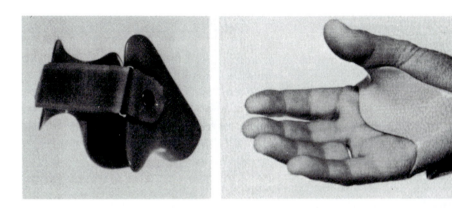

Figure 10-2. A short opponens. (*Source:* Becker Orthopaedic, with permission.)

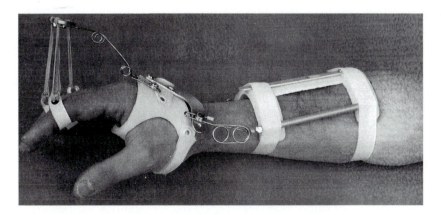

Figure 10-3. A spring wrist extension assist, with MCP extension assist. (*Source:* Becker Orthopaedic, with permission.)

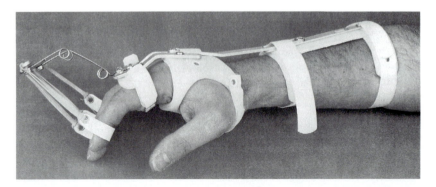

Figure 10-4. A dynamic long opponens, PIP extension assist with lumbrical bar or MCP extension stop. (*Source:* Becker Orthopaedic, with permission.)

lumbrical bar or MP extension stop may be added. Figure 10-4 shows the stop in place, using PIP assists, and long-opponens splint. Also a forearm-based dynamic PIP extension assist splint, this figure demonstrates the static wrist long opponens, PIP extension assist with lumbrical bar or MP extension stop. These are often used following major trauma to the volar wrist, when tendons, nerves, and bone may be cut or crushed. Thus, in addition to skin and joint tightness or contracture, flexor tendon and nerves may also be scarred following surgical repair.

Figure 10-5 demonstrates a long opponens, with dynamic wrist extension assist. This may be used when wrist-flexion contracture exists, when only wrist extension is interrupted (neurologically) or following scarring to the volar wrist, proximal wrist crease, area, when passive wrist extension is limited.

Figure 10-6 demonstrates the static progressive application of forces to produce increased flexion of finger joints, used following injury to the extensor or dorsal part of the hand. Gentle dynamic force over time will produce increased joint motion. This forearm-based static progressive flexion PIP/DIP splint may be adjusted by the therapist as the motion of the joints increases. Note the attachment of the force to a hook attached to the fingernail.

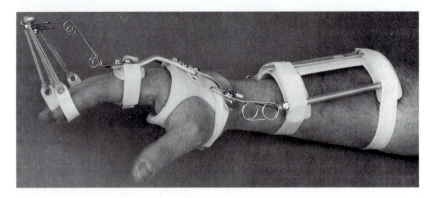

Figure 10-5. A long opponens with dynamic wrist-extension assist. (*Source:* Becker Orthopaedic, with permission.)

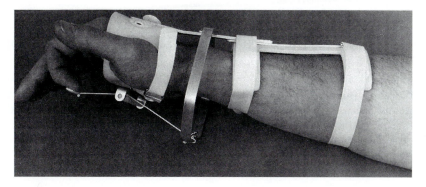

Figure 10-6. MP and PIP flexion assist. (*Source:* Becker Orthopaedic, with permission.)

Externally Powered Upper Extremity Orthoses. Since the development of the McKibben muscle, a carbon dioxide-filled latex rubber bladder, orthotists and therapists have attempted to provide externally powered upper extremity orthotic systems to cervical spine injured clients. Problems with air tanks and latex rubber bladders have given way to electric motors, but the problems of gadget tolerance or intolerance remain.

Beard and Long followed usage of externally powered devices for over 12 years, concluding that only one-third indicated that they used their device following discharge from the rehabilitation center. They cite the following problems:

> Poor quality of performance and the small number of activities which can be accomplished, due to limited range of motion and lack of forceful movement, lead to disuse. Without good proximal arm function, the externally powered hand splint is apparently of little value to these patients. The additional time required for application of the entire system is not justified. Poor quality of performance of activities was the reason most frequently cited by patients for disuse of externally powered orthoses.

Because of the aforementioned problems, Hoy and Guilford developed the functional ratchet system. This system, attached to a reciprocating wrist orthosis, or tenodesis splint, allows palmar prehension via wrist extension. The adjustable, spring-loaded ratchet maintains prehension of the object until the ratchet is released, at which time the wrist flexes and the hand releases the object.

State of the Art in Upper Extremity Orthoses

From 1975 through 1985, 21 articles concerning orthotics and the upper extremity appeared in *Orthotics and Prosthetics,* the official publication of the American Association of Orthotists and Prosthetists. Of these articles, none developed criteria from which clinical trials could be compared.

Crochetiere et al mentioned that 11 Granger orthoses had been fitted. However, no patient data was reported and no comparisons were made with any other orthoses, or reports of functional tests given. Katz et al presented a case report, providing a standard voluntary-opening terminal device for a C-6 quadriplegic. The report mentioned using functional tasks. No comparisons were made with other devices or with the absence of a device.

The fact that only two of twenty-one articles, through 1985, presented any clinical data demonstrates the lack of clinical interest in orthoses of the upper extremity. Twenty-one articles in 10 years also indicate less than enthusiasm about the upper extremity. Since 1991, only three articles have been published concerning upper extremity orthotics: one dealing with brachial plexus orthoses, and two with the needs of the quadriplegic. None presented data concerning a patient sample, and one described a case study. The lack of numbers of articles in the *Journal of Prosthetics and Orthotics* in the 1990s continues to demonstrate a void in the role and interest in the care of all patients with upper extremity injuries.

REFERENCES

1. Beard JE, Long C. Follow-up study on usage of externally-powered orthoses. *Orthot Prosthet.* 1970; 24(2):2.
2. Crochetiere W, Goldstein S, Granger CV, Ireland J. The "Granger" orthosis for radial nerve palsy. *Orthot Prosthet.* 1975; 29(4):27–31.
3. Evans RB, Thompson DE. The Applications of Force to the Healing Tendon. *J Hand Therapy.* Oct.-Dec.; 1993: 266–284.
4. Flatt AE, Personal communication; 1978.
5. Gribben M. Splinting principles for hand injuries. In: *Hand Rehabilitation.* Moran C, ed. New York: Churchill Livingston; 1986.
6. Hardy MA: Preserving function in the inflamed and acutely injured hand. In: Moran C, ed. *Hand Rehabilitation.* New York, NY: Churchill Livingstone; 1986.
7. Hoy DJ, Guilford AW. The functional ratchet orthotic system. *Orthot Prosthet.* 1978; 32(2):21–24.
8. Hunter J, Mackin EJ, Callahan AD. *Rehab of the Hand: Surgery and Therapy,* 4th ed. Saint Louis: CV Mosby; 1995.
9. Katz JA et al. A case study: Use of a terminal device to augment a paralyzed hand. *Orthot Prosthet.* 1983; 37(4):49–53.
10. Laseter GF, Carater PR. Management of distal radius fractures. *J Hand Therapy.* April-June 1996; 114–128.
11. Ingari JU, Pederson WC. Update on Tendon Repair. *Clinics in Plastic Surgery.* 1997; 24(1): 161–173.
12. Urbaniak JR, Cahill JD, Mortensen RA. AAOS Symposium on Tendon Surgery in the Hand. Saint Louis: CV Mosby; 1975.

CHAPTER 11

Foot Orthoses and Footwear

The polio epidemics resulted in many and various foot problems. Specialized centers were established around the world to care for the large number of polio patients who survived the disease. Deformities were common due to the imbalances created by the selective muscle weaknesses. Orthoses were eventually developed to treat the deformities, and in some cases to prevent them.

The left photo depicts a night splint to assist in keeping the feet and hips in neutral alignment and the ankle plantigrade while in bed. The photo on the

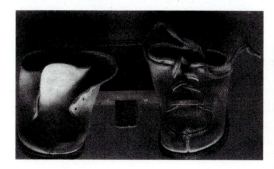

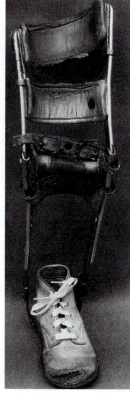

right shows a KAFO made of aluminum and leather worn by a polio survivor following the acute phase of the disease. Both devices were made in the laboratory at Warm Springs, Georgia, a well-known center for polio treatment during the epidemics of 1948 and 1950.

Following completion of reading this chapter, the student will be able to:

1. Differentiate between metatarsalgia and Morton foot structure and their relevance to foot pain.
2. Discuss the elements of diabetes, which lead to foot problems, disease, and ultimate amputation.
3. Discuss the concept of the total contact cast and its place in the treatment of the diabetic foot.
4. Describe the components of the shoe and their import in the treatment of foot problems in general and the diabetic foot in particular.

It shall be the purpose of this chapter to discuss the role of the Certified Orthotist (CO) in the delivery of patient services to the client with injury or disease to the structures of the leg, ankle, and foot. This effort will not be exhaustive because there are many conditions that are of sufficiently small numbers as to not merit discussion. However, these omissions do not intend in any way to diminish their importance to either the patient or condition.

INDICATIONS FOR PRESCRIPTION AND MEDICARE PAYMENT

Any aberration from normal can produce symptoms that could cause a patient to seek medical care. Such changes often produce pain. Similar changes, which may be attributable to trauma, often produce similar symptoms. A complete evaluation of the anatomy and biomechanics of the foot, coupled with an in-depth history leads to the assessment of the problem producing a prescription.

Irrespective of the medical specialist involved, orthotic services are best and most effectively delivered after an exhaustive evaluation of the medical problems involved and a plan of treatment has been established. This process often involves the input of the orthotist as the plan is being developed and the chronology established. In many managed care schemes currently in place, it is imperative that all parties are in touch with the insurance manager as many care coordinators are only tangentially experienced with even the more common problems of the leg, ankle, and foot.

The term orthotic has many connotations when considering the foot and ankle. Orthoses may be prescribed for structural or painful conditions caused by many diseases, including diabetes. It is interesting to note that it was not until 1994 that Medicare considered foot inserts, arch supports, and shoes to be medically necessary, and, therefore, paid for by Medicare.

The rationale stemmed from a long history of nonpayment, presumably based on the commercial insurers and Blue Cross who generally did not allow payments for such items. Medicare completed a study in late 1993 demonstrating a cost effective outcome from the inclusion of such orthoses and shoes in the reduction of inpatient stays related to diabetic foot ulcers. The most common reason for admission to an inpatient acute care bed is a diabetic foot ulcer. This change was intended to slow the growth of such admissions. Today, following the indication and rules set forth by Medicare, Certified Orthotists may treat diabetic foot problems under the prescription of a licensed medical doctor who is the physician responsible for treating the diabetes in a comprehensive medical program, which may include shoes and inserts or modifications as medically indicated. Current restrictions limit each Medicare beneficiary with diabetes to one pair of shoes and three pairs of inserts per year.

In 1999, Ramsey et al reported on a large (8,905) group of Type 1 and Type 2 diabetic patients who were followed for 3 years. 514 or 5.8 percent developed a foot ulcer over the 3 years, an incidence of 2 percent per year. Fifteen percent of those developed osteomyelitis, and 15.6 percent required amputation. Survival at 3 years was 72 percent for patients with foot ulcers, and 87 percent for patients without foot ulcers. The cost to the Medicare program for a 40 to 65 year-old male with a new foot ulcer was $27,987.

BIOMECHANICAL STUDIES OF FOOT PROBLEMS

Although there may be numerous causes of problems of the foot and ankle, biomechanical foot problems provide the need for orthotic solutions. One problem often seen is the Morton's foot structure (MFS) (Figure 11-1). Rodgers and Cavanagh, in 1989, found MFS pressures were significantly higher under the head of the second metatarsal, thought to be attributable to the shorter length of the first and its lack of incremental weight-bearing function. The authors concluded that although the loading distributions were similar, the amount of peak pressure was high enough to predispose these feet to problems usually associated with excessive localized pressure.

A rather simple, yet often seen problem, relates to shoeing and the relative size of the foot in the shoe with and without inserts. An injured or diseased foot and leg may remain swollen for many weeks or months following injury, especially if external fixation and/or multiple surgical procedures are done. The addition of even 1/8 or 3/16 inch inside the shoe is enough to alter the fit, if the shoe was not fitted with the insert in place, in consideration of the inflammation and subsequent edema. Care must always be taken to teach patients to check the feet following new shoe fittings, the addition of new inserts, or following episodes and/or the onset of foot edema.

Support for this premise was presented by Basford and Smith in 1989. Twenty-five of 96 subjects in their evaluation of insoles for reduction in symptoms of back, leg, and foot pain, rejected the insoles because they made their shoes fit too tight to be comfortable. Therefore, the insoles can't reduce pain (which the study proved the insoles did) because the subjects couldn't tolerate the shoe fit. Apparently it wasn't considered to seek a larger size, width, or depth of shoe. The situation needs to be well documented early in the orthotic treatment and communicated with the case manager and/or managing physician to allow for approval of both the inserts, any other modifications, and the accommodative shoe.

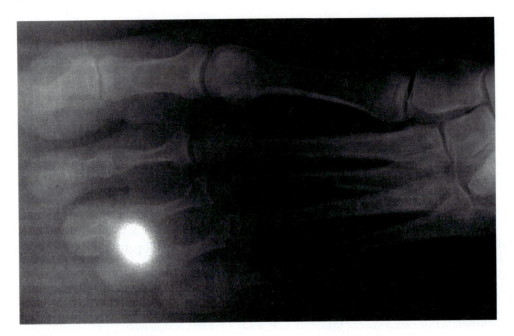

Figure 11-1. MFS.

In 1992, Sussman reported that 81 percent of cases leading to lower limb amputation in males and armed forces veterans were initiated by trauma secondary to poor shoe fit. The direct care cost to Medicare of hospitalization due to lower extremity complications exceeds $2 billion annually. The Centers for Disease Control and Prevention estimates that 85 percent of diabetic foot and leg amputations could be prevented by good foot care including properly fitting shoes.

McGuire provided a complete overview of the pathophysiology of the aging foot: included are discussions of the skin, musculoskeletal, neurological, and vascular systems.

In general, the skin thins due to the thinning of the stratum corneum, coupled with a reduction in fat and water content. Loss of metatarsal fat pad, either through migration or absorption, increases metatarsal head pressures.

Nail plate inflammation and infection are common due to reduced blood flow and neurological status. Nail hypertrophy and changes in contour result in frequent ingrowing. A generalized decrease in resistance to infection and a slowed response allow more frequent infection around the nails.

Other system slowing and degeneration produce numerous foot problems associated with arthritis, diabetes, and progressive stiffening of the connective tissues. Finally, changes attributable to age-related neurological diseases may produce foot and ankle sequelae. Included in these are strokes, Alzheimer's, Parkinson's, and conditions secondary to various tumors, all of which may alter the normal and aging foot and ankle.

Pes planus (Figure 11-2) may occur secondary to posterior tibial tendon dysfunction (PTTD) or rupture, arthritis, Charcot joints secondary to diabetes, or other problems causing ligamentous

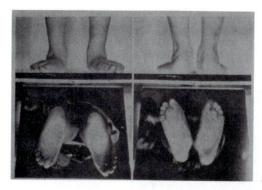

Figure 11-2. Pes planus.

laxity secondary to trauma. The foot often exhibits abnormal callosities from medial foot weight bearing, and shoes that are "run over" medially (Figure 11-3), yielding little midfoot support or forefoot weight bearing. Often these feet are unyielding into dorsiflexion or inversion, and the axes of the foot do not lead the patient toward the line of progression.

Metatarsalgia has many causes and effects patients in a variety of ways. Often post-traumatic injury to the foot produces an atrophy of the fat pads both heel and ball. An in-depth evaluation may yield evidence of both bony and soft tissue abnormalities making the pre-scription include both orthoses to alter the architecture and alignment, as well as strategies to reduce forces from weight bearing. Last, the shoe needs to include a lower heel, rocker sole, and sock liner to reduce local pressures in the absence of a formal insert. Posting may finally complete this work to alter or neutralize any existing anatomical differences from normal.

Wong measured shear forces on the plantar surface of the foot to determine whether cot-ton socks produced more shear than silicone-insole socks. Their conclusion was that silicone-insert socks are superior to cotton in reducing horizontal shear forces.

BIOMECHANICS OF DESIGN

Orthotists and physical therapists need to acquire a basic understanding of the biomechanics of both the normal anatomy and kinesiology in order to understand the pathological. Once the abnormal condition is established, the design of the orthosis develops. Included in the under-standing of the design must be the appreciation for the role of the chosen material, as proper-ties vary and can offer advantages to both the orthotist and eventually the patient. Captured in the negative impression of the custom orthosis must be the true, abnormal anatomy in order to provide the orthotist an accurate model with which to fabricate the finished orthosis.

Included in the repertoire of the professional orthotist is an appreciation for the ground reaction forces acting on the anatomy during both normal and pathological gait. These forces may be altered or augmented depending on the need. Fine-tuning of these forces may spell the difference between success and failure. Also included in this mix is the insistence that the shoe play its vital role to deliver the necessary forces during the gait cycle.

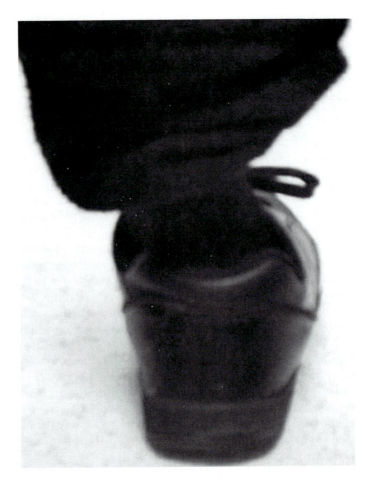

Figure 11-3. "Run-over" shoe.

PURPOSES

Orthoses of the leg, ankle, and foot provide assistance in the following ways:

1. Correction of deformity, whether fixed or flexible, that may include distal deformities presenting from abnormal more proximal joints
2. Control of motion, generally to allow motion and provide a stop
3. Augmentation of muscle weakness, either flaccid or spastic
4. Transferal of weight bearing proximally, or to better distribute pressure

Most orthoses of the leg and foot utilize one or more of these purposes. It is not unusual during this process to take away some normal motions, thus "robbing Peter to pay Paul." This is very common in even the most modern orthotic procedures.

FOOT ORTHOSES

There are many varieties of devices that would broadly fall into the category of foot orthoses. Recently, a patient was referred to the University of Iowa Hospitals and Clinics with a piece of newspaper in the shoe that had been shaped like the foot. Although some would argue that it represented the first "managed-care foot orthosis" (Figure 11-4), it also underscores that foot orthoses may be fabricated from many materials and made from vastly different designs.

Foot orthoses may be thought of as being modular, in that they can have modifications placed or removed and not disturb the original orthosis. This fine-tuning makes it very possible to follow the patient over a long period of time, making necessary changes as the patient improves or regresses. If, for example, a medial/posterior post (Figure 11-5) was added to an insert to further reduce the tendency to pronate, the addition could be removed or altered at any time if other indications emerge.

Designs of inserts need to fit the indications in order to solve the stated problems. The axiom of accommodating fixed deformities and correcting flexible ones is followed. Sometimes the correction of flexible deformities is more of an art than a science, particularly in cases where the deformity has taken place over a long period of time, and the changes have occurred very gradually. It is not uncommon to indicate an intermediate orthosis, followed by the more corrected definitive one, as the return to near normal may be more successful when done in steps or stages.

Figure 11-6 shows a soft insert, one made of Pelite that has been fabricated over a custom-modified positive model, and lined with Poron. Schaphoid pads and metatarsal pads may be added during the fabrication process if indicated, and posts used to reduce or augment floor reaction forces as necessary. These inserts are usually casted using a nonweight-bearing position. This technique is used with many diagnoses, particularly in flexible conditions or in situations where more rigid inserts have been tried and failed. Two layers of 4 mm Pelite is usually enough, especially if longitudinal support or metatarsal pads have been added.

The shoe fit may present a problem, particularly if the patient desires to wear thin, slip-on fashion-type shoes. Experience has taught to discuss the shoe issue at the time of the impression to clear up any misunderstandings before the insert is fabricated. Like so many other issues in orthotics, the insert is no good if the patient is unable to access a shoe. The shoe

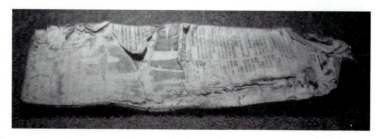

Figure 11-4. "Managed-care" orthosis.

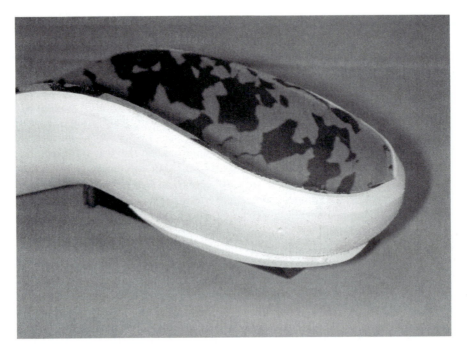

Figure 11-5. Med/heel posting.

fit is made easier when deep-lasted shoes are used. Many have been successful with the New Balance shoe line. Both the running and walking lines are manufactured in both deep and wide models, in some cases up to 6E (Figure 11-7). Using the running and walking models also allows access to the soles for modification. Many models utilize crepe covering with a friction layer, which is very easily alterable with wedges, rockers, or bars.

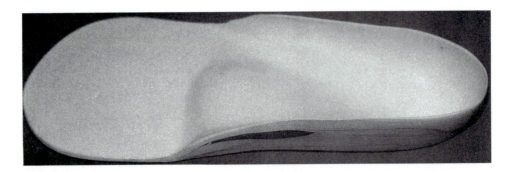

Figure 11-6. Soft insert.

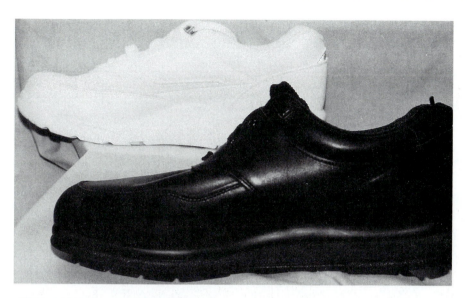

Figure 11-7. Deep and wide shoes.

The insert University of California at Berkeley (UCBL) (Figure 11-8) was introduced to help control hindfoot valgus, while staying below the ankle. This set of trimlines can assist with mid-foot pronation as well. Many early PTTD patients can benefit from the UCBL device, and some require a thin layer of polyethylene, or acrylic (Figure 11-9) to increase the overall stiffness and further assist in the reduction of pronation or valgus of the hindfoot. Shoe design can present more of a problem with the UCBL as a soft medial counter is often of no help to these patients. Additionally, the rigidity of the device makes saggital plane roll-over more difficult and may produce heel slippage in low-counter shoes. Often patients who need to stand on their feet all day can benefit from using a high-top boot, because it provides anti-pronation support and suspension preventing heel slippage.

The insensate foot presents different problems and therefore the need for different treatment. In the early stages of diabetes, calluses often form on the weight-bearing areas, usually on the metatarsal heads of the first, second, and fifth. Perry et al point out that the risk of amputation due to diabetes is 15 times greater than the general population. Therefore the type of shoes and inserts worn may influence this outcome. Their 1995 study concluded that leather-soled shoes produce plantar pressures equal to barefoot pressures while walking on hard wood floors. Inexpensive, crepe-soled running shoes reduced the plantar pressures by 31 percent, with the most relief occurring in the feet that had the highest pressures when unshod.

In 1996, Nyska et al studied the plantar foot pressures between high-heel and low-heel shoes. They found that the high-heel shoes decreased the forces on the heel, lateral forefoot, and mid-foot, and increased the pressures on the medial forefoot, and hallux. The magnitude of the increase was 40 percent from low heel to high heel. Additionally, they found the medial forefoot to be in contact with the floor 100 percent of the stance phase. The authors suggested that the high medial load aggravates and may further contribute to the deformity called hallux valgus.

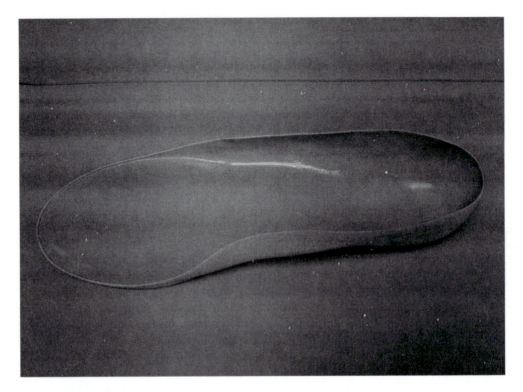

Figure 11-8. UCBL insert.

In an article by Clark, high-speed film evaluated 36 different shoes with varied midsole hardness, heel flare, and heel height, and their effect on hindfoot motion during running. Results showed that shoes with softer midsoles allowed more pronation and hindfoot motion than either the medium or dense midsoled shoes. Shoes without outflares allowed more motion than shoes with either 15 or 30 degrees of outflare. Heel height had no effect on frontal plane motion, as would be expected.

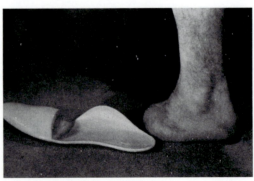

Figure 11-9. Acrylic insert.

Frey, Thompson, and Smith studied 356 women to evaluate trends in women's shoe wear and the effects on the development of foot deformities and pain. The majority of women in this study wore shoes that were too small, experienced foot pain and foot deformity, and had not increased in shoe size since age 20. Not surprisingly, few of the women had measured their feet prior to new shoe purchase in the past 5 years.

Perhaps the only more frequent diagnosis seen in foot clinics than heel pain is plantar fasciitis. Its treatment may involve both conservative and surgical modalities and involves many different approaches. Mizel in 1996 reported on 71 feet treated in 57 patients. The treatment consisted of the use of a night splint and shoe modifications consisting of a steel shank and an anterior rocker placed on their running shoe. The results reported at 16 months showed 59 percent symptoms gone, 18 percent better, 15 percent no change, and 7 percent worse. Although the methodology was not pristine, the results indicate that night splints and stiff-soled shoes can offer some relief. The other result of interest is that the resolution may take as long as 16 months and that the better satisfied patients were older, 68.4 years compared with 55.3 years.

TOTAL CONTACT CASTING FOR DIABETIC FOOT PLANTAR ULCERS

The concept of wound care has only recently begun to attract the depth of attention it deserves. Any wound involving a break in the skin presents even normal healthy people with great potential harm. Likewise, the older, immosuppresed, or diseased patient risks loss of limb, the longer the open wound persists.

In the clinical mix generally seen, the patient with diabetes and a foot ulcer is certainly the most common. There can never be a substitution for a complete history and physical examination prior to diagnosis and assessment leading to the recommendation for treatment. These components examine the sensation or lack of it, the presence or absence of infection, a recommendation to limit nicotine and/or caffeine that may act as vasoconstrictors, good diabetic control, and an evaluation of footwear, which are actually *worn* by the diabetic. Often the footwear worn to the clinic is not the footwear worn at home. Sometimes further questioning reveals that no footwear is worn. Once this information is complete, the managing physician determines the treatment plan and the team members proceed.

From the orthotic point of view, *examination* of the footwear offers an opportunity to both evaluate the foot together with the shoe or shoes to assure a proper match. If the patient is wearing several types of shoes, it is well to request to see all because the narrow and short dress shoes may undo a complete footwear program during a 60-minute trip to church.

As part of the neurological examination, a test for protective sensation should include the use of Semmes-Weinstein monofilaments in the 5.07 gradation. Lack of protective sensation must be treated with fitted shoes and inserts in an attempt to retard or reduce the processes that may lead to ulceration. Numerous options exist for leather, wide and deep toe box oxfords that are reasonably cosmetic and will accommodate both the foot, sometimes swollen, and the prescribed inserts. As stated previously, Medicare now allows payment for shoes for diabetics removing one more hurdle to attainment of properly *fitted,* protective footwear.

THE ROLE OF THE ORTHOTIST IN THE CASE OF DIABETIC FOOT ULCERS

There is never any absolute scheme for which caregivers provide orthotic services, clinic to clinic. Because there are many diabetics and many more foot ulcers, each clinic director may assign roles differently. At the University of Iowa Hospitals and Clinics, the Certified Orthotist plays an integral role in the delivery of services to diabetic patients. In addition to the director, patients are fortunate to be offered the services of a trained foot care nurse, a wound care nurse, a physical therapist, and a social worker. The physical therapist evaluates the loading of the foot using the latest in portable pedobarographs, and also provides a gait evaluation and the need for auxiliary walking aids.

The following represents a description of the more common approaches used for treatment of the diabetic foot. It is important to stress the philosophy of treating all patients individually, paying careful attention to honor or respect any individual wishes or concerns unique to each patient.

PLANTAR SURFACE ULCERS IN DIABETICS

Because the most common indication for admission to an acute care hospital bed in the United States is a diabetic foot ulcer, it comes as no surprise that these are also quite common in the outpatient clinics. Medical evaluations will dictate treatment and may include any of a number of orthotic interventions.

THE SUPERFICIAL PLANTAR ULCER

Superficial plantar ulcers occur often on and under the metatarsal heads of the first, second, or fifth. They may be produced from shear (friction), direct pressure, inadequate cushioning due to fat pad loss, or pressure ulcers due to muscle imbalance seen usually on the fifth secondary to supination. Treatment may include custom-molded inserts, designed to off-weight high pressures over the involved met heads(s), and accommodative footwear. The custom-molded insert is made from a nonweight-bearing cast (impression) and is fabricated from any of a variety of soft, heat-moldable foams of many densities. In clinics, the CO does not utilize many orthoses of hard plastic, acrylic, or graphites, because these are primarily used with slip-on shoes and have little to do with general patient acceptance of pressure-reducing goals.

If fabrication time of custom-molded inserts is a problem, or if a relatively longer-standing ulcer is present, a healing sandal may be prescribed (Figure 11-10). The sandals were first described by Dr. Paul Brand at Carville, Louisiana, due to ulcers of the insensitive foot in Hansen's disease. These sandals are attached to a custom-molded foot insert using Plastazote #1, a closed cell, softer foam than those used in definitive foot orthoses. A 1/4-inch plastazote combined with 3/16–inch polyethylene foam such as Pelite can afford an accommodative and reasonably durable insert. By utilizing the goal of total contact, the entire foot is able to be

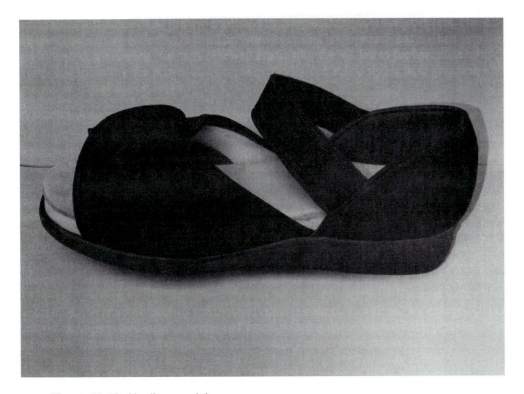

Figure 11-10. Healing sandal.

loaded with pockets built in and under the metatarsal head ulcers. The sandals require shorter steps, thus emphasizing foot flat and reducing heel strike and heel off and the friction association with those phases. Also, care should be taken to clearly explain to the patient that healing sandals *are not* to be used to mow the yard, or shovel the snow. Patients also need to know that nonweight bearing continues to be an acceptable treatment recommendation. Also, the sandal needs to include a rocker sole (Figure 11-11) to insure the off loading of the involved metatarsal heads.

The length of time these sandals need to be worn varies with the ulcer, the patient, the disease, and the compliance of each patient. Patients with chronic ulcerations and without Charcot changes are encouraged to keep the used healing sandal because chronic ulceration may require additional use in the future. Close follow up monitors the ulcer and degree of degradation of the materials over time.

Once healed, the patient may return to their custom-molded insert and accommodative shoes, careful to inspect the foot multiple times following reentry into more normal footwear.

Chronic superficial plantar ulcers may also be treated using a commercially available product with a unique plantar surface design. The Diabetic Healing (DH) Walker (Figure 11-12), marketed by Royce, allows geometrical pressure accommodation using a series of rubber hexagons. These six-sided, three-layer pieces may also be removed to allow a pocket for

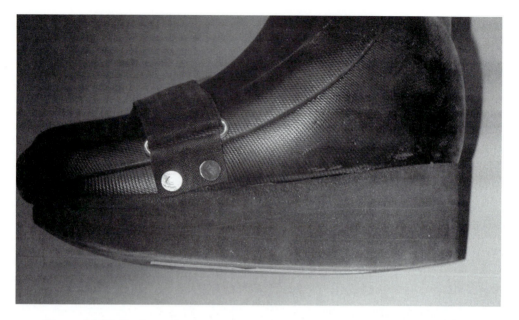

Figure 11-11. Rocker sole.

the ulcer or dressings. It has bilateral plastic bars, medially and laterally, that attach to the wide base via a stirrup. The soft lining has multiple Velcro closures and the base has a molded rocker sole. This walker may be removed to allow bathing and for dressing changes and may be used repeatedly if ulcers reappear. In published studies at The University of Texas Health Science Center, Lavery, in 1996, found the DH Walker to be superior to other similar products. Further research needs to quantify the degree to which these devices transfer load to the leg.

Armstrong studied the ability of these products to relieve plantar heel pressure. Using a repeated measure design, he reported on 25 patients with Grade 1A ulcerations and compared total contact casting, the Aircast (Figure 11-13) pneumatic walker, and the DH pressure relief walker, and depth inlay shoes. The total contact cast reduced the pressure better than the rest, but only 33 percent less than a baseline sneaker. The shoe was inferior to the Aircast and DH boots.

THE TOTAL CONTACT CAST

Any review of treatment of plantar surface ulcers wouldn't be complete without a section on the total contact cast (TCC) (Figure 11-14). In recent years, numerous articles have focuses on this technique and, like anything new, report the apparent successes without reporting the scientific explanation as to exactly why the casts work, if in fact they do.

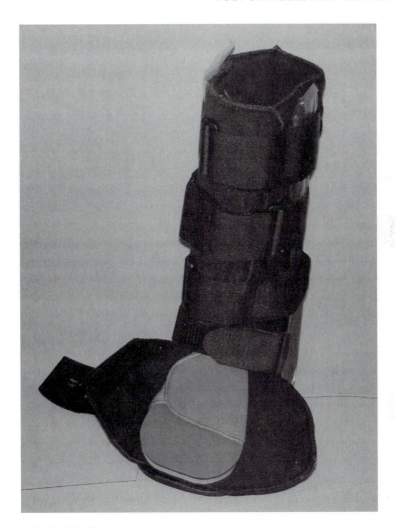

Figure 11-12. DH Walker.

Reports of clinical success using the TCC are numerous. In 1989, Mueller reported a 90 percent healing rate in 42 days compared to 67 percent in 65 days using conventional dressings. Birke, in 1985, reported up to 84 percent reduction in metatarsal head pressures using total contact casting. Conti, in 1996, compared plantar pressures using TCC and conventional short-leg casts. Results demonstrated reduction of plantar pressures using both types of casts. Although midfoot load increased, pressure did not. However, because ground reaction forces were not recorded, it was not possible to quantify load transfer to the skin of the leg.

In 1997, Shaw reported on the transfer of forefoot load using both pressure-measuring insoles and the Kistler 9287 force plate, during walking in a TCC, shoe, and

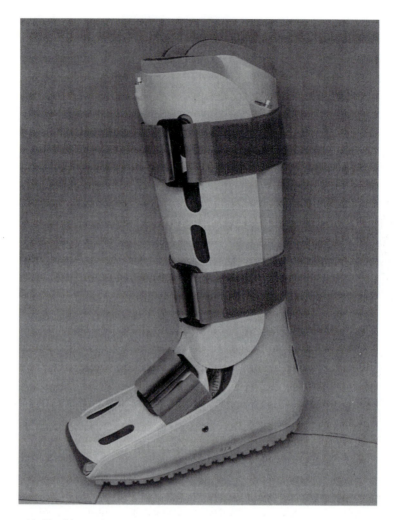

Figure 11-13. Aircast boot.

barefoot. Five diabetic subjects demonstrated reductions of 75 percent compared with bare-foot and 86 percent compared with hard-soled shoes. Peak heel pressures were not signifi-cantly reduced.

Shaw reported a 30 percent load transfer to the leg directly from the cast wall, a greater proportionate load sharing by the heel and a reduction of metatarsal head load via the cavity created by the soft foam used to cover the forefoot in the cast. This study explains, at least in part, the reasons for the off loading of the metatarsal heads, where the force is actually trans-ferred to, and raises the question as to the utility of this procedure in treating heel ulcers, in view of the consistent forces reported regardless of the type of treatment utilized. A clinically im-portant inference involves the use of loose short leg casts. Due to the mechanical principles in-volved, both would yield an increased midfoot pressure because the forces of a loose cast can't

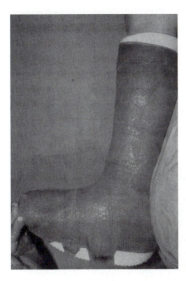

Figure 11-14. TCC.

be easily transferred to the cast walls. This demands careful attention to detail and observation of changing volume with concomitant, regular changes of casts. Additionally, when and if custom-molded ankle foot orthoses are used, the same concern for volume exists. The transfer of forces alluded to by Novick demand that regular follow-up visits to the orthotist occur to alter existing orthoses for volume changes to assure snug fit and necessary force transfer.

In 1995, Wertsch et al reported on plantar pressure measurements taken on six male subjects, using eight pressure transducers on the first, second, fourth, fifth, medial and later midfoot, calcaneal midline, and plantar aspect of the great toe. Each subject walked 720 meters using a self-selected walking velocity. The reduction in plantar pressure averaged 32 percent less under the fifth, 63 percent decrease under the fourth, 65 percent decrease under the great toe, and 69 percent decrease under the first metatarsal head.

Conti, in the most complete reference on the subject, credits Drs. Milroy Paul and Joseph Kahn for developing the first use of the total contact cast. They used the casts in Ceylon in the early 1930s for ulceration secondary to Hansen's disease. Any practitioner who is unfamiliar with the depth of this topic is referred to Conti's article. It is *must* reading prior to beginning a program of ulcer treatment using the total contact cast.

TOTAL CONTACT CASTING: THE TECHNIQUE

The preparation of the plantar ulcer should be done by the medical director or other physician using a sharp knife to carefully debride any and all dead tissue. In addition, there often exists a rind which usually needs to be cut away to allow the ulcer to fill in from the perimeter to the center. Once completed, haemostasis needs to occur prior to proceeding with the application of the lycra spandex knitted sock, with the toe sewn shut. The toes need to be separated by lambs wool to prevent maceration and further ulceration between toes.

Next a 1/4-inch felt is placed over the malleoli and anteriorally over the crest of the tibia to prevent anterior/proximal pressure and ulceration during late stance phase via the extension moment affecting the knee. The felt also allows easy removal with the cast saw without danger of burning or cutting the fragile skin of the diseased patient. Next a piece of 1/2-inch soft foam (such as Sifoam, from Omni Medical Specialties) is applied to the toes dorsally from the metatarsal phalangeal joint distal and around the toes and back under the met heads on the plantar surface in the way described by Birke. Cast padding is then rolled over all bony prominences including the tibilar head, the malleoli, the metatarsal heads, the navicular, if prominent, and the entire heel.

The first layer of casting material is Orthoflex, a plaster impregnated into an elastic cotton bandage. This elasticity allows the orthotist to obtain a snug, conforming wrap and to contain all under padding firmly and accurately against the skin and bony prominences. This first layer needs to be well molded being careful to preposition the foot and ankle in the position that ultimately will allow a normal plantigrade foot. Perhaps the most difficult concept for the new orthotist is the visualization of the final foot and ankle position. A poorly aligned foot can actually worsen the condition and potentially produce additional ulcers if not properly positioned. Often this process involves the visualization of the most recent X-rays to appreciate the current bony configuration.

Regular fast-setting plaster bandage is applied over the elastic plaster to reinforce the flexible material and to maintain the foot and ankle position already established. Depending on the weight and/or activity level, a 4-inch, five-layer plaster splint may be added to the posterior leg, around the heel and under the foot to the toes. This acts to reinforce the cast producing a solid ankle and preventing any cast breakage and ankle dorsiflexion. The final layer of plaster acts to incorporate the splint into the cast.

Once set, with the temperature of the cast peaked and reducing, a layer of fiberglass casting tape is used to reinforce the plaster wall and to secure the walking base to the cast. Not all patients are allowed to walk on their TCCs, as medical condition, namely the acute Charcot joint (end stage foot disease), usually precludes weight bearing. The walking base provides a durable, rocker sole base that allows easy and reasonably normal cast ambulation.

Because a plaster bandage is used, and because a layer of fiberglass covers the plaster, it is important to emphasize to the patient the need to refrain from weight bearing on the TCC for 24 to 48 hours and perhaps a bit longer in the hotter and more humid months, particularly if the patient does not have home air conditioning.

As stated earlier, the presence of acute Charcot symptoms, such as edema, or volume due to infection, must be evaluated and used as criteria for follow-up scheduling. Return visits of 1 week are routine for first-time TCCs or for edematous legs treated for the first time. Homegoing instructions include the warning about loosening of the cast or any discomfort associated with weight bearing. If the patient travels long distances, instructions include the change to nonweight-bearing status if question about slippage, volume reduction, or pain result.

It is important to remember that many diabetic patients have reduced or absent protective sensation and if Charcot fractures are present, may feel no pain at all. This further complicates the treatment because many patients report that they seem to have more available energy with the TCC in place. Caution needs to be stressed while quietly supporting the notions of exercise and return to normal home duties and activities.

The TCC is changed at either week 1 or 2, and following careful inspection of the wound and limb, a decision is made whether to continue. Generally, peripheral healing is quite visible, and further debridement may be needed in order to allow the healing to progress. Wounds of up to 1 inch in diameter may require four or five TCCs until completely healed. Careful attention to detail between casts can spell the difference between success and failure. Following the removal of each cast, a careful history and skin evaluation will identify any problems. This information then forms the basis for any changes necessary in subsequent application.

Lastly, a word about the remaining foot. Patients with diabetes present the potential for bilateral foot ulcers. The use of TCCs may reduce the forces required by the remaining limb and although less than if nonweight bearing, still presents forces in excess of bipedal normal walking. An evaluation of the remaining foot and footwear may alert team members to impending problems and head off further ulceration.

THE SHOE

Many patients in need of shoe inserts, whether custom molded or off-the-shelf, balk at the notion that these therapeutic devices may require special shoes in order to function properly. The phrase "special shoes" conjures up ideas of ugly, leather, orthopaedic shoes like those prescribed for polio patients in the 1950s or for children with congenital conditions many years previously. Therefore, the first role of the Certified Orthotist or physical therapist is to educate the patient about modern adult shoes and the components and designs that will assist the patient in the treatment of their problem.

Shoes, like many other parts of our lives, have changed for the better. Biomechanical studies and new materials have replaced the sleek Italian dress shoe for women to a lower-heeled, wiser shoe with a non-leather sole. Men no longer wear the all leather wing tip, with 3/4-inch solid leather (hard) sole, because these have been replaced with shoes of lighter weight uppers and EVA or crepe-soling materials. Many of today's truly therapeutic shoes have retained some of the traditional designs and supplanted others with newer, more-friendly materials.

The very few number of remaining leather shoe manufacturers left in the United States is testimony to how fast and how deeply the so-called running shoe has replaced the conventional shoe. Even children now can buy running shoes as small as 000. To dismiss all running shoes as "tennis shoes," and therefore bad, is a great misunderstanding of current technology and materials. It is also as incorrect to dismiss all "depth" shoes as ugly, and not to pursue these lines because many are both therapeutic and cosmetic, as well as quite comfortable.

SHOE DESIGN AND CONSTRUCTION

Much time and money has been spent in the research and development of shoes in order to satisfy basic biomechanical needs of both normal and diseased feet. Few patients make any attempt to educate themselves about these components, designs, or materials. This then becomes the role of the caregiver at the time the evaluation and impression taking occurs.

HEEL COUNTERS

Heel counters provide varying degrees of resistance to movement of the hindfoot. Squeezing the heel of the upper of the shoe gives one an idea of counter stiffness. Many shoes have no heel counter stiffness at all and when coupled with a very narrow heel and midfoot width, provide no resistance to pronation. Generally, these shoes may be found on patients with early PTTD or other pronation problems. Any attempt at orthosis use will fail because this shoe provides very little, if any, resistance to either varus or valgus when using an FO or an AFO.

The other issue concerning counter is height. The length of the counter upward to and approaching the height of the malleoli dictates the degree of resistance to heel varus or valgus. Standard dress shoe counter height stops distal to the malleoli. Cross trainer, running, or deck shoes often extend the height of the counter to offer additional support in the frontal plane. The extra height also allows more room in the shoe's midfoot and heel for the placement of inserts or heel lifts. It also provides additional resistance to heel slippage often seen with the stiffness secondary to inserts or sole stiffeners such as Springlites.

THE THROAT OR INSTEP

The design of the throat or instep, otherwise called the closure, is responsible for the available room into which any insert might fit. Those designs often used include the blucher, balmoral, lace-to-toe, and the slip on.

The blucher design offers the largest volume into which to add inserts. Additionally, should the foot volume increase, other volume is available without undue foot pressure. The presence of the laces allows each patient to individually tighten each foot so the shoe, with or without inserts and edematous or not, will remain snug on the foot. Also, in the occasional situation where one foot is extremely edematous, the utility of the blucher design affords the option to cut the throat (vamp) of the shoe to provide even more room into which to enter the shoe. This maneuver does not destroy the shoe because the vamp may be restitched once the volume has reduced.

The balmoral closure is not insert friendly or volume friendly and therefore is not a design that most orthotists recommend. It is a stitched throat design that limits the entry of the foot into the throat. Cutting this vamp, unlike the blucher, will produce an unusable shoe.

The lace-to-toe closure offers the easiest entry into any shoe design. Once the laces have been loosened down to the toe, a foot may be placed into the shoe with very little ankle or foot motion. Also, the donning of shoes over totally insensate feet, as in spina bifida, allows nearly complete visualization of the foot in the shoes. To assure that the toes are totally extended, one may manipulate the toes, with the use of fingers, to check for final toe position in the shoe.

Slip-on shoes have little to offer most biomechanical foot problems. They offer very little if any hindfoot or midfoot support, limited toe room, and no room for additional foot volume, even without an insert in place. Toe box room is usually inadequate and may cause dorsal rubbing and potential ulceration on the dorsal skin of the toes.

Lastly, a word about the counters of the walking and running shoes. Looking posteriorly at a running or walking shoe, the height of the posterior is greater than a standard dress shoe. This extra material allows a more secure grip on and above the calcaneus. By using the extra (proximal) eyelets provided, a snug closure is attained and heel slippage is reduced. These shoes also usually provide a removable sock liner that allows for the introduction of an insert with the resultant neutral change in volume within the shoe, without sacrificing suspension and secondary heel slippage.

In 1995, Perry studied plantar foot pressures when comparing leather-soled shoes with crepe-soled shoes and reported a 31 percent reduction. This data supports the use of crepe over leather. The art of orthotics includes the recommendation as to shoes that have soles firm enough to produce the necessary ground reaction forces while relieving undue plantar foot pressures.

Because moment derivation includes both force multiplied by perpendicular distance from the rotation center, the width of the heel and midfoot of the shoes become critical. Therefore, a shoe with a wider heel, wider mid sole and firm crepe sole will support many custom molded in prescription adequately. A too-soft soling material will be overpowered by the weight of the patient and will not allow the insert to produce its desired biomechanical effects.

In certain application, due to the pathological location of the axial load or the axis of the hindfoot, a longer lever is required to produce the desired neutralizing effect. In such cases, a lateral or medial outflare can be added to the sole. It is imperative that both the density of the soling material and the distance of the outflare be enough to offset the pathological moments. A point may be reached where any combination of shoe and outflare is too little; at that point, an AFO of some type may be required. Patients who are generally desirous of the least AFO possible will also welcome the educated opinion, because a useless foot orthosis and shoe buildup combination may be difficult to "sell" to the patient who must pay for something that will not work.

A note of caution: The size of the toe box includes two dimensions—the width and the height or depth. The other concern with the toe box is the true width of the shoe and its relationship to medial forefoot abduction, particularly if the heel is excessively raised.

The toe box of the shoe should be made of soft leather or lined with soft materials with no stitches over either the first or fifth metatarsal heads. This is related to the true width of the shoe, because the width is often too narrow for the aged and widening forefoot. Numerous studies have confirmed the prevalence of ill-fitting shoe, particularly through the forefoot. It is interesting to note clinically the number of patients who purchase shoes that are much too long in order to attain the larger width necessary for their forefoot. Proper fitting of shoes demands a heel-to-ball measurement, followed by a true width measurement *and* an available shoe that offers more than a "medium," particularly if an insert is to be used.

Also seen frequently are the small red or callused areas seen over the dorsal skin of the interphalangeal joints. This is diagnostic for a toe box that is too narrow, not deep enough, or a combination of both. Cock-up toes or any intrinsic-minus posturing will also require a larger toe box. The insensate foot can produce open ulcerations if new shoes are not carefully watched, particularly if inserts have been recently prescribed or if foot volume has recently increased.

The tapered toe box of many dress shoes presents potential problems for wide feet. The tapers come from both proximal to distal, as well as from the metatarsal heads to the toe. The more the toe is round and less pointed, as well as boxier from the lateral view, the more it provides a larger volume for the patient's feet. All these features should be considered when purchasing shoes for aged and/or diseased feet.

The bottom of any shoe should offer a friction layer to prevent slippage on wet or frozen surfaces. Many shoe soles have a friction layer that can be replaced when worn smooth. These running or walking shoe designs also offer the orthotist the ability to add a wedge or build up, and then to replace the friction layer. This allows the patient to not "wear off" the wedge or build up, and so offers friction to prevent slippage.

REFERENCES

1. Armstrong DG, Stacpoole-Shea S. Total contact casts and removable cast walkers. Mitigation of plantar heel pressure. *J Am Podiatr Med Assoc.* 1999; 89(1):50–53.
2. Basford JR, Smith MA. Shoe insoles in the work place. *Orthopedics.* 1989; 12:285–289.
3. Birke JA, Sims DS, Jr., Buford WL. Walking casts: Effect on plantar foot pressures. *J Rehabil Res Dev.* 1985; 22:18–22.
4. Centers for Disease Control Diabetes Surveillance Policy Program Research Annual Report 1990. Atlanta: U.S. Department of Health and Human Services.
5. Clarke TE et al. The effects of shoe design parameters on rearfoot control in running. *Medicine in Science and Sports Exercise.* 1983; 15:376–381.
6. Conti SF, Martin RL, Chaytor ER et al. Plantar pressure measurements during ambulation in weight bearing conventional short leg casts and total contact casts. *Foot Ankle Int.* 1996; 17:464–469.
7. Conti SF. Total contact casting. *AAOS Instructional Course Lectures.* 1999; 48:305–315.
8. Frey C et al. *American Orthopaedic Foot and Ankle Society Women's Shoe Survey.* 1993; 14:78–81.
9. Lavery LA, Vela SA, Lavery DC et al. Reducing dynamic foot pressures in high risk diabetics with foot ulcerations: A comparison of treatments. *Diabetes Care.* 1996; 19:818–821.
10. McGuire JB. Pathology of the aging foot. *Orthot & Prosthet Business News.* February 15, 1998; 9–14.
11. Mizel MS et al. Treatment of plantar fasciitis with a night splint and shoe modification consisting of a steel shank and anterior rocker bottom. *Foot and Ankle Int.* 1996; 17:732–735.
12. Mueller MJ, Diamond JE, Sinacore DR et al. Total contact casting in treatment of diabetic plantar ulcers: Controlled clinical trial. *Diabetes Care.* 1989; 12:384–388.
13. Novick LA, Birke JA, Graham SL et al. Effect of walking splint and total contact cast on plantar forces. *J Prosthet Orthot.* 1991; 3:168–178.
14. Nyska M et al. Plantar foot pressures during treadmill walking with high-heel and low-heel shoes. *Foot Ankle Int.* 1996; 17:662–666.
15. Perry JE et al. The use of running shoes to reduce plantar pressures in patients who have diabetes. *J Bone Joint Surg.* 1995; 77A:1819–1828.
16. Ramsey SD, Newton K, Blough D et al. Incidence, outcomes, and cost of foot ulcers in patients with diabetes. *Diabetes Care.* 1999; 22(3):382–387.
17. Reiber GE, Boycho EJ, Smith DG. Lower extremity foot ulcers and amputations in diabetes. In: *Diabetes in America,* 2nd ed. National Diabetes Data Group. National Institute of Diabetes and Digestive and Kidney Diseases. NIH Publication. 1995; 18:409–428.
18. Rogers MM, Cavanagh PR. Pressure distribution in Morton's foot structure. *Med Science Sports Exercise.* 1989; 21:23–28.
19. Shaw JE, Hsi WL, Ulbrecht JS et al. The mechanism of plantar unloading in total contact casts: Implications for design and clinical use. *Foot Ankle Int.* 1997; 18(12):809–817.
20. Sussman FE, Reiber GE, Albert SF. The diabetic foot problem-A failed system of health care? *Diab Res Clin Pract.* 1992; 17:1–8.
21. Wertsch JJ et al. Plantar pressures with total contact casting. *J Rehabil Res Dev.* 1995; 205–209.
22. Wong PY, Chene MD, Hong WH et al. Effects of silicon-insole socks on pressure distribution and shear force of the foot. *Chang Kong I Hsueh.* 1998; 21(1):20–27.

CHAPTER *12*

Pediatrics

As a result of the polio epidemics of the late 1940s and early 1950s, large numbers of survivors needed orthoses both acutely and for the remaining years of their lives. The center at Warm Springs, Georgia, became internationally recognized for their work in this area, providing medical treatment and rehabilitation for tens of thousands of people over the decades. Many orthotists who were trained there during this time returned to other parts of the country to provide similar care for these patients much closer to their homes. Among the best-known orthotists trained at Warm Springs were James Russ and Jack Conry, who became the inaugural faculty at the newly formed university programs and shared their expertise with subsequent generations of orthotists. Each set a positive example for all who followed, through prolific invention and publication.

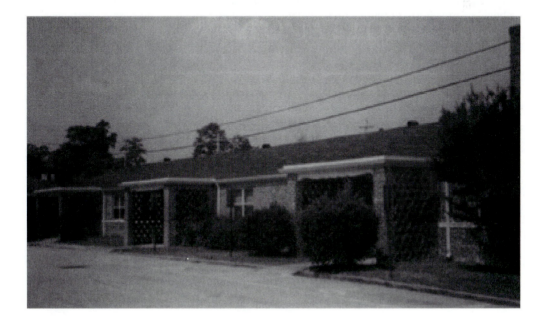

Following completion of reading this chapter, the student will be able to:

1. Differentiate between a child and an adult client and discuss the differences in orthotic and prosthetic treatment goals, components, and expectations.
2. Identify the problems in fitting small children compared to adults.
3. Discuss special concerns when treating juvenile amputees.
4. Discuss congenital transradial deficiencies including prevalence, associated physical or psychological problems, and the chronology of treatment.

The aphorism "The child is *not* simply a small adult" has become the sine qua non for modern prosthetic and orthotic care for skeletally immature individuals, as noted by Michael and many other authors. Of course, the biomechanical principles and mechanical components utilized are directly analogous to those applied to the adult. The key difference, however, is not in the technology itself, but rather in the manner in which the technology is provided. These key differences are highlighted in this chapter.

PHYSIOLOGICAL AND DEVELOPMENTAL FACTORS

The child is a dynamic, growing, and constantly changing organism, both psychologically and physiologically different from the aging, decelerating adult. It is *not* sufficient for the pediatric orthosis or prosthesis to be technically well designed and fitted. Long-term experiences by Aitken and other pediatric specialists demonstrate that it must also be provided when appropriate for the abilities and maturity of the child. Therefore, the pediatric clinician must be acutely aware of the developmental sequence of human maturation, and particularly of the developmental readiness of the individual child being treated.

Equally significantly, a child's neuromuscular and skeletal anatomy is constantly changing. This has two major implications for prosthetic and orthotic design. First, the relatively plastic nature of juvenile bones and soft tissues offers the potential for the device to "remodel" the anatomy gradually, by the careful application of controlled, low-level forces. Lonstein and Winter have summarized the well-documented effectiveness of plastic scoliosis jackets in modifying the natural history of idiopathic scoliosis, one example of the therapeutic use of this potential. On the other hand, it is also important for the clinician to minimize the forces applied as much as is possible and to monitor the long-term effect of the orthosis or prosthesis on the anatomy to avoid the risk of creating undesirable deformities.

The second implication of the changing contours of the juvenile body is the need to plan ahead for both linear and circumferential growth. Use of soft linings is one common strategy employed, because they can be easily removed after some months to accommodate increases in girth. Provision of the most extended trimlines possible is common to allow some linear growth without immediate loss of biomechanical support.

SPECIALTY CLINICS AND TEAMS

According to Lambert et al, the formation of a specialized pediatric clinic team to provide optimal prosthetic and orthotic treatment was first advocated following the conclusion of World War II. Particularly for children with complex deformities or pathologies, McCollough has observed that this has proven over the years to be an excellent model for comprehensive rehabilitation. Much of today's pediatric P&O treatment is provided by charitable institutions such as the Texas Scottish Rite Children's Hospital and the Shrine Clinics.

At a minimum, the clinic team consists of the physician, therapist, and prosthetist-orthotist. Such a "mini-team" can often be assembled in the private practice sector, too, even in relatively small towns and communities. The ongoing interaction between the team members facilitates both communication and attention to details. In larger cities and in charitable centers, the pediatric team is expanded to includes multiple physician specialties, social workers, psychologists, nursing personnel, and others, in addition to the core members, as advocated by Frantz and Aitken.

The Association of Children's Prosthetic Orthotic Clinics is the preeminent organization for clinicians who are interested in exchanging information or learning more about pediatric prostheses and orthoses. Their annual meeting and Web site (*www.acpoc.com*) are recommended sources for up-to-date information in this rapidly evolving area of rehabilitation.

OVERALL PEDIATRIC DESIGN PRINCIPLES

Cummings and Kapp have suggested four basic design principles for pediatric prostheses, which can also apply to orthoses as well:

1. Maximize durability
2. Minimize weight
3. Maximize performance
4. Protect against injury

Maximize Durability

Durability is an important aspect of pediatric devices, particularly during the "rough and tumble" years. In general, as emphasized by Sorbye, simpler designs are generally preferred over those that are more complex, because there are less associated mechanical problems.

Due to children's penchant for playing in sand, dirt, grass, and similar environments, any fabric and leather elements are easily soiled and will require periodic cleaning. The base plastic of modern prosthetic and orthotic devices can be washed with soapy water as needed, and is resistant to urine and feces as well.

As a general guideline, very basic orthoses and prostheses are preferred for infants and toddlers. The complexity of the design can be gradually increased in subsequent devices, as the child ages and becomes developmentally ready to utilize the added function offered.

Minimize Weight

The prosthetist-orthotist must balance the conflicting demands of creating a device that is sufficiently rugged for use by active children without making it too heavy. In general, it is better to err on the side of durability, because the child will become stronger and larger over time from normal growth.

The exception is when the child suffers from progressive neuromuscular weakness as is the case in pathologies such as Duchenne's muscular dystrophy. When the client has little or no energy reserve, as noted by Heckmatt et al, use of the lightest possible materials is in order. At this time, possible materials could include joints of aerospace alloys such as titanium and carbon fiber-reinforced elements as well.

Maximize Performance

Children are inherently active, eagerly exploring their universe as much as they are physically capable of doing so. Consequently, it is important to design their orthoses and prostheses to facilitate the highest activity level possible.

In recent decades, the use of dynamic response feet has become common for both adults and children. Despite the excellent clinical acceptance shown by Menard and Murray and others and supportive data collected by Hart et al and Schneider et al, this remains an area of some controversy with more conservative clinics arguing that use of advanced components for children needs further justification.

Protect Against Injury

The plastic nature of the immature musculoskeletal system has already been noted. Because even low-level forces applied over time can alter the anatomy of the child's body, it is important to consider the stresses applied to the bones and particular to the joints. Some clinicians recommend using hinges routinely to protect the knee against potential weight-bearing stresses. Most centers prefer to use low profile (transtibial level) orthoses and prostheses when indicated, but watch closely for any progressive deformity at the knee and then add knee hinges only when necessary.

When the skin is fragile, perhaps due to burn scarring or similar conditions, the prosthesis or orthosis can help protect against injury from contact with the environment. Some children with bilateral lower limb amputations, for example, choose to wear the soft inserts or flexible sockets from their prostheses whenever they are up and about—even when they choose not to wear the prostheses themselves.

UPPER LIMB ORTHOSES

Most pediatric upper limb orthoses are interim devices used for a few weeks or months to address a specific deformity or reconstructive surgical procedure. Typically made from low temperature thermoplastic material, such splints are usually provided by the occupational therapist or hand therapist.

The ABC certified orthotist most often is called in when a definitive orthosis, suitable for long-term use and able to withstand significant forces, is required. Fortunately, this need is rare in this population, except to treat such pathologies as radial club hand deformity.

Surgical correction of a severely deformed limb is sometimes necessary, and provision of a complex orthosis may sometimes be considered. In the great majority of cases, however, the sensation and mobility of even a significantly malformed limb that can reach the face and midline will offer greater practical function, so use training by the therapist is often the preferred method for increasing the patient's independence despite the presence of an anomalous upper limb.

SPINAL ORTHOSES

Pediatric spinal orthoses are commonly provided for postoperative protection during the healing phase, or as nonoperative treatment. In both cases, the orthosis is most commonly a custom-molded design, using high temperature thermoplastic material such as polypropylene or polyethylene.

Postsurgical body jacket orthoses for children are based on the same basic considerations as designs for adults, as discussed in chapter 9. Because such devices are necessary only for a few months, in most cases, no special provisions for growth are needed. The petroleum-derived plastics used are impervious to bodily fluids, and can be cleaned easily with soap and water to maintain good hygiene.

Nonoperative body jackets are generally provided to support the paralytic spine or to resist the progression of idiopathic scoliosis. As discussed in detail in chapter 9, it is now possible to identify the "window" for brace treatment of idiopathic scoliosis fairly precisely. Minor curves of less than 30 degrees are normally observed only, while larger curves beyond 45 degrees will likely require surgical stabilization. Intermediate curves between these limits have been shown to respond well to orthotic support.

Precisely why the orthosis can prevent the progression of the curve remains controversial, and continues to be studied by scientists worldwide. It has become quite clear, however, that a well-fitted orthosis can usually modify the natural history of this disease and, in many cases, eliminate the need for surgical fusion to stabilize the spine. In selected cases, an orthosis is used to delay the need for surgery so the child can grow taller, even if it is not expected to control the curvature completely.

LOWER LIMB ORTHOSES

As noted in chapter 8, children will generally use even complex orthoses without protest, in contrast to most adults. For this reason, prescription of bilateral KAFOs and higher-level orthoses for this population is common.

Although traditional minimal contact metal alloy orthoses can be used with children, the predominant trend worldwide is to use custom-made thermoplastic designs due to the light weight and total contact control they offer. However, these intimately fitting orthoses will need modification every 3 to 4 months in the case of the growing child.

Use of soft foam linings is ubiquitous, not so much to add comfort as to accommodate girth increases. Judicious remolding of the plastic shells with the addition of heat can also "open up" the orthosis as the child's muscles grow larger.

Due to the rapid linear growth that is typical in childhood, the clinic team must always reevaluate the congruency of the orthotic versus the anatomical joints and make adjustments as necessary. It is quite common to find that, on subsequent visits, the child's anatomic knee center is now 1 or 2 centimeters more proximal than when the orthosis was fabricated. The side bars must then be detached from the plastic shells and reattached at the new location.

Tone-Inhibiting Designs

In recent decades, much has been written about the possibility that special contours in the orthosis might be able to reduce the pathologic hypertonia common to many disorders, including cerebral palsy. Numerous clinical design variants have been reported, each with its proponents.

These theories are predicated on the work of Duncan and Mott, and postulate that the orthosis can:

1. Avoid stimulating undesired, primitive responses
2 Inhibit primitive responses, when feasible
3. Facilitate the functioning of antagonist musculature

No credible studies have emerged to date supporting the notion that internal contours of the device can have such effects. The current consensus is that an intimately fitted orthosis that supports the ankle-foot complex in a biomechanically sound position is beneficial for such children, even if the additional benefits remain conjecture.

Articulated Ankle Designs

Orthotic rehabilitation, like most health specialties, is sometimes subject to recurring trends. Use of articulated ankle joints in traditional minimal contact AFO and KAFO designs was typical in previous decades. As thermoplastic, total-contact designs gradually supplanted the heavier, earlier style of orthoses, there was a trend toward solid ankle configurations due in large part to the sleeker appearance, increased durability, and lighter weight they offered. This was particularly true in pediatric applications.

In the past decade, this trend has reversed and the use of articulated joints in thermoplastic orthoses is rapidly growing worldwide. Many different components are now available for this purpose, in both adult and pediatric sizes. As was the case with tone-reducing AFOs, there are at present no credible studies demonstrating objective criteria for the use of articulated designs, so this remains a subjective judgment based on the clinic team member's training and experiences.

As was discussed in detail in chapter 8, orthoses are rationally prescribed based on the biomechanical control needed by each individual. This principle is the determining factor in whether an articulated device is necessary or not. When the patient can control the joint through a given range of motion, or when such motion facilitates increased independence, the added cost and maintenance associated with an articulation are justified. Otherwise, the solid ankle designs are preferred due to their simplicity—particularly for small children.

JUVENILE PROSTHESES

Prosthetic management of the child with a limb deficiency has gradually evolved to become an area of specialized knowledge and practice. Understanding the basic principles in this area of rehabilitation, as defined by Frantz and Aitken, will help the clinician working with this population.

Etiology

Aitken defined the juvenile amputee as a skeletally immature person with an amputation or congenital limb deficiency. As director of the Grand Rapids, Michigan, Area Amputee Project for many years, Aitken reported that juvenile upper limb absences are more often congenital than acquired due to trauma, disease, or tumor.

Congenital Amputation

Congenital means present at birth, and may be either a limb deficiency, due to underdevelopment of a limb segment, or a true congenital amputation, where the distal part was once present but was severed sometime prior to birth. (These differences, although subtle, will become more important as further classifications emerge later in the chapter.) In Aitken's study, 372 of 1,210 (30.7 percent) patients who had true congenital amputations had two or more affected limbs. Of the 372 congenital amputees, 111 were affected in all four limbs. Although Aitken's group may represent a skewed sample, the fact remains that congenital limb deficiency often affects multiple limbs (Figure 12-1).

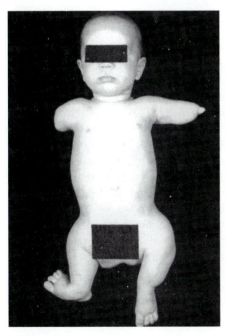

Figure 12-1. Congenital quadramembral amputee. (From Shurr DG, Cooper RR, Buckwalter JA, Blair WF. Juvenile amputees classification and revision rates. *Orthot Prosthet.* 1982; 36:24, with permission.)

Acquired Amputation

In Aitken's study, 850 of 923 (92 percent) acquired amputations affected only one limb. Aitken's data indicated that vehicular accidents led the list of causes for acquired amputations. The next three most common causes were power equipment (often farm machinery), gunshot/explosion injuries, and railroad injuries. Together these four causes accounted for 75 percent of acquired amputations in children.

Disease-Related Amputation

Tumor is the largest single cause of disease-related amputation in children. Other reasons might include vascular compromise, often in the form of thrombi secondary to disease, and other miscellaneous etiologies.

Surgical Conversion

The concept of surgical conversion involves a surgical "correction" to change an existing anatomical entity into one that can be more realistically fitted with a functional prosthesis. A common example is an ankle disarticulation procedure done in the case of a poorly developed or contractured foot. In this example, the foot is surgically converted into a more usable residual limb, one that can be more easily and cosmetically fitted with standard prosthetic components.

Aitken reported that 50.8 percent of congenital lower limb deficiencies required surgical conversion, in contrast to only 7.9 percent of upper limb deficiencies. Oftentimes, even severely malformed upper limbs can provide adequate function despite the unusual anatomical configurations that are often present. Additionally, even malformed upper limb remnants provide sensibility, something modern prostheses cannot, as yet, offer.

The Young Amputee

The juvenile amputee is not simply a miniature version of an adult amputee. Therefore, juvenile amputees should not be fitted with miniaturized prostheses that were designed for adults. The juvenile amputee is a growing person whose residual limb, especially its length, is always changing. The juvenile amputee is continually dependent on parents, society, and the prosthetic clinic team because growth spurts can render a prosthesis too small and/or too short in a matter of weeks. The juvenile is malleable both physically and emotionally, often making certain aspects of treatment easier than with some adults. Because the child's physical body is changing so rapidly, the socket is often less intimately fitted than with adults, making it possible to extend the useful life of a the prosthesis as the child grows into the socket. Rarely do juvenile amputees complain of pain or develop stump ulcers and most can comfortably tolerate rubbing or skin irritation that might cause a serious problem for an older dysvascular amputee.

Emotionally, juveniles adapt readily to various situations, allowing prosthetic fitting and gait training to occur with few complications. As compared to adults, children can often be walking independently with a prosthesis within a few days of initial fitting, whereas many adults may require much longer to adapt to the loss of a limb.

Growth

In order to anticipate the eventual growth of the long bones, the relative contribution of the epiphyses is important. In the leg, 70 percent of the length of the femur depends on the distal femoral epiphysis, while about 60 percent of the tibia and fibula come from the proximal epiphyses. Therefore, the epiphyses around the knee contribute 67 percent to the overall length of the lower limb. In the arm, 80 percent of the length originates from the proximal epiphysis, whereas the distal epiphyses of the radius and ulna provide overall growth to the arm and forearm. Loss or absence of these epiphyses may alter the eventual length of the limb, resulting in significant length discrepancies by adulthood.

Classification of Juvenile Amputees

Parents of juvenile amputees often request information from medical personnel concerning the anticipated nature and frequency of surgical and prosthetic modification that may be necessary due to bony overgrowth. Ideally, classification of the juvenile amputee by type, age and bones involved, and an analysis of patients with such classifications, should help to answer these questions.

Many children with acquired diaphyseal amputations will need revision surgery, particularly of the humerus and fibula (Figure 12-2). True congenital amputations that need revision, although rare, were reported by Lambert and Aitken, but were not described in detail. Shurr et al reviewed 120 patients with major limb deficiencies or amputations prior to skeletal maturity and developed a five-part classification scheme (Table 12-1).

Type I cases included acquired amputations. The amputees in this group ranged from 3 months to 14 years at the time of amputation. Seven cases were skeletally mature. The

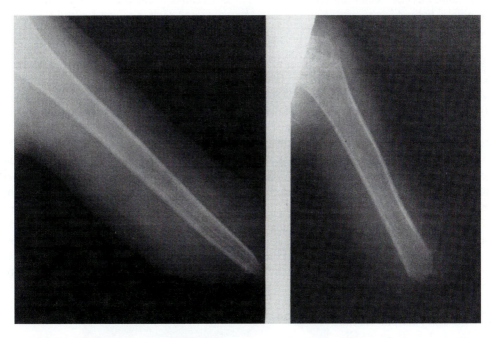

Figure 12-2. Bony overgrowth of the humerus, before, on left, and after surgical revision. (*Source:* From Shurr DG, Cooper RR, Buckwalter JA, Blair WF. Juvenile amputees classification and revision rates. *Orthot Prosthet.* 1982; 36:23, with permission.)

TABLE 12-1. CLASSIFICATION OF JUVENILE AMPUTATIONS

Type	Description	Number of Cases
I	Acquired amputations (infection, trauma, etc)	26
II	Congenital amputations through long bones	8
III	Congenital deficiencies surgically converted by amputation through bone	3
IV	Congenital deficiencies surgically converted by disarticulation	4
V	Congenital deficiencies treated nonsurgically with prostheses	79
		120

Source: From Shurr DG, Cooper, RR Buckwalter, JA, Blair, WF, Juvenile amputees: Classification and revision rates. *Orthot Prosthet.* 1981; 36:24, with permission.

humerus was found to show bony overgrowth most frequently and required as many as six surgical revisions, demanding a total of 14 procedures on four of the patients. The fibula was revised in three cases, the tibia/fibula twice, and the tibia once. Only one of these occurred at the above-elbow level and only one case required separate revisions of the tibia and fibula on an amputation that had been acquired at age 10. These revisions were done at age 15 and 16, respectively. Individuals acquiring an amputation after age 12 needed no revision, regardless of the bone involved.

Type II cases, true congenital amputations, are defined as amputations through the long bones that are present at birth. Shurr et al excluded from this type the classic terminal transverse transradial deficiency, with vestigial hand or nubbins, and all other congenital limb deficiencies not through the long bones. This latter group (Proximal Femoral Focal Deficiencies or PFFD, phocomelias, and amelias) is included in Type V. The distinction between Type II and Type V amputations is important. Type II includes only true congenital amputations through long bone and may result from defects such as constriction ring syndromes.

Of the eight Type II cases reviewed, seven underwent at least one revision. One fibula was revised five times, and two humeri were revised twice. Over a 20-year period, the patient depicted in Figure 12-3 with bilateral PFFD and bilateral transhumeral deficiencies had undergone two revisions for the right TH residuum but no revisions for the left side.

Type II congenital, through bone, amputations were found to overgrow. The humerus, the most common bone involved, required six revisions in four patients. Two tibia/fibulae were revised a total of four times: three in one case and one in another (Table 12-2). Because all patients in Type II had at least three limbs involved and had at least simple syndactylys, this group

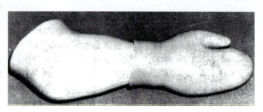

Figure 12-3. Below-elbow level first fitting with passive mitten. (*Source:* From Shurr DG, Cooper RR, Buckwalter JA, Blair WF. Terminal transverse congenital limb deficiency of the forearm. *Orthot Prosthet.* 1981; 35:23, with permission.)

appears to respond differently than the classical limb deficient patient with only one limb involved. From the data, patients with congenital amputations of the humerus and fibula react much like Type I or Type III, even though they appear to be true congenital amputations.

Type III cases are those in which surgical conversion of congenital limb deficiency required cutting through a long bone. In the group studied by Shurr et al, all were at the TT level. Two had congenital pseudarthroses of the tibia and fibula, and one a congenital absence of the fibula. Like the Type I amputations, Type III required surgical revision. Of the TT amputees, two needed revision of the tibia, one at age 12 and one at age 15, and one required revision of the fibula. All amputations had been done prior to age 5 and, predictably, acted similarly to Type I amputations.

Type IV encompasses congenital deficiencies converted surgically by disarticulation. PFFD and single or double ray feet without a hindfoot are examples. Surgical conversion in this group usually enhanced prosthetic fitting without concomitant loss in function. No bony overgrowth occurred in this group.

Type V comprises the largest sub-group of congenital deficiencies, treated nonsurgically. Type V includes the classic terminal transverse TR amputation that occurs more often in females, and on the left side. A vestigial hand or nubbins are usually present. In review of 33 unilateral cases with no other abnormalities, no cases of bony overgrowth were found.

After reviewing this group of juvenile amputees, Shurr et al concluded that the above described classification system is valuable for prognostic purposes. The known tendency of acquired amputations (Type I) to require revision, sometimes multiple revisions, was confirmed. Twenty-six patients underwent 21 revisions. The younger the patient at the time of amputation, the more likely the need for revision. The humerus was most often revised, followed by the fibula, tibia/fibula, and tibia. The analysis indicated that congenital transverse amputations (Type II) through long bones frequently require revision, occurring 14 times in seven patients and thus confirming the opinions of Aitken and Lambert. For prognostic purposes, the transverse congenital amputation (Type II) should be considered an entity distinctly different from non-surgically treated congenital terminal transverse deficiencies (Type V), in which revisions were not required.

TABLE 12-2. TYPE II CONGENITAL AMPUTATIONS THROUGH THE LONG BONES

Level	Follow-up (Years)	Number of Revisions	Age (Years) at Revision		
			Humerus	Fibula	Tibia/Fibula
AE	8	1	7		
AE	8	2	8, 10		
AE	3	1	2		
BK	14	3			2, 4, 14
(L)AE	20		3, 7		
(R)AE		2(R)			
BK	7	1			5
BK	9	5		1, 3, 6, 7, 9	

Note: AE = above elbow; BK = below knee.
Source: From Shurr DG, Cooper, RR, Buckwalter, JA, Blair, WF. Juvenile amputees Classification and revision rates. *Orthot Prosthet.* 1981; 36:27, with permission.

When congenital deficiencies were treated by amputation through long bones (Type III), they behaved, relative to surgical revision, as a congenital amputation through long bone. The congenital deficiency treated by amputation through long bone changed from an entity in which revision was unlikely to one in which revision was nearly predictable. If the congenital deficiency was surgically treated by disarticulation instead of amputation (Type IV), revision was not necessary, reaffirming that, when possible, disarticulation is the preferred surgical procedure.

Terminal-Transverse Congenital Deficiency of the Forearm

Birch-Jensen examined the records of over four million patients to determine the incidence of this common below elbow limb deficiency. In this classic study (Table 12-3), a total of 161 patients were identified as congenital below elbow amputees; 69 male and 92 female. Of that number, 108 occurred on the left and 53 occurred on the right side. Aitken and Franz reported a total of 49 patients; 22 males and 27 females, 37 left sided and 12 right sided. In a series published by Aitken and O'Rahilly, a total of 331 cases were reviewed. Of these, 156 were male, 175 female; 212 were left sided and 119 were right sided. Shurr identified 48 patients with this below elbow amputation. These patients were placed into two groups: Group 1, having unilateral below elbow congenital amputation, and Group 2, patients with associated anomalies including four bilateral upper extremity amputees. There were 19 males and 29 females. To complete the series, one patient with a below elbow amputation also had a contralateral elbow disarticulation, making a total of 52 amputations. Of 51 below elbow amputations, 35 were on the left and 16 were on the right. The data in each of these studies agrees in regard to relative incidence, indicating a predominance of females and a left-to-right ratio of nearly 2 to 1. The congenital below elbow terminal transverse amputation appears to be a distinct entity, well defined in its unilateral presentation.

Early, aggressive fitting of prostheses at about 6 months of age is well accepted by both parents and children.

Initiating Lower Limb Fitting

As noted previously, many experts agree with Krebs, Edelstein, and Thornby that it is important to provide prosthetic devices only when the child is developmentally ready to benefit from their use. For those with a lower limb deficiency, initial fitting when the child begins to pull to

TABLE 12-3. OCCURRENCE OF CONGENITAL BELOW ELBOW AMPUTATIONS

	Shurr (1980)	Birch-Jensen (1949)	Aitken and Frantz (1955)	Aitken and O'Rahilly (1961)
Total number of patients studied	48	161	49	331
Male	19 (40%)	69 (43%)	22 (45%)	156 (47%)
Female	29 (60%)	92 (57%)	27 (55%)	175 (53%)
Left	35 (69%)	108 (67%)	37 (76%)	212 (64%)
Right	16 (31%)	53 (33%)	12 (24%)	119 (36%)

Source: From Shurr, DG, Cooper, RR, Buckwalter, JA, Blair WF. Terminal transverse congenital limb deficiency of the forearm. *Orthot Prosthet.* 1981; 35:23, with permission.

stand at about 9 to 12 months of age is usually recommended. As emphasized by Kitabayashi, the actual time of fitting must be individualized, because many children with disabilities reach developmental milestones at a later age than the average while others reach them earlier.

Infant designs emphasize simplicity, light weight, and reliability. The basic SACH foot is used almost exclusively at this age, and articulations are generally avoided until the child is several years older. Because the toddler typically walks with a wide-based gait and a flexed-hip/flexed-knee posture, the initial prosthesis is aligned in a similar fashion. Suspension is kept as simple as possible, and the socket design must often accommodate the bulk of disposable diapers at this age.

Initiating Upper Limb Fitting

Fitting of children with upper limb deficiencies is more varied, and more controversial. When prosthetic fitting is desired, the initial device is usually offered when the child begins to develop sitting balance between three and six months of age. Traditionally, this has been a passive mitten device that is very lightweight and can serve as a "prop" for balance while the child explores the environment with the contralateral arm and hand (Figure 12.3).

Some centers have had good success with the early fitting of a simplified myoelectric device, as noted by Patterson, McMillan, and Rodriquez, reporting good acceptance by infant and parents as well as the development of functional grasp and release at an earlier age than is normally anticipated. Meredith, Uellendahl, and Keagy have suggested that the simplified control scheme of the so-called "cookie-crusher" myoelectric hand is easy for the child to master, perhaps even easier than the much more complex multiple finger control needed to use the human hand (Figure 12-4).

This system uses a single muscle site such that any EMG signal causes the hand to open while the lack of a signal results in automatic closure via the electric motor. The strength of the grip is always the maximum possible (but set at a very low rate by the manufacturer); hence, the name cookie-crusher. Advocates postulate that children fitted with electronic arms from infancy will become virtuoso users over time. There is some clinical evidence that this may be so, including the passionate support of parents of children who have grown up with such devices such as Leingang.

As MacNaughton has noted, the third option is to fit a body-powered terminal device, usually a small hook, but not to harness it for active use. Due to shoulder-strength limitations,

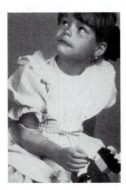

Figure 12-4. In recent decades, the widespread availability of reliable, light weight electric prostheses for children and infants has led to a significant number of clinically successful fittings, particularly in unilateral cases of transradial absence. (*Source:* Otto Bock Orthopedic Industries, Inc.)

Shaperman, Leblanc, and Setoguchi have shown that, due to shoulder strength limitations, the typical amputee child cannot be expected to operate a body-powered device actively until they are a few years old. Traditionally, the mother can place objects into the hook fingers where they are stabilized by the rubber band. The child can then remove the objects from the hook, thus learning about the "release" of objects even at an early age. When the child eventually develops sufficient shoulder strength to voluntarily open the terminal device, the harnessing is added and active grasp and release can begin. (Figure 12-5).

It is now apparent that although early fitting is generally preferred, motivated children can adapt to the use of a prosthesis at many times throughout their lives, with the possible exception of during the "terrible twos" or while in the throes of pubescent crises. Despite the best efforts of experienced and caring clinic teams, it remains very difficult to predict in advance which prosthesis will be preferred by which child. In addition, it is not uncommon for children to abruptly choose to stop wearing a prosthesis for some years or forever, or to suddenly decide to begin wearing one despite years of disinterest previously. Most clinic teams listen carefully to the wishes of pediatric patients and their families, supporting whatever decisions each individual and each family makes regarding use of a prosthetic device.

Independence Training Without a Prosthesis

It is well established that use of an upper limb prosthetic device is *not* essential for functional independence. Edelstein reports the use of the contralateral arm and hand is virtually always sufficient for all activities of daily living, particularly if use training by a knowledgeable therapist has been offered.

In addition, Marquardt and Fisk have reported that clinical experience with the complex high-level loss associated with the Thalidomide drug has confirmed that very few, if any, chil-

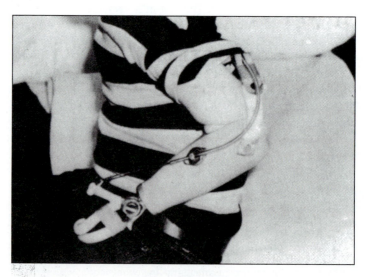

Figure 12-5. Below elbow level fitting with split-hook TD. (*Source:* From Shurr DG, Cooper RR, Buckwalter JA, Blair WF. Terminal transverse congenital limb deficiency of the forearm. *Orthot Prosthet.* 1981; 36:23, with permission.)

dren born with severe, high-level bilateral deficiencies will use prostheses long term. Virtually all become much more independent by developing their foot skills, and these appendages offer more grasp options and exquisite sensory feedback than do even the most sophisticated artificial arms.

Because the child who is born with a limb deficiency has not "lost" anything—as would be the case with an acquired amputation—Baughn has argued that provision of prosthetic arms creates an unnecessary technological dependency. Others argue just as passionately that early provision of prosthetic devices allows the child to most easily master the available technology, and this often does seem to be true in the case of lower level and unilateral deficiencies.

It is perhaps most accurate to say that there are no absolute guidelines in the management of upper limb loss, and this is particularly true in the case of children. Dillon has suggested that although the "rules" of earlier eras have been rendered moot by advances in available technology, we do not yet have sufficient collective clinical experience to identify the "new rules" objectively.

REFERENCES

1. Aitken GT. The child amputee: An overview. *Orthop Clin North Am.* 1972; 3:447–472.
2. Aitken GT, O'Rahilley R. Congenital skeletal limb deficiencies. *J Bone Joint Surg* 1961; 43A: 1202–1224.
3. Baughn B. Caveat Emptor? *J Prosthet Orthot.* 1992; 4(4):180.
4. Birch Jensen A. Congenital Deformities of the Upper Extremity. Commission: Andelsbogtrykkeriet i Odense und det danske forlag; 1949. Thesis.
5. Cummings DR, Kapp SL. Lower limb pediatric prosthetics: General considerations. *JPO* 1992; 4(4):196–206.
6. Dillon SS. New technology and the status quo. *J Prosthet Orthot.* 1992; 4(4):178–179.
7. Duncan WR, Mott DH. Foot reflexes and the use of the "inhibitive cast." *Foot Ankle.* 1983–4; 4:145–148.
8. Edelstein J. Rehabilitation without prostheses: Functional use training. In: *Atlas of Limb Prosthetics,* 2nd ed. Bowker JH, Michael JW (eds). CV Mosby; St. Louis 1992.
9. Frantz CH, Aitken GT. Management of the juvenile amputee. *Clin Orthop.* 1959; 14:30–49.
10. Hart TJ et al. Below-knee child amputee gait: Dynamics of an energy storing prosthesis (abstract). *J Biomech.* 1992; 25: 660.
11. Heckmatt JZ et al. Prolongation of walking in Duchenne muscular dystrophy with lightweight orthoses: Review of 57 cases. *Dev Med Child Neurol.* 1985; 27:149–154.
12. Kitabayashi B. The physical therapist's responsibility to the lower extremity child amputee. *Phys Ther Rev.* 1961; 41:722–727.
13. Krebs DE, Edelstein JE, Thornby MA. Prosthetic management of children with limb deficiencies. *Phys Ther.* 1991; 71:920–934.
14. Lambert CM, Pellicore RJ, Hamilton RC et al. Twenty-three years of clinic experience. *ICIB.* 1976; 15(3/4):15–20, 25.
15. Leingang AF. Myoelectrics for children: Sine qua non? *JPO* 1992; 4(4):181–183.
16. Lonstein JE, Winter RB. The Milwaukee brace for the treatment of adolescent idiopathic scoliosis: A review of one thousand and twenty patients. *J Bone Joint Surg (Am).* 1994; 76:1207-1221
17. MacNaughton A. The role of the occupational therapist in the training of the child arm amputee. *Physiotherapy.* 1966; 52:201–203.

18. Marquardt E, Fisk JR. Thalidomide children: Thirty years later. *J Assoc Child Prosthet Orthot Clin.* 1992; 27:3–10.

19. McCollough N. Conception, birth, infancy and adolescence of the juvenile amputee program in North America. *J Assoc Child Prosthet Orthot Clin.* 1988; 23:50–56.

20. Menard MR, Murray DD. Subjective and objective analysis of an energy-storing prosthetic foot. *J Prosthet Orthot.* 1989; 1:220–230.

21. Meredith JM, Uellendahl JE, Keagy RD. Successful voluntary grasp and release using the Cookie Crusher myoelectric hand in 2-year-olds. *Am J Occup Ther.* 1993; 47:825–829.

22. Michael J. Pediatric. Prosthetics and orthotics. *Phys Occup Ther Pediatr.* 1990; 10(2):123–146.

23. Patterson DB, McMillan PM, Rodriquez RP. Acceptance rate of myoelectric prosthesis. *J Assoc Child Prosthet Orthot Clin.* 1990/1991; 25:73–76.

24. Schneider K et al. Dynamics of below-knee child amputee gait: SACH foot versus Flex foot. *J Biomech.* 1993; 26:1191–1204.

25. Shaperman J, Leblanc M, Setoguchi Y et al. Is body powered operation of upper limb prostheses feasible for young limb deficient children? *Prosthet Orthot Int.* 1995; 19:165–175.

26. Shurr DG, Cooper RR, Buckwalter JA, Blair WF. Juvenile amputees: classification and revision rates. *Orthot Prosthet* 1982; 36(2):22–28.

27. Shurr DG. Terminal transverse congenital limb deficiency of the forearm. *Orthot Prosthet* 1981; 35(3):22–25.

28. Sorbye R. Myoelectric prosthetic fitting in young children. *Clin Orthop.* 1980; 148:34–40.

29. Watts HG. Differences between a child and an adult amputee. *Contemp Orthop.* 1992; 24:33–40.

Index

A

Abdominal support, spinal orthoses, 205–214
Abdominal support apron, 207, 209
Above-elbow harness, 159–160
Above-knee amputation, levels of, 107
Ace wrap, 90
Aegis system, 80, 82
Alignment, knee socket, 117
Alignment, residual limb, 125–126
Alignment, of transtibial prosthesis, 94–95
   dynamic, 94
   heel height, 95
   static, 94
Alpha system, 79
Aluminum, 31–33
Ambulation, lower limb functions during,
     42–59
   foot-ankle functions, 43–52
   hip functions, 57–59
   knee functions, 52–57
American Academy of Orthopaedic Surgeons
     (AAOS), 16, 17
American Academy of Orthotists and Pros-
     thetists (AAOP), 17
American Board for Certification (ABC) in Or-
     thotics and Prosthetics, Inc., 4
American Orthotic and Prosthetic Association
     (AOPA), 17
Amputation
   adjustments to, 10
   causes of, 6–10
   congenital malformation, 9–10
   disease, 8
   economic factors, 13–14
   individual reactions, 14
   knee disarticulation, 107
   level of, 6, 7, 107
   physical factors, 10–12
   population, 6–7
   psychosocial factors, 12–13

   reactions to, 10–14
   transfemoral amputation, 108–109
   trauma, 6–7
   tumor, 8–9
   vocational factors, 13–14
Amputation, transtibial, 66–69. *See also* Pros-
     thesis, transtibial amputations and
   amputee training, 95–99
   ankle disarticulation, 64–66
   comfort liners, 77–82
   energy expenditure, 99–101
   feet and, 69–74
   ICEROSS fitting, 78, 83
   levels of, 62–69
   long, 67–68
   medium, 68
   partial foot, 62–63
   preparatory prostheses, 84–85
   prosthetic skin, 83–84
   PTB socket, 74–76
   short, 69
   surface-bearing design, 76
   Syme amputation, 64–66
Amputation, upper limb, 144–146
   elbow disarticulation, 148
   forequarter, 149
   interscapularthoracic, 149
   levels of, 146–149
   partial hand, 146
   rehabilitation for, 149–150
   shoulder disarticulation, 149
   transhumeral, 148–149
   transradial amputation, 147–148
   wrist disarticulation, 146–147
Amputee training, 95–99
   definitive prosthesis, 98–99
   gait training, 97–98
   preparatory prosthesis, 97–98
   pre-prosthetic care, 96–97
   transtibial amputations, 95–99
Amputees, distribution by site, 5